Reference. R1.
39

PERSONAL CONSTRUCT THEORY AND MENTAL HEALTH

Personal Construct Theory & Mental Health

Theory, Research and Practice

Edited by Eric Button

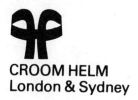

CROOM HELM
London & Sydney

© 1985 Eric Button
Croom Helm Ltd, Provident House, Burrell Row,
Beckenham, Kent BR3 1AT

Croom Helm Australia Pty Ltd, First Floor, 139 King Street,
Sydney, NSW 2001, Australia

British Library Cataloguing in Publication Data

Personal Construct theory and mental health:
   theory, research and practice.
   1. Personal construct theory   2. Mental illness
   I. Button, Eric
   616.89   RC343
   ISBN 0-7099-3250-2

Printed and bound in Great Britain
by Billing & Sons Limited, Worcester.

CONTENTS

To Frances and Andrew

LIST OF CONTRIBUTORS

Joyce Agnew
Principal Clinical Psychologist (Child Health)
Stratheden Hospital
Cupar
Fife
Scotland

Eric Button
Lecturer in Clinical Psychology
Department of Psychiatry
Royal South Hants Hospital
Graham Road
Southampton, S09 4PE

Willem Claeys
Psychology Department
University of Leuven
Tiensestraat 102
B – 3000
Leuven
Belgium

Cliff Cunningham
Senior Lecturer
The Hester Adrian Research Centre
The University of Manchester
Manchester, M13 9PL

Hilton Davis
Senior Lecturer in Clinical Psychology
Department of Psychiatry
The London Hospital Medical College
Turner Street
London, E1 2AD

Andrew Dawes
Department of Psychology
University of Cape Town
Rondebosch 7700
South Africa

Paul De Boeck
Psychology Department
University of Leuven
Tiensestraat 102
B – 3000
Leuven
Belgium

Fay Fransella
The Director
The Centre for Personal Construct Psychology
132 Warwick Way
London SW1

Hugh Koch
Principal Clinical Psychologist
Severalls Hospital
Colchester
Essex CO4 5HG

Alvin W. Landfield
Department of Psychology
University of Nebraska
Lincoln
Nebraska
USA, 68588-0308

Greg J. Neimeyer
Department of Psychology
University of Florida
Gainesville
Florida, 32807
USA

Robert A. Neimeyer
Department of Psychology
Memphis State University
Memphis
Tennessee, 38152
USA

Harry Procter
Senior Clinical Psychologist
Southwood House
13 King Square
Bridgwater
Somerset, TA6 3DQ

P. Clayton Rivers
Department of Psychology
University of Nebraska
Lincoln
Nebraska,
USA, 68588-0308

Charles Stefan
Binghamton Psychiatric Centre
Binghamton
New York State
USA

Omer van den Bergh
Psychology Department
University of Leuven
Tiensestraat 102
B – 3000
Leuven
Belgium

Linda L. Viney
Department of Psychology
University of Wollongong
PO Box 1144
Wollongong
New South Wales, 2500
Australia

Judith Von
State University of New York at
Binghamton
Binghamton
New York
USA

David Winter
Principal Clinical Psychologist
Napsbury Hospital
Nr. St. Albans
Herts

PREFACE

In 1955, the late George Kelly, an American psychologist, published a two volume book entitled *The Psychology of Personal Constructs*. He presented what is arguably the most elaborate psychological theory that exists even to this day. It is a theory of *people* and, in particular, of how people interpret their experience and seek to *anticipate* what lies ahead, through what he conceptualised as a 'personal construct system'. Although the theory can be and has been applied to all aspects of human experience (e.g. education, politics, business), its 'focus' was the clinical context, as reflected by one whole volume devoted to 'Clinical diagnosis and psychotherapy'. Kelly's ideas were both a challenge to the then predominant behavioural school of psychology, as well as to the psychiatric system of classification and treatment. Kelly, above all, believed in taking people seriously and invited us to explore the *questions* people were asking with their behaviour, rather than just dismissing them as symptoms or the result of faulty learning.

Kelly's book has proved an inspiration to many, although some, like myself, have discovered the value of his ideas initially from others who have carried through his thinking. For me this was through *Inquiring Man*, first written by Don Bannister and Fay Fransella in 1971. Having since spent over a decade putting the theory into practice in the clinical context, the idea for editing this book came to me towards the end of 1982. It seemed to me that clinical psychology, having been relatively dominated by the aim to change behaviour, had now discovered that there were thoughts or 'cognitions' to change as well. Kelly had, of course, discovered this three decades earlier, but somewhat surprisingly the current cognitive trend seems to have emerged independently of his thinking. It may be, however, that revolutionary thinking, like music, initially threatens and is not appreciated fully until some years hence. I believe, therefore, that the time is right to bring personal construct theory into the centre of the stage as far as mental health is concerned.

Fortunately at the time when these ideas were developing, I also had sitting on my desk a letter from a publisher who responded positively to my plans. Although the theme of mental health is central in Kelly's original work, his book is neither widely available, nor can it, of course, provide an up to date account of its applications. Whilst recent general books, such as Adams-Webber and Mancuso's *Applications of Personal Construct Theory* (1983), give credence to the wide scope of the theory, there is also a need for more specific books focusing in depth on a particular area of application. I have been deeply gratified by the enthusiastic response of my fellow contributors who have joined me in this venture.

Personal Construct Theory and Mental Health is in three parts:

In Part One, I introduce the concepts of Personal Construct Theory, as well as ways of exploring personal constructs. Both the concepts and the techniques are explored by reference to examples directly relevant to mental health.

The largest section of the book is Part Two, in which there are eleven chapters focusing on particular types of 'disorder'. This is not a comprehensive list of disorders, but an attempt to explore a fairly wide range of problems that might come the way of the mental health worker. In fact, some of the titles (e.g. mental handicap) don't fit easily into the term disorder at all, although in all cases there is the potential for people to be construed as 'disordered', 'ill' or the like. Although we have chosen terms like 'schizophrenia' or 'neurotic disorders' because they are likely to be familiar to you, you will find that there are recurrent themes irrespective of the presenting problem. We are, therefore, offering what may to you be a different way of construing your 'patients' or 'clients', a way we hope you may find meaningful and constructive. Each author sets about this in a slightly different way but in each case we present a theoretical stance, relevant research evidence and, in particular, an account of what we see as the *practical* implications of the approach.

Part Three focuses on 'change'. Here the emphasis is on more general principles of helping people to change. Although therapeutic examples are extensively provided in Part Two, here we aim to spell out an approach to helping people irrespective of the presenting problem. There are chapters on individual, group and family therapy. In the final chapter, I attempt to go beyond the clinical context and explore societal and institutional change which may be consistent with mental health.

There is no easy recipe for mental health. Life is risky and often disturbing. We believe, however, that the greatest obstacle to mental health is a failure to continue 'elaborating' our construing. I hope that this book is consistent with this aim for you.

Eric Button
University Dept. of Psychiatry
Southampton

ACKNOWLEDGEMENTS

We wish to express our thanks to the *British Journal of Medical Psychology* and the *International Journal of Group Psychotherapy* for the reproduction of figures.

I wish to express my gratitude to Julie Hamer and Eileen Reeves for their help and patience in typing parts of this book.

I also wish to express my thanks as editor to all my fellow contributors who have helped me make this possible by meeting my deadlines, following my guidelines and above all for producing such an interesting and varied collection of chapters.

Last but by no means least, my thanks to my wife, Frances and my son, Andrew for bearing with me during my many hours of being hidden away 'working'.

Eric Button

PART ONE

THEORY AND METHODS OF EXPLORATION

Part One is particularly directed at newcomers to personal construct theory. The key concepts are introduced as are a range of methods of exploring personal constructs, with particular reference to the mental health context.

1 PERSONAL CONSTRUCT THEORY: THE CONCEPTS

Eric Button

In deciding how to start this book, I find myself engaged in a process at the very heart of George Kelly's personal construct theory (Kelly, 1955).[1] Essentially I see myself as trying to anticipate the views, needs and expectations of other people, in this case, you the readers. On the basis of my previous experiences, I have certain hunches both about the kind of people who are likely to read this book and also of what they might expect and hope to get out of the experience. These hunches don't necessarily start off in a very explicit form, but the very act of putting pen to paper forces me to try and verbalise them and use this as a basis for action. For example, I am guessing that many of you are mental health professionals and that most of you have heard of personal construct theory, but that you may still be left with many questions both about the theory and whether it can be of any practical value to you in your work. It also seems reasonable to expect that you will hope to learn or discover something new and that if we are to achieve that we will need to be both challenging and relevant. I may, of course, be way off the mark in my predictions. Although this may be a little disappointing for both me and my publishers, I would not dream of attempting this enterprise if I could accurately predict all possible readers and expectations! The point I am trying to make here is that this business of trying to anticipate things (whether it be . . . Who will read my book? Will there be a nuclear war? Will I get my breakfast in bed today?) is the kind of activity with which personal construct theory is concerned. In fact, anticipation is the very cornerstone of the theory as stated in Kelly's 'Fundamental Postulate'.

Basic Assumption of Personal Construct Theory

Kelly uses the term 'Fundamental Postulate' to state his basic assumption as follows: *A Person's Processes are Psychologically Channelised by the Ways in which he Anticipates Events*. Put simply, Kelly is suggesting that it may be useful to try and understand human behaviour and experience as the consequence of our attempts at anticipating future events. (This term 'event' is used very broadly by Kelly to include everyday actions and experiences like dreams, headaches and smiles.)

Kelly is indirectly emphasising that man is not static but in motion and making predictions about the future on the basis of his previous experience. This is not to suggest that Kelly sees us all as crystal ball gazers. Anticipation neither has to involve conscious thought nor does it merely relate to the far-off future. Some experience requires very immediate, virtually instant action, whereas at other times we have almost unlimited time to ponder various eventualities. At all points on this spectrum, however, it is argued that we proceed according to our anticipations. Much of the time we may be success-ful in our anticipations. We manage to avoid bumping into that low ceiling, we get the customary reply to our greeting of 'Good morning', our loved ones are there to turn to. Occasionally, how-ever, we get it wrong: a casual off-the-cuff remark leads to a catastrophic reaction, we go into the back of a car, we are struck for the first time in life by an all-pervasive sense of panic. A central theme which will become evident throughout this book is that what we sometimes call mental illness may be re-conceptualised as occur-ring within the context of the need to anticipate. This may be a two-way process between the person and his associates. Faced with a breakdown in his ability to anticipate events, the potential patient may engage in unusual or uncharacteristic behaviour as part of his attempts to make sense of his experience. At the same time, how-ever, people around the potential patient, having been 'thrown' by this new behaviour, may eventually latch on to the possibility that he may be 'ill'. In my experience, however, the most popular construction offered by potential patients is 'Am I going mad?' Doctors may prefer, however, not to use this term and offer the more socially acceptable — 'It's an illness.' Thus the process of becoming mentally ill seems to be an essentially social process in which the client and/or his associates may come to a negotiated view of his behaviour as reflecting the fact that he is ill. Such a construc-tion is more than mere labelling but may actually help the patient and others around him to be more successful at anticipation. Rather than risk surprise and invalidation, a wider range of behaviour may now become 'understandable' since he is mentally ill. Of course, the 'patient' doesn't always share this construction and may offer some other explanation such as,[1] There's a conspiracy against me.' Such a theory holds great possibility for successful anticipation if the patient chooses to perceive everyone as involved in the conspiracy — he can hardly go wrong.

The 'Corollaries'

Kelly chose to elaborate his main assumption into a system called 'The Psychology of Personal Constructs' (Kelly, 1955). He does so by presenting a series of eleven propositions or 'corollaries' — a word which few people can pronounce let alone understand. I have therefore chosen to omit the term below, although you will find in the remainder of the text that I and my fellow contributors return to it quite often.

Construction: A person anticipates events by construing their replications

We are able to anticipate because we succeed in inferring some sort of pattern and order in our experience. From our origins as part of the unending and undifferentiated stream of life we notice recurrent themes: days, songs, breakfasts, disappointments are never identical but share common features which tend to recur or 'replicate'. Instead of a monotonous flow we separate our experience into chunks or 'events'. Such differentiation of our experience involves both an awareness of likeness and difference: the resultant contrast (e.g. 'yesterday — today'; 'nice — nasty'; 'mine — somebody else's') is termed a 'construct'. Once we are able to structure our experience in this way, we are able to anticipate or make predictions. Such replications, however, are less usefully viewed as 'realities' than as reflections of our personal interpretation ('construction'). Faced with similar experiences, a wide range of constructions is possible. Let us take a pertinent example which should be familiar to most of you — admission to a psychiatric ward. It is likely that prior to one's first experience of such an event, most people will have heard stories, seen films or even had first-hand experience with a relative. Such experience will lead us to anticipate the sorts of behaviour that will lead to such an event (i.e. admission) and its consequences. The behavioural implications of our anticipations (fear, violence, relief) will, of course, vary according to our particular constructions, but what is important is that unless the event is a completely novel one, the patient is likely to have his own expectations of what will ensue.

As recently re-emphasised by Tschudi (1983), Kelly sees constructs as 'hypotheses'. As such, they are put to the test by our actions and experiences. Kelly went as far as suggesting that people may be looked upon as 'personal scientists', in developing theories which are put to the test by 'behaviour', which might be seen as a kind of experiment. Although this metaphor might have served to highlight the importance of taking the 'subject' seriously in social science research, we don't need to view the professional scientist's behaviour as a kind of ideal for mankind. In fact, the cautious way some scientists seem to go about their work seems to me to be a distinctly unappealing prospect.

Individuality: Persons Differ from Each Other in their Construction of Events

This may seem like stating the obvious, but at the time when Kelly advanced his theory (the early 1950s), psychology was still heavily under the influence of 'stimulus-response theory' which ignored the personal interpretations we place on our experience. In fact, an implicit assumption that events have some inevitable outcome seems to have run through much of psychological and psychiatric theory and practice as well as in the field of social work. Nowhere has this been more pronounced than in the field of child psychology, where the pendulum seems to have swung back and forth with its alternating remedies of freedom or discipline as a way of producing a healthy adult. We even see evidence of it in recent times in the field of life events (Paykel *et al.*, 1971), where much research has been conducted on the assumption that mental illness (such as depression, schizophrenia and suicide) can be the outcome of too many 'events'. Not surprisingly, more sophisticated recent research has highlighted the fact that individual differences account for a much higher proportion of the variance than the events *per se* (Andrews, 1981). This is not to ignore the importance of adverse or even positive experiences as potential precipitants of disturbance, but to emphasise that it is what we make of these 'events' that matters: getting pregnant could mean a dream come true, just another mouth to feed or the end of a career.

Organisation: Each Person Characteristically Evolves, for his Convenience in Anticipating Events, a Construction System Embracing Ordinal Relationships Between Constructs.

It follows that, if you are to anticipate events successfully, then you will have detected some relationship between events. Like the elements of the physical world (or universe for that matter) in which we live, our constructs are inter-related. Kelly is suggesting here that there is a hierarchical aspect to this organisation.

For example Figure 1.1 illustrates a possible segment from a system of constructs.

The characteristic way in which our constructs are organised, Kelly goes as far as suggesting, is what constitutes our 'personality'. Thus, the term 'personal construct system' may represent our particular way of viewing the world. As we shall see later, people vary in terms of how their constructs are arranged — some arrangements are more complex, flexible and all-embracing than others. The exploration of personal construct systems, both as a clinical procedure and in the context of research, has arguably proved to be the most popular of applications of the theory (see Chapter 2).

Finally, it should be emphasised that the term personal construct system is, of course, an abstraction and does not necessarily exist in a concrete sense like the central nervous system. Nevertheless, it seems likely that there must be ultimately some sort of physiological representation of constructs and their inter-relationships. Both the formation and 'destruction' of construct systems will be sensitive to maturational and disease processes. It is even possible that particular styles of construing may have a genetic basis, but this for the present can remain a matter of speculation.

Dichotomy: A Person's Construction System is Composed of a Finite Number of Dichotomous Constructs

This corollary has proved to be one of the more controversial aspects of the theory, given its challenge to classical logic. For example, rather than viewing goodness as a category in its own right, its meaning would be defined in terms of what it was being contrasted with — e.g. 'badness'. Similarly, it is hard to imagine how a construct such as 'dark' would mean much if we had not experienced 'light'. Thus, although we often refer to constructs as if they were unipolar, there is always an implicit opposite pole. When a psychiatrist is using the term 'schizophrenic' he is likely to be implicitly contrasting the person with other patients he might call 'manic-depressive', 'neurotic' or the like. The lay person, however, is unlikely to share such fine gradations and might simply have an implicit contrast such as 'normal' or 'sane'.

Figure 1.1: An Example of a Hierarchical Segment from a Construct System

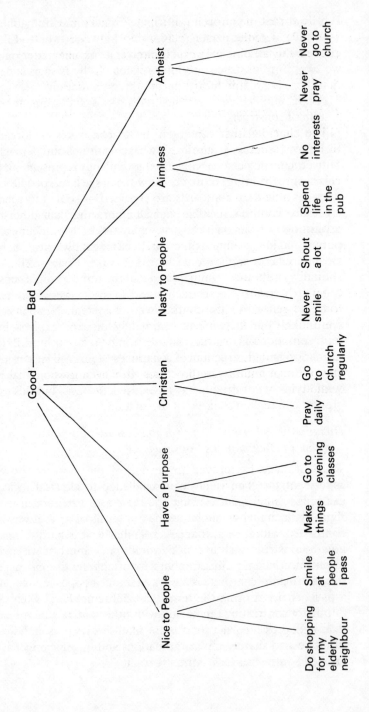

Sometimes the implicit pole of a construct may be 'submerged' (see p.9), e.g. the person who says, 'Nobody can be trusted' has presumably at some time experienced trust which went wrong.

Choice: A Person Chooses for Himself that Alternative in a Dichotomised Construct Through Which he Anticipates the Greater Possibility for Extension and Definition of his System

Given the idea that constructs are bi-polar (good-bad, honest-dishonest, success-failure), it follows that we have to choose between the poles of constructs in line with our anticipations. Some choices might be no more than the toss of a coin with little risk, whereas others have wide-reaching implications. Broadly speaking, a person may either seek to 'extend' his system (he might opt for the adventure) or 'define' it (he may play safe). Whichever choice a person makes Kelly suggests an 'elaborative choice' is made. People, of course, don't always make the choices we think they should. They carry on smoking, they don't 'pull themselves together', they won't go out and meet people. Why do they choose to be so awkward? Kelly suggests that the over-riding issue is the continuing need to anticipate events. Life as a smoker, an ill person or a criminal might at least be predictable. In short, what we can most do without is too much uncertainty. Thus, we may choose to stay with our misery rather than risk the uncertainty of living without it.

Range: A Construct is Convenient for the Anticipation of a Finite Range of Events Only

A construct's 'range of convenience' consists of all elements to which it could be reasonably applied: constructs concerned with love-making are not usually very relevant to golf courses; constructs concerning soil texture will not help us to predict our gas bill! Constructs are, thus, more or less tied to contexts, but of course, some are more widely applicable than others. Consider, for example, the almost universal construct 'good-bad', which could be applied to anything from behaviour to apples. At the other extreme, however, there are constructs such as 'isosceles-scalene' which are fine for triangles but not much use for anything else.

In addition to a construct's 'range of convenience', there is also its 'focus of convenience', i.e. those situations where it is maximally useful. For example, any of you who have played chess will be familiar with the term 'check-mate'. Although having a wide 'range', its 'focus of convenience' would be the chess game.

Experience: A Person's Construction System Varies as he Successively Construes the Replications of Events.

The process of living continually invites us to reconsider our assumptions. What worked well yesterday may not work too well today, leave alone tomorrow: the experience of bereavement is a painful reminder of this fact. As pointed out above, constructs are basically hypotheses and, as such, are capable of revision. When I leave the house for work on Monday it is a reasonable assumption that my car will start, I'll have at least one traffic hold-up, parking will be a problem and I'll feel like a cup of coffee when I eventually get to my office. Each day, however, we are confronted with new, sometimes unwelcome and surprising experience. Although these surprises are usually fairly trivial, occasionally they may challenge us to alter radically our expectations and goals. Kelly's view of experience, however, is not of something that *happens* to us but as the successive *interpretation* and *re-interpretation* of what happens.

This variation or change in our construct system, of course, can be potentially very threatening. It follows that new experience can be at the root of much that we call mental disorder. In its extreme form there is the risk of disintegration as suggested by Bannister (1963) in schizophrenia (see Chapter 3). It is no wonder that people don't always readily accept the implications of their experience. They may instead distort the facts, ignore it, or put it to the back of their minds. It is tempting, in fact, to invoke Freud's concept of defence mechanisms to describe such processes, but as we shall see later, Kelly proposed his own 'diagnostic constructs'.

Modulation: The Variation in a Person's Construction System is Limited by the Permeability of the Constructs within Whose Range of Convenience the Variants Lie

The 'permeability' of a construct refers to the extent to which it can make sense of new events. If it can only be applied to that which has already been experienced, it is said to be 'impermeable'. Of course, in practice, permeability can be regarded as a dimension and constructs are more or less permeable. Furthermore, both extremes have their uses depending on the context. For example, in a psychotherapeutic context, a degree of permeability will help the client to assimilate new perspectives on his problem. A client with too permeable a system, however, will be in danger of being disturbed by virtually every occurrence.

Fragmentation: A Person May Successively Employ a Variety of Construction Subsystems Which are Inferentially Incompatible with Each Other

This corollary is closely linked with the modulation corollary. If we took a snapshot of a person in a variety of situations, we might have difficulty in seeing any connection between the various bits of behaviour. Such 'inconsistencies' are not regarded as undesirable in construct theory. We do need, however, to maintain some degree of continuity. This is achieved by means of relatively permeable, more 'superordinate' (see pp. 20-21) constructs which can transcend the contrasting aspects of our experience. For example, a construct such as 'working-playing' might help to reconcile the very different behaviours a person might show on the football pitch compared with when interviewing someone for a job.

Commonality: To the Extent that One Person Employs a Construction of Experience which is Similar to that Employed by Another, his Psychological Processes are Similar to Those of the Other Person

The previous corollaries have been primarily concerned with the individual. This individualistic approach is consistent with the major focus of psychology. Kelly did, however, have something to say about what goes on between people. Having emphasised his view that people interpret experience in differing ways, he is here adding that they can also share similar interpretations. There is no doubt that people tend to form groups on the basis of some similarity, whether it be occupation, religion or sex. The emphasis here, however, is on the similarity in construing, not the experience in itself. For example, members of a religious sect may have come from widely differing backgrounds, but have come to view the purpose of life very similarly. Furthermore, although different in their outlooks in general, two people may in some contexts look at things similarly (e.g. a bank manager and a bricklayer at a football match). Kelly further points out that similarity doesn't just rest with similar constructs, but also refers to the similarity in the way the person makes something out of his experience.

In case it is not already obvious, I would like to sound a note of caution. We should be wary of assuming that similar verbal labels imply similar constructions. Human experience is littered with examples of the misunderstandings which can result from such assumptions.

Sociality: To the Extent that One Person Construes the Construction Processes of Another, he may Play a Role in a Social Process Involving the Other Person

Although a degree of similarity of construing between people may be a prerequisite for the formation of a relationship between people (see Duck and Spencer, 1972) this in itself would not be regarded as sufficient. The ability to have constructive social experience depends on whether we can see things from the other person's point of view. We don't necessarily have to agree with him, but we do need to try and understand his outlook. This doesn't mean that we have to understand him as a whole. In many situations such as driving a car or playing a game of tennis we only need to understand specific aspects of his construct system. In some relationships, however, such as marriage, we need to be able to construe a much wider range of the person's constructions. This would, of course, not just include the verbalised aspects of our partner's construing, but would extend to more active pursuits such as love-making and washing up. This understanding is not necessarily reciprocal. Some relationships are very one-sided. A patient may have a good idea of what the doctor is after, without any guarantee that the doctor is really in touch with his patient's real concerns. It is all too easy just to try and fit the person into our construct system (whether we see him as 'deficient in social skills', a 'problem patient' or a 'hysterical personality'). If we are to offer a truly therapeutic relationship to the mentally disturbed, we need to take them seriously and try to understand them as people. One important implication of this point of view is that the training of the caring professions should place a major emphasis on this very process of 'stepping inside somebody's shoes'. Understanding is not just one-sided, however, and it is just as incumbent on us to help our clients and their families to do similarly. Otherwise, we are in danger of fostering the very sorts of non-reciprocal relationships we may be seeking to minimise!

It can be seen that Kelly's notion of 'role' is rather different from that often applied in social psychology. Rather than seeing a role as a socially prescribed set of expectations, he brings the individual and society close together. In fact, he suggests (Kelly, 1966a) that role behaviour may not just be something to *act out*, but may also be a means of understanding the world.

This task of trying to understand another human being seems to be one of the potentially most problematic we face. The very diversity of our individuality presents us with the challenge of reconciling the many different values and expectations of those we encounter. We may feel confused, angry and in despair when people don't conform. More often than not, this is because we don't understand. Understanding is not easy: we may fail, but we can keep trying.

To Summarise so far

Personal construct theory assumes that people strive to *ANTICIPATE* 'events' (whether other people's behaviour, our own behaviour, or 'physical' events like the rising of the sun or a red traffic light). They do so by their detection of recurrent themes or 'replications' within their experience *(CONSTRUCTION)*.

The interpretations he places on events are termed 'constructs' and are considered to be bipolar in nature *(DICHOTOMY)*. Constructs are applicable to some things and not others *(RANGE)*. In any particular situation a person has the choice (not necessarily made explicit) as to which pole of a construct is more appropriate *(CHOICE)*.

A person's constructs are inter-related in the form of a system. This system is hierarchial in nature, with constructs being relatively 'subordinate' or 'superordinate' to each other *(ORGANI-SATION)*. Some aspects of our system ('sub-systems') may be inconsistent with others *(FRAGMENTATION)*. Our personal construct system is capable of changing as we interpret new experience *(EXPERIENCE)*. The degree to which we change is limited by the extent to which we utilise constructs 'permeably', i.e. in such a way as to be open to new experience *(MODULATION)*.

People may interpret similar events in different ways from each other *(INDIVIDUALITY)*, but may also share similar outlooks *(COMMONALITY)*. Social interaction involves the need to understand other people's personal construct systems *(SOCIALITY)*.

Diagnosis and Disorder in Personal Construct Theory

Although personal construct theory can be applied in a wide variety of settings (e.g. Pope and Keen, 1981 — Education; Stewart and

Stewart, 1981 — Business; Honikman, 1976 — Environmental Design), its original focus was the clinical context. Kelly was both an academic and a clinician and it was out of his experiences as a clinical psychologist and psychotherapist that he offered a number of 'diagnostic constructs', 'designed to help the clinician assume professionally useful role relations with his clients' (p.452). Unlike the diagnostic constructs of psychiatry (thought disorder, delusions, hysterical personality etc.), Kelly did not assume disease entities. He proposed his diagnostic constructs as axes (like 'north-south' for a sailor), which may be useful for plotting changes in a person's psychological processes. In other words, people need not be seen as fixed on a particular axis, but as potentially capable of movement or change just like the sailor. It is not suggested that these diagnostic constructs are intrinsically superior to the traditional psychiatric diagnostic system. This mainly depends on one's purposes. If one is concerned with more than just categorisation, however, then one may find Kelly's diagnostic constructs helpful in exploring avenues of change.

Before examining the diagnostic constructs, I should like to turn to the question of what is a 'disorder'. I have chosen the term disorder in preference to the term ill, although I would not wish to take issue with those who prefer the term mental illness. Far more important than the precise verbal label is the meaning we ascribe to such terms. Some mental health professionals have shied away from the term mental illness because of the connotations of biological aetiology and lack of personal responsibility that might be implied. It seems to me, however, that psychological formulations like 'low reinforcement' or 'maternal deprivation' are just as capable of being sterile as are 'illness' formulations. What seems of more interest, however, is whether our categories have any implications for constructive change. In using the term psychological disorder, therefore, I shall not be presenting a list of fixed states or traits. In fact, Kelly resisted the temptation to define disorder categorically and instead chose a very flexible definition:

> From the standpoint of the psychology of personal constructs we may define a disorder as any personal construction which is used repeatedly in spite of consistent invalidation. (p.831)

He goes on to say:

. . . it represents any structure which appears to fail to accomplish its purpose . . . Appears to whom? . . . we are content to let 'disorder' mean whatever is ineffectual from the viewpoint of his stuffy neighbours, from the viewpoint of history, or from the viewpoint of God. (p.835)

The point being made here is that describing someone as having a disorder is essentially a construction. Like all constructs, the term disorder is useful to the extent that it aids anticipation. Presumably, the persistence of terms like 'neurotic' means that they have helped some people to predict some of the sorts of things to expect of certain people. That does not preclude the possibility that at some point the term might be abandoned as relatively meaningless. We don't have to look back too far in history to find various constructions of mental illness in Western societies which have subsequently been abandoned. Nowadays, the prevailing models invoke science and illness conceptualisations. Who knows when it will change? It may be preferable, therefore, to apply our concepts of disorder in a 'propositional' way, i.e. as *ways of viewing* certain behaviour and experience. They don't have to be the only way, nor necessarily the best way. Neither do we have to be committed to them as sacred and permanent.

A further implication of what has been said is that we don't necessarily all agree with each other about who should be regarded as exhibiting a psychological disorder. Although in a particular society there might be a fair amount of agreement about the kinds of behaviour and experience which could be construed as disordered there is also plenty of room for difference of opinion. The teenager who stays in bed all day may be regarded by some as typical of his peers and by others as behaving abnormally. Similarly there may be a discrepancy between the subject and the observer as to whether the subject is ill etc. This can work both ways. There are those who won't accept everyone else's view that there's something wrong with them: they may go as far as suggesting that there's something wrong with everyone else! At the other extreme there are those who *want* to have something wrong with them, but no one will let them! Neither has to be seen as right or wrong, but in all such situations people are trying to find some way of making sense of their experience. Whatever our professional explanations might be, it is clear that some people are presented or present themselves as having something wrong with the way they think, feel or act. Let us now turn to some of the ways we can look at such people from the standpoint of the psychology of personal constructs. Kelly's Dimensions of Diagnosis will be subdivided into four broad categories, namely 'Covert Construction'; 'Content of Construction'; 'Dimensions of Transition' and 'Cycles and Processes of Construction'.

Covert Construction

Kelly offers a number of constructs relevant to what is sometimes called 'the unconscious'. Although the latter term has had a controversial history, few would disagree that not all of our behaviour is governed by consciously verbalised ideas: such phenomena were described by Kelly as covert construction'. The first form of 'covert construction' that shall be described is as follows.

Preverbal Constructs. A Preverbal Construct is one which continues to be used even though it has no consistent word label. I have already emphasised that constructs need not have a word label. Children seem to be engaged in construing, well before they have the grasp of their native language. From an early age, a child is seen to discriminate successfully between different aspects of its world (familiar people — unfamiliar people; food — not food; comfort — discomfort), to anticipate (e.g. the sight of food) and to test out his anticipations (e.g. throwing toys out of prams). No-one would suggest, however, that a 9-month old baby has a set of verbal labels tucked away in his head. Similarly, dumb people are not prevented from forming concepts simply because they cannot speak. Because 'preverbal constructs' are often formed before a person has the command of speech, we should not be suprised if they often need to be 'acted out'. This might involve anything from crying to dribbling. We should try and avoid being impatient at such behaviour. Although it might prove helpful later to try and attach a verbal label to such experience, we should not assume that the person concerned has the verbal constructs which we as therapists are applying to his behaviour. Thus in personal construct psychotherapy one may often be dealing with the client's actions rather than his words. One type of behaviour which might express itself non-verbally is 'dependency'. Therapists often feel uncomfortable about such behaviour in clients. It should be recognised, however, that preverbal constructs might form a kind of last line of defence. Faced with the virtual collapse or deficiencies of his current constructs, rather than face total unpredictability, the person might seek validation in terms of more infantile constructs. Crying might lead to cuddles, naughtiness might lead to smacks. Although we might not wish to play the role of Daddy or Mummy, such behaviour is likely to persist until the person has developed some alternative way of construing his current situation.

Preverbal constructs are not all formed in childhood, however, and particularly when facing a new situation we may be confronted with vague feelings and thoughts which can't yet be put into words. In such situations we might grope with incoherent verbalisations until, perhaps sometimes with the help of others who know what we mean, they eventually crystallise into more structured ideas.

Submergence. The submerged pole of a construct is the one which is less available for application to events. When one pole of a construct is markedly less available than the other this is referred to as the 'submerged' end. For example, we have all met the sort of person who says he has never been angry or claims that he likes everybody. Given that constructs are bipolar, then we may be interested in what the contrast end of the construct is.

One might explore a number of directions in trying to identify the contrast. The person who says he has never been angry may be implying that although he has never been angry, someone else was once very angry and look at the consequences of that! Alternatively, it may be that although he has never been angry *yet* in his life, one day someone might make him angry and what would be the consequences? Although not going as far as using the term defence mechanisms, Kelly clearly implies that such construction might serve the purpose of avoiding construing himself at the 'submerged end'. This may be because for that person the submerged end carries unacceptable or incomprehensible implications, which he is unwilling to put to the test. If, for example, he was prepared to construe himself at the angry pole, he may fear far-reaching and devastating effects which could threaten both his identity and the whole integrity of his construct system.

Suspension. A suspended element is one which is omitted from the context of a construct as the result of revision of the person's construct system. Kelly's concept of 'suspension' is akin to the Freudian concept of repression. When aspects of a person's construct system are 'rejected' or 'forgotten' because they are no longer compatible with the person's current construing, this would be described as

'suspension'. Given that people change, their newly formed outlook may not be able to handle some aspects of their previous
experience. For example, as 'mature adults' we may wish to disown
the way we acted when we were in our youth. The old way of
looking at things is not lost, but held in a kind of abeyance and
sometimes may be returned to when the person has developed a
more comprehensive construct system which can incorporate the
old outlook without being threatened. We don't just see this with
individuals. Societies that go through revolution typically seek to
deny all evidence of the old life style, even to the point of having to
destroy buildings and people. Thus in contrast to the Freudian
notion of repression, suspension implies that we 'forget' that which
is *unstructured*, rather than just in terms of 'pleasantness — un-
pleasantness'.

Level of Cognitive Awareness. Finally, in this section on 'covert
construction', Kelly introduces the dimension of 'level of cognitive
awareness'. Preverbal constructs, submergence and suspension are
seen as representing a relatively low level of cognitive awareness.
The concept of cognitive awareness is offered as being particularly
appropriate for understanding changes that may occur in psychotherapy. One might aim for a higher level of cognitive awareness by
making constructs more verbalisable, with both poles of the construct accessible and render the construct more compatible with
other aspects of a person's construing. In some schools of therapy
this process might be called achieving insight.

Content of Construction

Propositionality. Although not classified by Kelly under his heading
of Dimensions of Diagnosis, this concept is an important one within
the theory and is particularly applicable to the clinical context. I
earlier referred to 'propositional' construing when discussing the
concept of psychological disorder, but the concept deserves further
elaboration. *Propositional* constructs are contrasted with two other
forms of construct — *pre-emptive* and *constellatory* constructs.

A pre-emptive construct is one which doesn't allow its elements
to be construed in any other terms: in other words it 'pigeon-holes'.
For example, if we were using the construct 'schizophrenic-not-
schizophrenic' we would be construing pre-emptively if people we
called schizophrenic were seen as 'nothing but' schizophrenics.

Pre-emption, in practice, however, is a matter of degree and few constructs are used totally pre-emptively. Although there might be a time and place for pre-emptive construing (e.g. on detecting a fire), the very essence of constructive alternativism invites us to question the usefulness of the 'nothing but' kind of construing.

A constellatory construct is one which, although allowing elements to be construed in other terms, fixes what those terms are. Applied to our schizophrenic example, such a person would be construed as also, let's say, completely incomprehensible, dangerous and not to be trusted. He would not be allowed to be also construed as a gardener, a great lover or a creative person. We could equally apply such thinking to the staff in psychiatric settings. A psychiatrist who in his working role allows himself to be concerned, professional and competent, but under no circumstances to have a good laugh or feel despair also construes in a constellatory manner (constellatory construing is, thus, similar to the concept of 'stereotyping').

A propositional construct, however, is much more flexible. Used propositionally, the schizophrenic construct would allow someone so construed to be open to any number of alternative constructions. He might be anything from a hard worker, a visionary, a good golfer to a neighbour. Like pre-emptive and constellatory construing, however, propositionality is a matter of degree. It may be comparatively rare to construe things completely propositionally, but we may be more or less open to construing things in other ways. Although Kelly does not suggest that propositional construing is a panacea in all situations, there is more than a hint in Kelly's writing that greater use of propositional or 'as if' construing might free individuals, groups and societies from the dangers of being too sure and committed to their version of reality.

Tight and Loose Constructs. Tight constructs are those which lead to unvarying predictions . . . Loose constructs are those which lead to varying predictions but which, for practical purposes, may be said to retain their identity. When a construct is 'loose' an event may sometimes be construed at one pole and at other times at the other pole. For example, in applying the construct 'trustworthy-untrustworthy', the person keeps changing his mind about which people are to be trusted or not. Similarly, this inconsistency might also apply to one's construing of oneself. In very loose construing, a person shows very little consistency in how elements are construed.

The person jumps about from one pole to the other with the same elements. The most clear example of loose construing in everyday experience is dreaming. Loose construing is like a rough sketch in which the precise configuration of its elements is still left undecided. In tight construing, however, we are more decisive and consistent. For example, some nurses seem to have very 'tight' construction about how to run a ward. Things have to be exactly in their place, patients must get out of bed at precise times, visiting and non-visiting time is very clearly defined. Amongst psychiatric patients, there is no better example of tight construing than the obsessive-compulsive neurotic, who within the area of his rituals creates an extremely predictable world. It may be, however, that outside his rituals, his construing is much looser (Fransella, 1974). In addition to being applied to individual constructs, the term term 'tight-loose' has also been applied to whole systems and sub-systems of constructs, so that a person may be seen as relatively tight or loose in his construing in general. More likely than not, however, a person will construe 'tightly' in some contexts and 'loosely' in other situations. A person may, for example, seek certainty and precision in his work, but look for excitement and uncertainty in his love-life.

Neither tight nor loose construing is superior. Both may be appropriate at different times. In fact, as we shall see later, Kelly envisaged a healthy individual as moving from one to the other in a cyclical manner.

This dimension is arguably one of the most useful in the clinical context and forms the basis of the extended work of Bannister (1960, 1963, 1965a) on his serial invalidation hypothesis of schizophrenia. It is also relevant, however, to other disorders and is particularly relevant to the conceptualisation of the process of change in psychotherapy.

Superordinacy. We have already seen in the Organisation Corollary that construct systems are hierarchical, with each construct capable of subsuming or being subsumed by another. For example, the construct 'good-bad' might be applied to the constructs 'winner-loser', 'kind-unkind' and 'believes in God-Atheist'. In this respect, 'good-bad' would be 'superordinate' to these constructs. However, at a higher level of abstraction 'good-bad' and 'strong-weak' might be subordinate to the construct 'evaluative-descriptive'. Thus constructs are not superordinate or subordinate *per se*, but may be either, depending on the context.

Although a construct may be 'superordinate' to another, in itself this does not carry any restriction on the relationship between the constructs. Kelly describes one form such relationship might take. He calls a construct *Regnant* over another, if it applies its elements to a category on an 'all or none' basis. For example — 'doctors are always right' or 'all schizophrenics are dangerous'. Although undoubtedly helping to simplify things, when applied to people, the consequences of such construing hardly need spelling out.

Comprehensive and Incidental Constructs. 'Comprehensive' constructs are those which subsume a relatively wide variety of events. Incidental constructs subsume a small variety of events. Good-bad is an example of a construct which can be applied to a wide variety of things, whereas 'positively charged-negatively charged' is generally applied in a more restricted range of situations.

Core Constructs and Peripheral Constructs. Core constructs are those which govern a person's maintenance processes — that is, those by which he maintains his identity and existence. Peripheral constructs are those which can be altered without serious modification of core structure. Some constructs are thus more central to a person than others. This may range from the kind of food we eat to our nationality, although what's 'core' for one person may be more peripheral to another. For one person whether he is regarded as intellectual or not may be crucial to his very identity, whereas for another it may be a peripheral matter compared with whether he is resolute as opposed to fickle. When a person's identity is at stake there are considerable risks for a person. We are on dangerous ground when we challenge a person's cherished beliefs about himself, whereas when dealing with more peripheral matters we may take more chances. Core constructs are, thus, of direct relevance to the notion of the *Self*. In construct theory the 'self' is in many ways no different from any other element, i.e. it is 'constructed', it needs to be anticipated and it is capable of various interpretations. It is likely, however, that we will have a lot more invested in those constructs which are central to our view of ourselves. The self is, after all, an element which it is difficult to ignore or cast to one side. It is not surprising, therefore, that some people place enormous restrictions on themselves for the sake of preserving consistency. At the other extreme, however, if we are too unpredictable we may end up wondering who we really are. The chances are, therefore, that most of us have a view of ourselves which is in some respects open to negotiation, whereas, in other ways we may have a continuing sense of 'me-ness' which we will be reluctant to abandon.

We would do well to be on the lookout for a person's core constructs.

Dimensions of Transition

A person's construct system is never completely at rest, although some changes are more disturbing than others. In fact, it could be argued that 'emotion' represents, in effect, a construct system undergoing change or disruption. This state of transition doesn't have to be regarded as bad. Although there is sometimes something to be said for predictability, when life becomes too predictable we are faced with the prospect of a kind of 'psychological death by boredom'. Thus, 'emotion' may be an inevitable consequence of the human search for variety and novelty. Rather than treating emotion as a separate subject (versus 'cognition, or 'behaviour'), however, Kelly instead described some of the kinds of experience we typically call feelings, in terms of transitions in personal construct systems. The first of these dimensions is what Kelly called 'threat'.

Threat. Threat is the awareness of imminent comprehensive change in one's core structures. Like all of Kelly's Dimensions of Transition, threat is a term applied commonly in everyday life, including the field of mental health, although his particular meaning for the term does not necessarily coincide identically with any dictionary definition. Kelly stresses that, in order for threat to be significant, the change has to be substantial. Imminent death or a close bereavement are obvious examples, but almost any experience where a person's most basic assumptions about himself and the world are called into question might be described as threat. The loss of use of his hands for a pianist, the last child leaving home for a parent or a loss of faith for a Christian, may all signal change of massive proportions. As Landfield (1954, 1955) has pointed out, we may also feel threatened by our past. A return to 'old pastures' might make us all too aware of how easily we could slip back into a way of life we thought we'd outgrown. The reformed alcoholic who takes a drink knows all too well the path he could so easily follow.

Kelly wrote extensively about the importance of managing threat in psychotherapy. This is not just because one may be treading on dangerous ground, but reflects the fact that change for the better can also be threatening. 'Getting better' or reaching one's ambitions can prove very threatening as a person becomes aware of the ramifications of what this change will mean for his life. The reader may be reminded here of Paykel's 'entrances' (Paykel *et al.*, 1969) as a class of 'life events' which may be stressful even though generally regarded as pleasant. Of course, in personal construct theory there is no assumption that 'life events' can be threatening unless they imply comprehensive change for that person.

Fear. Fear is like threat, except that, in this case it is a new incidental construct, rather than a comprehensive construct that seems about to take over. Kelly points out that the 'incidental' construct is still a 'core' construct and hence the person's 'maintenance processes' are also at stake as in threat. In both cases, disturbance may ensue as we face the need to reconstrue the core of our personality. But the Kellyian definition of fear does not involve radical restructuring of our construct system. When paying a visit to the dentist, most of us feel afraid of possible pain, but it is unlikely that there will be far-reaching ramifications. A knock on the door by a policeman, however, might be more than just fear-inducing, as thoughts flash in front of our mind which may threaten our whole identity and existence. 'My child's been killed?' . . . 'They've finally caught up with me?' Furthermore, what starts off as fear may turn into a feeling of threat as we digest the full implications of the immediate event.

Anxiety. Anxiety is the recognition that the events with which one is confronted lie outside the range of convenience of one's construst system. When we fail to make sense of what happens we may experience anxiety. My favourite personal example is my first day at school: unlike my own son, I had not had the benefit of a prior visit. I can still recall that feeling of strangeness — of being 'lost': I neither knew what to do or where to go. You might think of your own example — perhaps when you first went to a foreign country or moved to a new home. Kelly emphasised, however, that it is a *partial* failure to anticipate: something totally unconstruable would neither be perceived nor lead to anxiety. Note that in contrast to threat and fear, there is no stipulation for 'core' constructs' to be involved, so that we may feel anxious where relatively peripheral matters are at stake. Going to dinner with relative strangers, watching a science fiction film or failing to find one's car in a car park may all be difficult to construe, without necessarily involving your identity or threatening your existence.

Kelly's definition of anxiety although broader in its range, seems particularly relevant to describing what is sometimes called 'free-floating anxiety'. The subjective experience of anxiety without an object of concern may be a sure sign that a person is confronted with events which are relatively meaningless to him. For example, a woman may have no clear idea of what it will be like when her child starts school. She doesn't necessarily make this connection, however, and may just focus on the alien nature of her 'symptoms'. The chances are that if she can retreat into some area of her life which is familiar and safe, the anxiety will recede, albeit probably only temporarily.

Guilt. Perception of one's apparent dislodgement from his core role structure constitutes the experience of guilt. When discussing the 'Sociality Corollary' we considered the concept of 'role': a course of action based on one's interpretation of the thinking of other people. The 'core role' involves those aspects of a person's role construing by which he maintains himself as an integral being: more 'peripheral' role constructs are not included in one's 'core role'. Core role is thus not a superficial thing. We act out our 'core role' as if our life depended on it. When we fail to live up to ourselves as a social being, Kelly calls the resulting experience 'Guilt'.

Some people seem capable of the most despicable acts without experiencing remorse. At the other extreme, we find the depressive who is tormented with guilt over some seemingly innocuous act. Kelly's definition of guilt offers a clarification of this potentially puzzling matter. In the case of the brutal mass murderer who feels no remorse, he presumably sees his actions as consistent with his view of himself: he may argue that he was putting them out of their misery or doing society a favour. He is thus at odds with the prevailing popular view of what is right or wrong at that time. The depressive, however, may share the social expectations of his peers, but may have over-defined the meaning of good-bad.

We may also feel guilt when we experience something generally regarded as 'positive'. Doing something nice, even though enjoyable, may make us feel guilty if in retrospect it seems like it was 'not me'. The shy person who speaks up for the first time, the frigid person who eventually has an orgasm, the failure who has a success may all feel none too at ease about the new experience. Rather than watching a science fiction film or failing to find one's car in a car face the uncertainty of wondering what sort of person they really are, they may instead choose to retreat to the 'old me'.

Aggressiveness. Aggressiveness is the active elaboration of one's perceptual field. Kelly's concept of 'aggression' is not the same as the hitting people over the head view of aggression and is certainly not viewed as simply an anti-social impulse. In fact, there is more than a touch of the 'positive' in Kelly's use of the term. The Kellyian aggressive person is actively doing things, always precipitating himself and others into situations where choices and action are required: he certainly doesn't rest on his laurels. Of course, such behaviour may sometimes be perceived by his associates as unwelcome. Those who are seeking a quiet life may not take too kindly to the person who is constantly challenging, questioning and pestering.

'Aggression' should, however, not be seen as a trait. At some stages of our life (e.g. during adolescence) we may be more actively 'elaborating', whereas at other times we may be content just to 'tick over'. Furthermore, in some contexts we may be more aggressive than others: the 'dynamic' businessman may be pretty un-dynamic in his home life.

Hostility. Hostility is the continued effort to extort validational evidence in favour of a type of social prediction which has already proved itself a failure. When faced with mounting evidence that we are wrong we may go to extraordinary lengths to hold on to that crumbling theory. The mother who has devoted much of her life to her maternal role may find that her teenage children are increasingly failing to adhere to her expectations about the mother-child relationship. Rather than face the inevitability of this change, she may seek to force her children into continuing to depend on her and prove that they really do still need their Mum.

The concept of 'hostility' is particularly relevant to the problem of resistance. Patients may triumph at proving that they can't change . . . 'Didn't I tell you it wouldn't work?' This might extend into trying to force people into one's expectations. The person who believes that no one really cares for him, when faced with the caring therapist, may go out of his way to annoy the therapist, whether by sending him threatening letters, ringing him up incessantly or by turning up late for appointments. It is not just our patients who behave in a 'hostile' manner: therapists also have their theories! One such theory might be, 'If you follow the steps in the behavioural programme then you will eventually develop a sense of control over your symptoms'. When patients don't conform to such expectations, we may try to bully them into proving we're right. We may search around for some crumb of evidence that they are improving, or perhaps try and prove that they or we haven't followed the programme properly . . . anything rather than face the possibility that we may be wrong.

Cycles and Processes of Construction

Dilation and Constriction. When, following a series of alternating uses of incompatible systems, a person broadens his perceptual field in order to reorganise it on a more comprehensive level, the adjustment may be called 'dilation' . . . When one minimizes the apparent incompatibility of his construction system by drawing in the outer boundaries of his perceptual field, the relatively repetitive mental process that ensues is designated as 'constriction'. Although classified by Kelly under 'content of construction', the concepts of 'dilation' and 'constriction' seem to me to fit better in this section as a process, along with Kelly's 'Cycles of Construction'. When 'dilating', a person may jump from topic to topic, he may see connections between a vast array of events. When taken to extremes, as for example in the manic patient, virtually every event may be seen as relevant to his concerns. An extreme example of constriction would seem to be catatonic withdrawal, where the person seems virtually to switch off.

Both dilation and constriction may be therapeutically wise depending on the context. A narrowing of focus ('constriction') may prove helpful for the person who is hyperattentive whereas the person who is locked into a very narrow view of his problem might be helped to see links between that problem and other facets of his life ('dilation').

The C-P-C Cycle. The C-P-C cycle is a sequence of construction involving, in succession, circumspection, pre-emption, and control leading to a choice which precipitates the person into a particular situation. This cycle describes the sequence which precedes choice and action. Firstly, we consider a range of possible ways of viewing a situation (*circumspection*). After the circumspection phase, we opt for one particular issue (*pre-emption*), e.g. like Hamlet who concluded . . . 'To be or not to be — that is the question'. The 'question' might be anything from what to have for lunch to marrying as opposed to remaining single. Eventually, we decide or choose which pole to go for (*control*).

The man who has his finger on the dreaded nuclear button may one day be faced with the situation where there is some evidence of something happening. He could look on this from a number of standpoints (from the standpoint of his family, his mortality, as an event in history, his competence as a signal detector or as an interesting moral issue). If his training has prepared him 'well', he will presumably decide eventually that there is only one issue to consider . . . 'Do I or don't I press the button?'

This cycle doesn't necessarily proceed through each stage in an orderly and consistent manner. In some people the circumspection phase is fore-shortened or non-existent — Kelly calls this *Impulsivity*. In others, circumspection may be a way of life, such that any real action is impossible. Without decision and choice of course, there can be no development and change. Action without circumspection, however, may mean a life devoid of any pattern, order or direction.

The Creativity Cycle. The Creativity cycle is one which starts with loosened construing and terminates with tightened and validated construction.

Kelly is using the term 'creativity' here in a much broader sense than is often the case. Put simply, he is indicating that one can't create anything new without first questioning our assumptions. By making 'tight' predictions in which one is consistent and precise we may appear to be quite productive. The chances are, however, that it is 'more of the same'. If we are ever to go beyond going over the same tracks, we will need to loosen our construing, i.e. consider alternative predictions.

For example, the problem drinker might reconsider his assumptions about drinking. Having always regarded non-drinkers as 'boring' as opposed to 'fun', he might start to wonder if, in fact, some of his drinking mates are bores and some of his sober acquaintances are actually having fun. Eventually this 'loosening' needs to be followed by a revised tightened construction in which a new formulation can be put to the test. He may instead decide that perhaps 'honest' people get some real 'joy' out of life. He might put this prediction to the test by endeavouring to start being more honest with people. The matter doesn't rest there of course: in life there may be continuing series of cycles of this sort as we successively revise our understandings.

The management of loosening and tightening is given a prominent place in Kelly's approach to psychotherapy. Excessive loosening (when most of a client's predictions have been challenged) may lead to a near-psychotic state. Although potentially therapeutically constructive, the loosening may get out of hand because the therapist has failed to anticipate the repercussions of his interpretations or whatever technique he has applied. At the other extreme, however, excessive reliance on tight construing might make the therapy sessions feel safer, but with little chance of progress. Optimum intervention, therefore, might facilitate the client's ability to move more freely from vagueness to precision and so forth.

Implications for Mental Health

Having outlined the main concepts of personal construct theory, I would like to turn to the other focus of this book, namely 'mental health'. You will doubtless have your own opinions on what sort of implications this wide-ranging theory may have for mental health, but I will share with you some of my personal views on this matter.

Firstly, you might be interested in the very fundamental issue of what is mental health? This question has indirectly been addressed in the section on 'disorder': mental health might be regarded as the opposite pole of 'psychological disorder' or 'mental illness'. It should be clear by now that there is no attempt to define mental health in absolute terms within construct theory. The term 'mental health — mental illness' may thus be seen as a construct invented by people as one way of understanding and predicting certain sorts of behaviour and experience. Previous attempts at defining mental health have, not surprisingly, come up with no clear consensus. Although the language of psychiatry has developed an extensive language for defining what might be called mental illness, there is ample evidence that psychiatrists don't always agree about the matter, leave alone considering the socio-cultural factors which influence such labelling.

Furthermore, the difficulties in deciding what is mental illness, are mild compared with the problems of defining its opposite.

This is not to say that attempts have not been made to spell out what we may be aiming at in the field of psychotherapy. In fact, Kelly wrote an essay entitled 'A Psychology of the Optimal Man', a theme eleborated by Epting and Amerikaner: both articles appear in Landfield and Leitner (1980). Thus terms like 'coming alive', 'actively elaborating one's construct system', 'invention', 'more effective anticipation', 'continually re-defining one's potentials', have been applied to describe the process of growth and evolution that might characterise what we might call 'healthy living'. Such concepts thus emphasise the open-ended nature of life and invite us to view it as something of an exploration in which we can never be quite sure where it will all end up — or even if it will end at all! Perhaps the crucial thing about life is that 'it goes on': when people effectively grind to a halt or keep going round in circles we sometimes call them mentally ill. Whilst they keep moving, we might, if we care to think about it, call them mentally healthy.

So what is personal construct theory's contribution to these matters. In my view its main strength is in taking people seriously. Rather than dismissing a person's behaviour as being a reflection of forces beyond his control and which can be 'treated' without reference to him as a *person*, we are invited to try and understand him, to try and enter into his world. Of course, this kind of approach is not unique to construct theory. This kind of theme runs through a number of notable alternatives to a medical model of mental illness (e.g. Laing, Szasz, Rogers). What is different about personal construct theory is that it focuses on one particular aspect of a person's psychological processes, namely his need to try to *anticipate*, his reaching into the future. Rather than see symptoms as the outcome of some experience or some biological event, we may see him as trying to make something out of both his social and biological experience. The chances are that if he has come the way of the psychiatric services then he and/or his associates are entertaining one possible explanation of his predicament. We can choose to collude with that version and offer to take control of his life until he's 'better'. Alternatively, we can take the more challenging approach of viewing mental health services as a kind of 'personal laboratory' or 'college of living' rather than act as if we can 'cure' people of their problem or living. I find it hard to see how we can achieve this, however, without recognising that, more than anything else, we as professional helpers, are basically *people* and that our most powerful tool is likely to be our concern, care and respect for people and our willingness to try and help people achieve the understanding they have failed to elicit in their life. Perhaps once they have found some way of being able to make sense of themselves and others, they then turn to the business of 'living' and not just 'existing'.

Summary

An approach to the understanding of people has been described which places its main emphasis on man's need to anticipate. Human lives are seen as constructed and reconstructed on the basis of people's anticipations of what might follow. In addition to this main assumption of the theory, a series of related concepts have been offered as ways of understanding the various pathways and changes open to people. A number of 'diagnostic constructs' have been introduced which may be particularly relevant to those working in the field of mental health. The reader should not feel, however, that these concepts are real entities which have to be remembered or recited at all times. You may find some of them useful, others less so. You may also conceivably even dream up a few more of your own!

Note

1. Throughout this book references to Kelly without a date should be taken to imply Kelly (1955).

2 TECHNIQUES FOR EXPLORING CONSTRUCTS

Eric Button

Having examined the basic concepts of personal construct theory, we can now move on to the 'how' of it. In later sections of this book we shall be considering applications to specific psychiatric disorders and helping people to change. In this chapter we will focus on methods of 'exploration'. This term is chosen in preference to alternatives such as 'assessment'. The term 'assessment' tends to imply that the 'assessor' knows in advance what parameters to assess (e.g. assertiveness, level of hostility or neuroticism). In contrast, personal construct theory offers an approach to psychological enquiry in which we as investigators are not pre-judging the parameters. This is what we will want to 'explore' together with our client.

So what might be the focal point of enquiry from a personal construct theory standpoint: whereas the doctor might be interested in symptoms, the behaviourist in 'behaviour', we would be interested in, surprise-surprise . . . 'constructs'. There are other books specifically concerned with ways of exploring constructs (e.g. Bannister and Mair, 1968; Fransella and Bannister, 1977), including at least one book on applying this approach in a specific context (business applications, Stewart and Stewart, 1981). My aim here is to illustrate some of the basics which will allow the mental health worker to try out some of the techniques on the sorts of questions which might particularly interest him. Whatever the particular purpose of your enquiry, you are likely to start out by seeking to identify or 'elicit' a person's or group of person's constructs.

Eliciting Constructs

The Elements

Normally when we wish to find out about a person, rather than expecting to cover everything, we usually have some particular focus in mind, although this might still be relatively broad. We thus have a *context* in mind. This might be drinking bouts, family members, sexual relationships or anything you *and your client*

31

choose: I emphasise 'and your client' intentionally. The client is
likely to get more out of the exercise if he is involved in the choice of
what to investigate. Thus, a client who is complaining that she can't
go out, might be invited to say something about the various places
she might go to. We would start by identifying a set of 'elements; —
in this case, places or journeys outside the house.

At this point, I am going to complicate things somewhat by telling
you that 'elements' are also constructs! For example, delusions,
hallucinations and anxiety at one level would be elements which
would help us to define constructs, such as schizophrenia or depression. At another level, however, delusions etc., could be regarded
as convenient constructs for making sense out of statements like —
'I am evil', 'It tells me I'm evil' or 'I feel as if I'm going mad'.
Although nothing is, thus, just a construct or just an element, it is
convention to refer to the things one is considering or 'abstracting'
from as 'elements'.

In our above example the set of elements might be as provided by
a lady I recently worked with:

1. Going to the newsagents.
2. Going to the butchers.
3. Going to the post office.
4. Going to my mother's house.
5. Going to the 'nearly new' shop.
6. Going to my daughter Alice's.
7. Going to the local shopping centre.
8. Going to the supermarket.

You may be struck with the rather limited range of situations
selected. This highlights the fact that selecting the elements is a
form of 'sampling'. We are rarely likely to be able to identify all the
elements in a particular context. We are, therefore, required to
select some method of sampling from amongst a potentially vast
range. In a clinical context, we don't have to be constrained to a
narrow statistician's definition of 'representative sampling'. We
will, however, want to consider a variety of elements which are
important or 'meaningful' to our client in this particular context.
One way of doing this is by selecting a list of 'role titles'. For
example, in the context of people, the subject might be asked to
name 'a liked person', 'your best friend', 'a person you find difficult
to get on with' etc. Whilst this has the advantage of standardising a

procedure (e.g. in a research context), it has the disadvantage of imposing the investigator's own constructs on to the subject. An alternative is to ask the client the following kind of question: 'Since we have decided to look more closely at (trips outside your home) I'd like you to start by giving me a list of the various trips outside your home you have made in the past and would like to make in the future. You can include whichever ones you like, but try and cover a number of different sorts of trips'. One might go as far as restricting the number of elements (e.g. 10 is a popular number), although there are no hard and fast rules. Having suggested usually asking the subject to provide his own elements, there is no reason why the investigator can't also supply some of his own. It is wise, however, to sound the subject out about this rather than present it as a *fait accompli*. You might say, for example: 'Well, you've given me quite an interesting list — I wonder if I could add a few more which I'd be interested to hear about from your point of view — the ones I had in mind were 'travelling to town on a bus', 'going to the cinema' and 'going to a wedding'. Sometimes the subject might reject the supplied elements. They might not seem relevant to him or sometimes he may not wish to disclose what he feels about them. For example, in my work I am often interested in how clients construe their parents. Usually, they will spontaneously include them, but sometimes mother or father is conspicuously absent. On questioning, I find that some people quite clearly don't want to include one or other of them. Although sometimes, in a research context, having pushed people, I now feel this is unwise.

The Constructs

Constructs can be selected in a number of different ways, although certain methods have proved particularly popular. The most well known is the 'triadic' method.

The Triadic Method. From our total set of elements a set of three is selected. The triad may be either selected 'randomly' or on the basis of some pre-determined groupings or 'sorts'. One popular way of facilitating this task is to number the elements and write the name of each element on its own small index card. The cards may thus be shuffled or otherwise divided into groups of three. In any particular case a number of triads would be selected in order to allow for a range of constructs to emerge: this might involve anything up to ten or more triads. Once a triad has been selected, the cards would be placed in front of the person and the question asked — 'I'd like you to think of ways in which these elements (e.g. people) are different from or similar to each other. Is there any way in which you would say that two of them are alike and different from the third?' For example, I was recently asked to assess 'Brenda', a 30-year-old married woman who had been admitted to an acute admission ward of a psychiatric unit. She had tried to commit suicide after finding her husband in bed with a friend of hers. She responded positively to my invitation to her to tell me something of how she saw herself and the other important people in her life. The first triad I presented her was as follows:

Me   My mother   Ella

She said that she and 'Ella' were 'together', whereas she and her mother were 'not together'. I then made a note of this as follows:

Construct 1: 'together-not together'

Note that both poles have been identified. I was not just content to know how two people were similar. I also wanted to know in what way the other one was different. In this case the term 'not' seemed to suffice for this client, whereas often people have a specific verbal label which describes the opposite. For example, in another of the triads Brenda came up with the construct 'hard' as opposed to (perhaps surprisingly) 'feminine'.

Although reports of construct theory applications often give the impression that only one construct occurs in any particular triad, I find it is not uncommon for people to offer several constructs from a triad. In Brenda's case, for example, she re-arranged the elements so that 'me' was now placed together with 'Ella' and separate from her mother. She said that her mother 'relies on people' whereas she and Ella 'don't need people'.

Having exhausted the most obvious contrasts in the first triad, another triad is selected. In Brenda's second triad the following elements were included:

My husband   My first husband   My step-father

She said that her first husband and her step-father were 'unable to show happiness in the family', whereas her present husband was 'more able to show happiness in the family'.

This process of presenting new triads is repeated until the same constructs keep repeating themselves: in a research context, however, one might have a fixed number of triads in order to achieve a degree of standardisation. Depending on factors like a person's degree of articulateness one might run out of new constructs from as few as 3-4 to as many as 50 or more. For most people, however, about 10-20 is more typical. In Brenda's case, the following 12 constructs emerged:

1. 'Together – not together'.
2. 'Happy with their families – not happy with their families'.
3. 'Can show happiness in the family – can't show happiness in the family'.
4. 'Rely on people a lot – don't need people'.
5. 'Nice looking – plain'.
6. 'Slim – fat'.
7. 'Confident – not confident'.
8. 'Hard – feminine'.
9. 'Have a brick wall around them – happy'.
10. 'Able to cry – can't cry'.
11. 'Can talk about problems – can't talk about problems'.
12. 'Can be loving – can't be loving'.

Dyads. Although the triadic method has proved particularly popular, there is absolutely no reason why one should be restricted to it. One alternative is to present the elements in pairs (or 'dyads'). For example, the elements 'Me now' and 'Me before I became ill' might be presented and the subject asked to state any differences or similarities. One would, of course, still seek to identify both poles of any construct elicited. Thus, if our subject said that although he has 'lost confidence' compared with before his illness, he is still 'considerate', he might be asked what was for him the opposite of considerate. He might say, 'couldn't care less about anybody'.

Singly. Although, not much reported, elements could be presented one at a time and the subject asked to describe the element. The disadvantage with this approach is that the subject may reel off a whole list of 'constructs' or even go into a kind of story about the element. This might be very illuminating, but it can be very difficult to identify the contrasts he is making in any orderly way. On the other hand, I find it can prove intrusive to stop a person in midstream to ask him for the opposite poles.

Free Sorts. A method I find particularly useful is to present all the elements to the person at once. The full set of cards are placed in front of the subject and he is invited to sort the cards in any way he likes. This is a bit like the object sorting tasks that have been used to study concept formation. It is also similar to a method Kelly described called 'The Full Context Form'. In my use of this form, I allow any number of elements to be grouped at a time. For example, one of my clients split her set of elements into two piles: those who 'drift aimlessly' and those who 'have a vague sense of direction in life'. I generally use this method in combination with and after using the triadic method: I find that triads help people to get used to thinking in terms of contrasts. By switching to free sorts, I am allowing the subject to select in a flexible way the element combinations which most strikingly illustrate the contrasts he sees. I find it particularly appealing in giving more say to the subject, so that the exercise becomes more collaborative. Furthermore, one has the advantage of seeing the person in action, with some clear evidence as to whether he is able to switch spontaneously from one perspective to another. One might even see it as an exercise in 'elaboration', which might be therapeutic in its own right. In fact, all methods of exploring constructs have therapeutic possibilities and should not be viewed as assessment totally divorced from a helping relationship.

Essays and other less structured techniques. Sorting tasks are not appropriate for all groups. Children and handicapped people, for example, may require a degree of flexibility and ingenuity if one is to discover their constructs. One popular approach is to ask the subject to write a short essay or story. For example, Honess (1979) asked children to write about children they liked and disliked. Where writing would prove difficult, an alternative may be to elicit constructs from a conversation or interview.

Typical of this less structured approach to eliciting constructs is Kelly's technique known as 'Self Characterisation' in which the person is invited to write a short autobiographical sketch of themselves with the instructions: 'I want you to write a character sketch of (Harry Brown), just as if he were the principal character in a play. Write it as it might be written by a friend who knew him very *intimately* and very *sympathetically*, perhaps better than anyone ever really could know him. Be sure to write it in the third person. For example, start out by saying, 'Harry Brown is . . . '

Kelly offers a number of suggestions for 'analysing' self characterisations and the technique has undoubted considerable possibilities in the therapeutic context, as illustrated, for example, by Fransella (1981) and in Chapter 14.

For some groups, however, both written and spoken language may be lacking. For example, Fransella and Bannister (1977) cite an unpublished study by Baillie-Grohman (1975), who used mime and artistic sketches as a way of allowing deaf children to communicate the meanings of their constructs to each other. We don't thus need to be restricted to strictly verbal means of eliciting constructs. In fact, there would seem to be enormous potential for using music and other forms of artistic expression. Essentially, construct elicitation is a form of communication which has the potential for aiding the achievement of understanding. Although we rely a lot on words, there are other ways!

Grids

Having elicited a sample of the subject's personal constructs, one may wish to have some way of measuring the inter-relationships between a person's constructs. 'Repertory grid technique' is the term used to describe a methodology which derives a mathematical representation of part of a person's construct system. The original form described by Kelly is known as the Role Construct Repertory Test (Rep Test). Many of the forms of 'grid' in use today are basically extensions of the 'Rep Test'. Rather than describe the precise method described by Kelly, however, I shall present a general methodology for arriving at what I shall call 'standard grids'. Readers interested in knowing of Kelly's precise method should consult Kelly (1955, pp. 267-77) or Fransella and Bannister (1977, pp. 23-30).

'Standard' Grids

In its standard form, a repertory grid consists of a matrix of the type illustrated in Table 2.1. Basically, the grid might be seen as a form of 'sorting' in which a series of elements have been sorted in terms of a number of constructs. The usual procedure is to take one construct

Table 2.1: An Example of a Grid on 'Brenda'

ELEMENTS

Construct (Left Pole)	HUSBAND	BELLA	DIANE	VERA	STEP	FATHER	MOTHER	SISTER	ME	IDEAL SELF	Construct (Right Pole)
Together	3.5	3.5	7.0	8.0	10	9.0	5.0	6.0	1.5	1.5	Not together
Happy with family	6.0	3.0	8.0	7.0	10	9.0	4.0	5.0	1.5	1.5	Not happy with family
Can show happiness in the family	3.0	4.0	5.0	7.0	9.0	9.0	6.0	9.0	1.5	1.5	Can't show happiness in the family
Relies on people	1.5	7.0	6.0	9.5	3.0	4.0	5.0	9.5	1.5	1.5	Don't need people
Nice looking	4.0	6.0	1.0	8.5	8.5	8.5	3.0	8.5	2.5	1.5	Plain
Slim	6.0	5.0	1.5	8.5	8.5	8.5	6.0	8.5	1.5	1.5	Fat
Confident	5.0	3.0	4.0	8.5	8.5	8.5	6.0	8.5	1.5	1.5	Not confident
Hard	7.5	3.0	7.5	7.5	2.0	7.5	4.0	1.0	1.5	7.5	Feminine
Have a brick wall around	6.5	6.5	6.5	6.5	2.0	6.5	6.5	1.0	6.5	1.5	Happy
Able to cry	3.0	6.0	4.0	8.5	8.5	8.5	5.0	8.5	1.5	1.5	Can't cry
Can talk about problems	3.0	5.0	6.0	8.5	8.5	8.5	4.0	8.5	1.5	1.5	Can't talk about problems
Can be loving	6.0	4.0	3.0	8.5	8.5	8.5	5.0	8.5	1.5	1.5	Can't be loving

Note: Elements were ranked with ties. Left Pole 1, Right Pole 10.

at a time and ask the subject to assign each element a position in terms of that construct. There are several forms of scoring.

Dichotomous Scoring. Let us return to the example of Brenda's grid and consider her first construct . . . 'together-not together'. If using a dichotomous method of scoring we would simply ask her to indicate which elements were 'together' and which elements were 'not together'. In practice this might be best achieved by presenting one element at a time and recording her choices as say '1' for the left-hand pole and '0' for the right-hand pole. Although not actually done in Brenda's case, her choices for this construct might have been as represented in Table 2.2.

Table 2.2: An Example of Dichotomous Scoring on one of Brenda's Constructs

	HUSBAND	ELLA	DIANE	VERA	STEP FATHER	MOTHER	FIRST HUSBAND	SISTER	ME	IDEAL SELF	
Score 1											Score '0'
Together	1	1	1	0	0	0	0	1	0	1	Not Together

(ELEMENTS)

It can be seen that the elements have been evenly distributed between both poles with 'Me' contrasted unfavourably with 'Ideal Self'. It doesn't have to follow that elements are evenly split between poles. Bannister (1959), however, does suggest the possibility of doing this sometimes, by means of the 'split-half' method. Although there might be something to be said for this from the standpoint of simplifying the mathematical analysis of the grid, the resulting constraints imposed may present a rather distorted picture of the person's contruing.

This procedure would be repeated for every other construct in turn and the responses numerically recorded in the form of a matrix with each element having been construed in terms of every element. One problem that can arise with all grids is the matter of 'range of convenience'. In other words some constructs may not be very relevant for some elements. Although one may take steps to minimise this in one's choice of elements, this problem inevitably crops up. One way of dealing with this is to allow subjects to indicate that the construct is irrelevant to the elements in question. This might be recorded in the grid with a symbol such as an *X*. All such cells in the grid would then be ignored in any statistical analysis. It should be noted, however, that if one is planning to analyse the grid by computer, that not all programs allow 'irrelevant' or 'not applicable' categories.

Ranking. A finer degree of discrimination between the elements is offered by ranking. In this method, the elements would be presented to the subject who would be asked to order them from most to least (in our above example) 'together'. The most 'together' would get a rank of '1', the next most 'together' would receive rank '2' and so on up until the least 'together', which would be ranked 10. In Brenda's case (Table 2.1), I used this method with the modification of allowing 'tied ranks': this permits some elements to be judged as equally, in this case 'together'. In Table 2.1 it can be seen that 'Ella' is joint equally most 'together' with 'Ideal self' (ranks 1.5 each rather than 1 and 2). In fact, it can be seen that Brenda makes this choice for most of her constructs.

Rating (or Grading). Possibly one of the commonest forms of scoring currently used is to sort elements on a rating scale. Various kinds of scale are possible (e.g. 0 to 100, plus 3 to minus 3, 1 to 5), although the most popular seems to have been the 1 to 7 scale. Rating is the most flexible of the scoring methods in that it provides more freedom of choice concerning the differentiation of the elements. When using a rating scale the two poles would be allocated numbers such as 1 and 7. The subject would be told that he could assign elements any number along this scale depending on how far towards either extreme the elements seemed. On a 7-point scale 4 would be the mid-point. Some people choose to assign verbal labels to the various points on the scale (e.g. 'extremely' or 'moderately'), but this is very much a matter of discretion.

The use of rating scales, however, is not without controversy, particularly in terms of the meaning of mid-point ratings. For a penetrating discussion of such issues, the reader is directed to an article by Yorke (1983).

Dyad Grids

It has already been pointed out that there is no restriction as to what might constitute the elements in a grid. One very useful application of this principle is to centre the grid on the construing of relationships. In this context the elements become pairs of people. This method, known as the 'Dyad Grid' was first introduced by Ryle and Lunghi (1970). This is particularly relevant where one is interested in a person's interpersonal relationships. One might be particularly interested in relationships involving the 'self' (e.g. my relationship with my wife, my boss, etc.). For each element, Ryle and Lunghi suggest two versions — self to other and other to self. For example, I might not see my relationship with my boss as the same as his relationship with me. You may, like me, find this form of wording confusing and prefer instead to choose such expressions as 'how I feel towards my boss' and 'how my boss feels towards me': whatever the wording the basic principle is the same.

The procedure for obtaining a dyad grid is the same as in conventional 'standard' grids, although Ryle and Lunghi recommend that constructs should be elicited from pairs of elements, rather than three at a time, which proves too difficult. It is also fair to say that the interpretation of the results of a dyad grid can be particularly complicated, although the insights may often more than compensate for the effort involved. Ryle and Breen (1972b) have described a fascinating extension of this method known as the 'double dyad' grid, in which a couple may construct the dyad grid together. This would involve each person completing two versions of the same grid: one from their viewpoint and the other as they imagine their partner would see things. This is a clear example of Kelly's concept of 'sociality', with the opportunity for each partner to exchange their understandings of each other. Readers interested in the clinical application of dyad grids are advised to consult Ryle's (1981) article, in which he compares dyad grid 'dilemmas' in psychotherapy referrals and control subjects.

Dependency Grids

For Kelly, 'dependency' was not an all-or-none affair, but more appropriately investigated in terms of how the person distributes his dependencies. Kelly offered a means of investigating dependency, originally labelled the Situational Resources Repertory Test, latterly known as the Dependency grid. The precise content of the grid is entirely open but one might choose a set of 'situations' (e.g.

problems with your neighbours, the death of your mother, suicidal thoughts). The subject would then be asked to indicate which people he could turn to in such situations (e.g. wife, best friend, his social worker). The person's responses to these questions could be recorded in the form of a grid, just like 'standard grids'. In other words, the 'situation' could be the rows and the people the columns. One could record the responses as ticks and blanks, so that the resulting matrix could be analysed as a dichotomous grid. Alternatively, one could use ranking or rating, thus representing degrees of likelihood that the subject would turn to the various people available. Illustrations of the clinical use of dependency grids are provided in an interesting article by Beail and Beail (1982).

Implications Grids

Implications grids (often known as Impgrids) were devised initially by Hinkle (1965) as part of his doctoral thesis on a 'theory of construct implications'. Hinkle was concerned with exploring the meaning of a construct in terms of both its subordinate and superordinate implications. Although the focus is on construct interrelationships, Impgrids differ from 'standard' grids in that there are no elements: both rows and columns in the matrix are represented by constructs (see Figure 2.1).

The instructions for the Impgrid are rather complicated. The reader can find the full details of both Hinkle's original method and a modified 'Biopolar Impgrid' devised by Fransella (1972) in *A Manual for Repertory Grid Technique* (Fransella and Bannister, 1977). The essence of the Impgrid is that the cells of the grid represent the person's judgement as to the relationship between each pair of constructs. For example, in Figure 2.1 the subject is indicating that she expects that someone who is 'genuine' (Construct 1a) is also likely to 'get on well with people' (6a). On the other hand, the reverse is not true: someone who gets on well with people is not expected to be genuine.

Impgrids are ideally suited to the detailed exploration of the implicative network of a person's constructs. They do, however, have the disadvantage of being rather cumbersome and time-consuming to administer. They are also not amenable to analysis by the more widely available methods of analysis. Both Honess (1982) and Fransella (1972), however, have devised computer programs for their analysis and Impgrids have been applied in interesting ways to clinically related problems, e.g. stuttering (Fransella, 1972), eating disorders (Button, 1980) and depression (Sheehan, 1984).

Figure 2.1: An Example of a Bi-Polar Implications Grid

		1a	1b	2a	2b	3a	3b	4a	4b	5a	5b	6a	6b	7a	7b	8a	8b	9a	9b	10a	10b	11a	11b	12a	12b
Genuine	1a																								
Artificial	b																								
Bad-tempered	2a																								
Not bad-tempered	b																								
Feels sorry for self	3a																								
Prepared to help self	b																								
Shy	4a																								
Extroverted	b																								
Honest	5a																								
Acting	b																								
Gets on well with people	6a																								
Does not get on well with poeple	b																								
Has a weak character	7a																								
Has a strong character	b																								
Less self-assured	8a																								
Too pleased with self	b																								
Like I would like to be	9a																								
Not at all like I would like to be	b																								
Like me	10a																								
Not at all like me	b																								
Like me at my thinnest	11a																								
Like me at my heaviest	b																								
Like me as I'd be at normal weight	12a																								
Not at all like I'd be at normal weight	b																								

Source: Button, E.J. (1980). Construing and Clinical Outcome in Anorexia Nervosa, Unpublished PhD Thesis, University of London.

Resistance-to-Change Grids

This form of grid was also developed by Hinkle (1965) and was used by him partly to test his hypothesis that people were more resistant to changing on those constructs which were relatively 'super-ordinate[1]' in the person's construct system. In a similar way to Impgrids, constructs are taken in pairs and the subject is asked to indicate which are his preferred poles, i.e. how he prefers to construe himself. For example, with the constructs 'content-discontent' and 'prefers rock music – prefers classical music', the subject might say that he preferred to be 'content' and to be someone who 'prefers rock music'. Having identified the preferred poles for all constructs, pairs of constructs are taken and the subject is asked to imagine changing to his non-preferred side. He is faced with a choice, however, in that the imagined change would be on only one pair of constructs. In our example, therefore, the subject would be required to choose between becoming 'discontent' or 'preferring classical music'. We wouldn't be surprised if he said content, but if music was extremely important to his self definition (a 'core' construct) he might surprise us and opt for being discontent. Each choice would be represented in a grid in similar fashion to Impgrids, with the 'resistant to change' construct being represented by a tick in the appropriate cell. One can then add up all the ticks for every construct and use this as a measure of the relative superordinacy of the constructs in the grid.

Like the Impgrid, this is a lengthy procedure, but it is much easier to interpret and it can clearly prove invaluable in highlighting areas of intransigence which would have important implications in a psychotherapeutic context. An example of a Resistance to Change Grid can be found in Fransella and Bannister (1977).

Analysing Grids

Having produced a grid, the next question is obviously what to do with it. Several possibilities arise:

1. To leave the grid to gather dust.
2. To attempt some limited 'eyeball' analysis, without recourse to formal statistical analysis.
3. To carry out some sort of formal analysis, possibly using a computer program.

No Analysis

As pointed out previously, much can be gained from the process of eliciting constructs, so that one isn't bound to complete a grid in the first place. If one does decide to do a grid, then one might find that the process of completing the grid can itself be reconstructive. In fact Kelly suggested that doing a grid might be seen as a form of tightening of construing and there are certainly indications that during the process of construing the elements, the subject may change his mind about the elements. While he is completing the grid the subject may, in fact, be reflecting on his own construing. He might start to see patterns and links of which he had not previously been aware: in short the client may have completed his own analysis of the grid while he was doing it. Such 'insights' may set the client off in a direction which may well render further analysis superfluous or even retrograde. In fact, grid computer programs have been devised solely for use in the 'interactive mode' (Thomas and Shaw, 1977). In this form the client is able to sit opposite his friendly computer and type his responses to a series of simple questions. The program both elicits elements, constructs and grids and gives feedback such as . . . 'Did you realise that when you say someone "has a drinking problem" you tend also to say that they are "good company", whereas "non-drinkers" are generally "bores".' Although statistical analysis can be applied to grids generated by this program, the primary aim is to provide feedback as part of a learning experience.

Eyeballing

Provided our grid is not too large, we can get a lot out of it by the 'eyeball' method, i.e. just by looking at it. In fact, formal statistical analysis is no more than a sophisticated form of 'eyeballing'. Essentially, in both cases there is a search for order and pattern. In this sense, grids are similar to projective techniques in that they are open to varying interpretations, although they do hold the popular appeal of having numbers to back up such impressions. In fact, it might be more accurate to regard grid analysis as a form of exploration or hypothesis testing, rather than imagining that there is one and only one 'analysis' or interpretation of the grid.

For example, if we visually examine the hypothetical grid in Table 2.3 we can see that the constructs 1, 2 and 3 all have similar patterns of element sorting. They would thus seem to be essentially similar in meaning for the subject. Furthermore, constructs 4 and 5 also show similar patterns to each other. Construct 6, however, seems to be unlike all the other constructs and, thus, seems to have very little 'meaning' in this grid.

We may also be interested in *contrasts* rather than just looking for similarities. You may notice that the 'cluster' of constructs (1,2,3) has a virtually opposite pattern to that of 4 and 5. Thus, we may infer that there is one major contrast in the grid between constructs 1,2,3 and 4/5, with 6 'isolated' from the rest.

We may also be interested in the elements and by examining the columns we can make analogous inferences as with the constructs. For example, it is quite clear that element 1 is rated virtually oppositely to element 2.

Thus, at a glance we can form some sort of idea about 'identification', 'self-image', or whatever other question we have about the set of elements in question.

Table 2.3: Hypothetical Grid Illustrating 'Eyeballing' Analysis

		Elements					
C		1	2	3	4	5	6
O							
N	1	6	1	2	3	4	5
S	2	6	2	1	3	4	5
T	3	6	1	3	2	4	5
R							
U	4	1	6	5	3	4	2
C	5	1	6	4	3	5	2
T							
S	6	4	2	3	5	1	6

We may also be interested in how individual elements are construed. For example . . . Does our subject construe himself more favourably than his father on construct X?

As in the other levels of grid analysis, this kind of process can most usefully be carried out between client and researcher/clinician. Both you and your client may exchange impressions as part of a counselling relationship.

Formal Statistical Analysis

If we are dealing with relatively large grids, the array of numbers may be too complex a visual task and we are inevitably confronted with the need to step into the world of statistics and computer programs. With a little guidance, however, this does not have to be too painful. Although some computer programs concentrate on a visual analysis (e.g. FOCUS — Thomas and Shaw, 1976), there will always have been some form of numerical analysis of the grid. If you intend to use grids systematically (e.g. if you want some concrete evidence of change in repeat grids) then numerical measures can be very useful, provided they are treated with caution, if not downright scepticism. Measures derived from psychological scaling make many mathematical assumptions and there is also always the possibility of error; for example, the subject may have got confused about the ends of the scale.

The best way to illustrate the kinds of measures derivable from grids is to illustrate from the above clinical example of Brenda's grid.

Correlational Methods. The simplest form of statistical analysis is to examine the degree of similarity or dissimilarity between pairs of elements or constructs. A number of statistical measures can be applied, the most commonly used being 'correlational' methods, although some such as Thomas and Shaw (1976) prefer what are

Table 2.4: Correlations between Constructs derived from 'INGRID' Analysis of Brenda's Grid

											CONSTRUCTS
	2	3	4	5	6	7	8	9	10	11	12
1	.94	.90	.09	.66	.63	.87	-.24	-.40	.85	.92	.80
2		.75	-.13	.49	.56	.76	-.07	-.30	.67	.79	.72
3			.24	.83	.74	.94	-.51	-.62	.94	.94	.89
4				.27	.26	.19	-.24	-.19	.36	.36	.16
5					.92	.86	-.52	-.54	.92	.81	.91
6						.83	-.35	-.54	.83	.76	.91
7							-.38	-.54	.91	.90	.97
8								.79	-.52	-.40	-.39
9									-.54	-.54	-.54
10										.96	.91
11											.87

technically known as 'distance' measures. In fact, Rathod (1981), in his extensive review of the technicalities of analysing grids, claims to have come across at least 40 different measures. Although the methods may differ, the underlying principle is similar, i.e. to obtain a measure of degree of similarity in meaning.

I shall illustrate with the commonly used correlational method as applied to Brenda's grid (Table 2.1).

For those of you who are unfamiliar with measures of correlation, coefficients of correlation can range from +1 to −1. The closer the coefficient is to 1 the stronger will be the relationship. Constructs which correlate at levels closer to zero may be said to be unrelated. Positive correlations indicate that variation on one construct is similar to that of the other. Negative correlation indicates that variation on one construct tends to be opposite to the other. Most computer programs for the analysis of grids tend to include a correlation matrix of all the inter-correlations between the constructs. Table 2.4 illustrates the correlation matrix for Brenda's grid.

For instance, we can see that construct 1 (together-not together) is correlated highly and positively with a number of other constructs: 2 (happy with family – unhappy with family); 3(can show happiness in the family-can't show happiness in the family); 7(confident not confident); 10 (able to cry – can't cry); 11 (can talk about problems – can't talk about problems); 12 (can be loving – can't be loving). Thus, for Brenda, 'together' is closely linked to being happy with family, confidence, ability to cry, to talk about problems and loving. Conversely, being 'not together' is associated with the opposite poles of these constructs.

It can be seen that there are no very high negative correlations. This reflects the fact that in Brenda's grid the 'positive' or 'desirable' poles of Brenda's constructs are mainly on the left poles. If the poles had been more 'mixed' in this respect then there would have been more of an equal balance of high negative and high positive correlations. Thus, the polarity of the constructs affects the direction of the correlation. A correlation of −0.9 is as strong a relationship as one of +0.9, although the interpretation of the meaning of the relationship would be quite different in the two cases. If Brenda's above correlations had all been high negative, we would infer that 'together' means 'not happy with their family' etc.

You may be rightly wondering about how you decide whether a correlation is 'high' or not. The commonest method is to invoke some criterion of 'statistical significance'. We might, for example, choose to ignore those correlations which could easily have occurred by chance. If we decide to do this we can make use of statistical tables of the 'significance' of correlation coefficients. In such tables, we should regard 'n' as the number of elements. For example, at the 0.05 level with 10 elements a product moment correlation (as used in the above analysis) of −0.63 would be regarded as significant. If we were more cautious, the 0.01 level would be 0.77. Using the latter more conservative criterion, we would pick our correlations (negative and positive) above 0.77 as 'significant'. Thus, in our example we would regard the correlation between constructs 1 and 12 (0.80) as 'significant' but not that between 1 and t (0.66). It should be emphasised, however, that such criteria of statistical significance should be treated as a guide and not as a God! Furthermore, it should be borne in mind that statistical significance only helps us to judge whether a relationship exists, not about the strength of a relationship: the chances are that a correlation of, say, 0.92 reflects a stronger relationship than one of 0.54 although both might be 'significant'.

Correlational measures don't have to be restricted to constructs. We can also compare the relationships between elements in a similar way. In Brenda's grid, for example, (Table 2.1), we can see that Me (element 9) is construed relatively similarly to Mother (element 6), but quite dissimilarly to Ella (element 2).

There are many possible uses to measures of correlation from grids. One possibility might be to focus in on particular elements (e.g. Who's like and unlike the ideal self?) or particular constructs (e.g. What are the implications of the construct 'slim-fat'?). Alternatively, one might want just to scan through and pick out all the high correlations. The varying clinical possibilities of such analysis will be examined in the final section of this chapter.

Multi-Dimensional Analysis. As can be imagined, a correlation matrix is still a rather complex set of numbers. With 10 constructs there are just 45 inter-correlations! With 20 constructs there are 190! Scanning such large arrays of numbers is no easy task. It is no surprise, therefore, that a number of methods of 'simplifying' or summarising such data have been devised. These include principal components analysis (e.g. Slater, 1977), multi-dimensional scaling (e.g. van der Kloot, 1981) and cluster analysis (Thomas and Shaw, 1976). Readers interested in the technicalities of such methods of analysis should refer to Rathod (1981) or Slater (1977). It goes without saying that such analyses can only be carried out with the help of a computer. Although calculated in various ways and based on contrasting assumptions, all these methods attempt to break down the data in a grid in terms of a number of groups representing the major contrasts in the grid. Each group will summarise a number of closely related constructs and/or elements. Although such groupings are numerically derived, it is usually preferable to have some sort of visual representation. From any one grid, such analysis might reveal several groupings, although 2 or 3 is usually adequate. The best way to illustrate what this means is by example and I shall return again to Brenda's grid. In this case I have analysed the grid by means of Slater's 'Ingrid' programme (part of the Grid Analysis Package — see Slater, 1977), which utilises principal components analysis. It can be seen (Figure 2.2) that the first grouping (technically called a 'component') mainly contrasts 'Ideal Self' and 'Ella' with 'Mother', although 'Me', 'Step-father' and 'First husband' are closely grouped at the 'negative' end. We can also examine which constructs define this contrast. In this case all but three of the constructs 'load' highly, i.e. ideally (in contrast with mother etc.) she would like to be 'together', 'happy and able to show happiness with their family', 'nice looking', 'slim', 'confident', 'able to cry', 'can talk about problems' and 'can be loving'.

The second grouping mainly contrasts 'Me' with 'First husband', although there are a few other people who 'load' more moderately at either end. Me is seen as 'don't need people', whereas First husband 'relies on people a lot'. Interestingly, for these elements, relying on people is associated with being 'feminine', whereas not needing people implies being 'hard'.

The third grouping mainly contrasts 'Step-father' with 'Mother'. Mother is seen as 'relying on people' and 'hard' whereas Step-father 'don't need people' and is 'more feminine'. This is a clear example of the kind of contradiction and dilemma which can be revealed through grids: whereas on the second grouping, First husband, 'relied on people' and was 'more feminine', on the third grouping Mother 'relied on people' and was 'hard'. As revealed by the first grouping, however, neither seems to have achieved her ideal.

Although I have represented the three components as separate axes, some prefer two-dimensional plots in which two components are placed at 90 degrees to each other, much as maps represent spatial configurations in the north-south, east-west axes. Slater (1977) has also suggested a three-dimensional means of plotting using a geographer's globe. Whichever method one chooses, it is important that the representation makes sense to you and that you

Figure 2.2: Principal Components Analysis of Brenda's Grid (Constructs and Elements Loading Highly)

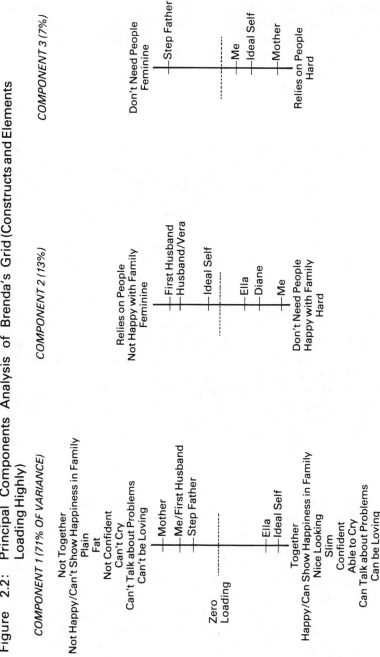

can communicate this to others, notably your clients. Once again, I should also emphasise that mistakes can be made in the original grid, so that one should not automatically assume that surprising results are 'interesting' — check the original grid and check out with your client!

Clinical Uses of Grids

It hardly needs emphasising that grid technique can be particularly useful in the clinical context. After all, Kelly did devise the technique primarily as a way by which a clinician might gain a clearer understanding of his client's problem. During the succeeding 30 years, applications of the technique have been far-ranging, although the clinical context remains as much its 'focal point' as ever. Grids have been extensively applied as a research tool in a number of areas of psychopathology (e.g. schizophrenia, depression, suicide, anorexia nervosa, alcoholism . . .). There is no doubt, therefore, that they have proved useful as a means of testing hypotheses about the nature of psychological disorder. In addition to this more formal use of grids, many psychologists and other mental health workers also use grids in their everyday clinical practice, both as a way of assessing a problem and as a means of monitoring changes in a person's construing.

It is not my intention here to produce an exhaustive list of clinical applications, but to suggest some general ways of using grids in the clinical context. More detailed examples can be found in other texts (e.g. Fransella and Bannister, 1977; Slater, 1976; Ryle, 1975; Beail 1985).

Self Image

Psychological disorders often involve some disturbance in a person's 'self image'. The study of 'self', so prominent amongst the Freudians, was rejected for many years by scientific psychology. Recently, however, there has been a revival of interest in this subject and a variety of methods have emerged for studying and measuring the self concept (Wylie, 1961). Repertory grid technique has found favour amongst many clinicians and researchers in view of its ability to combine subjectivity with objectivity and at the end of the day to produce measures of psychopathology etc. In seeking to explore someone's self image, one would normally start with an element set which included the self as well as various other important figures in the person's life. It is also common practice to include more than one view of the self: these might include 'ideal self', 'me as seen by others', 'me in the future' etc. Thus a person's self image will be understood in terms of how the person contrasts it with other people and other perspectives on himself. Constructs would then be elicited and/or supplied and a grid produced which could be analysed by any of the above general methods. If restricting one's focus to 'correlational' methods, then one would examine measures of relationship between the self and other elements. Measures of particular interest might obviously include self-mother and self-father, as well as clinically pertinent measures such as self-ideal self or 'self isolation'[1].

As well as using a correlational approach one may seek some visual representation of self image. As an example Figure 2.3 is taken from a study of patients with rheumatoid arthritis by a student I supervised (Plant, 1984). It can be seen that for this group there

Figure   2.3:   Loadings of Self and Other Elements on First Principal Component for a Group of Rheumatoid Arthritis Sufferers

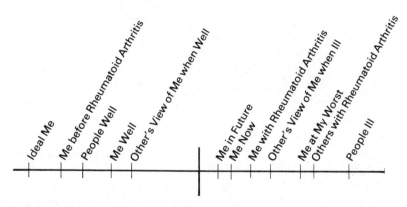

Source: Plant, R.D. (1984).   Belief and Illness: A Study of Patients with Rheumatoid Arthritis, Unpublished MSc Dissertation, Faculty of Medicine, University of Southampton.

was a tendency to idealise themselves before they developed rheumatoid arthritis, with their view of themselves now relatively negative.

Relationships

It is usually the case that as well as a disturbance in self image, psychological disorder involves a disturbance in the quality and/or quantity of a person's relationships with others. Once again, repertory grid technique has been extensively applied to measuring such problems. As we have seen earlier, 'dyad' grids are ideally suited to the investigation of relationships. One may both explore a client's own construing of his significant relationships as well as taking more than one perspective on relationships (how I see my wife's view of my relationships, how I think my wife views my relationships etc). Furthermore, such grids can be exchanged between partners, thus providing the opportunity for testing out one's understanding of others.

In making use of such grids on an individual, one may be interested in what kinds of constructs the person applies to his relationships. For example, one person might see all his relationships in terms of 'rejection-acceptance', whereas another might predominantly use 'comfortable-at ease'. We may also be interested in the degree of reciprocity: many patients might find it easier to construe other people's relationship to them, than in terms of what they might mean to others. One may also be interested in how the elements are dispersed: e.g. relationships with females might be quite different from those with males.

Grids involving relationships may thus provide a useful starting point for therapy, whether with an individual, a couple or a group such as a family. The question of relationships and their assessment will, of course, be explored in depth in Chapter 10.

Exploring a Problem or Complaint

Grids can be constructed around the person's 'complaint'. We saw an example of this possibility earlier, when I was illustrating the choice of elements of trips out for an agoraphobic. In similar vein, Fransella (1972) has constructed grids with stutterers in which the elements were stutter-provoking situations. Watson (1970a) also provides an example of this type of grid with a patient inclined to self-mutilation. In this case the elements were various feelings (e.g. being with my mother) and the constructs were possible consequences (e.g. make me cut myself).

Another general approach to the use of grids is to look for what have been variously described as 'dilemmas', 'conflict', 'contradictions', 'snags' etc. Such an approach is typified by Ryle (1975) in his book *Frames and Cages* in which he provides a number of clinical examples of such factors. As in the case study of an arsonist by Fransella and Adams (1966) or a depressed lady by Rowe (1971), grids can help to identify reasons for hanging on to symptoms as well as helping to clarify issues which need to be resolved prior to change. Slade and Sheehan (1981) have gone as far as producing a computer program which purports to identify and measure areas of 'conflict' within a grid.

Structural Measures from Grids

Some of you may have already come across Bannister's measure of 'Intensity' in the Grid Test of Schizophrenic Thought Disorder (Bannister and Fransella, 1967). This is just one of a large number of structural measures which have been derived from grids. For example, Fransella and Bannister (1977) list, among others, 'cognitive complexity' (Bieri, 1955), 'ordination' (Landfield and Barr, 1976), 'saturation' (Fransella, 1972) and 'articulation' (Makhlouf-Norris, Jones and Norris, 1970). This is a broad and potentially very confusing topic and could quite easily fill a book in itself and I shan't attempt to analyse the subtle differences between such measures. Readers wishing to pursue such technicalities should consult Fransella and Bannister (1977). I would like, however, to suggest that it may often be clinically relevant to measure structural changes in a person's construing, irrespective of the content of the constructs and elements.

For illustrative purposes I will choose just one possible measure derivable from grids. The same principle could apply to whatever measure you use. In Slater's Ingrid programme (Slater, 1977), the percentage of the total variance accounted for by the first principal component has frequently been used in psychiatric grid studies. In principal components analysis, the first component always accounts for the greatest proportion of variance, although individual grids vary considerably on the measure. For example, in my study of anorexia nervosa (Button, 1980) I found wide individual differences on this measure. Patients *a*, *b*, and *c* had first components of 89 per cent, 34 per cent and 57 per cent. A high percentage of variance for the first component (as with patient *a*) arises when most of the constructs are highly correlated with each other. This might be viewed as akin to 'tightness' of construing, or described as virtually one-dimensional thinking. At the other extreme, patient *b* shows much 'looser' or multi-dimensional construing. Patient c, however, shows a more intermediate position on this dimension. There is no absolute cut off which might be considered pathological, although a person with a first component of about 90 per cent is clearly operating in quite a different way from someone with a first component near 30 per cent. It is probably more useful to use such figures to monitor change. We might, for example, be looking for evidence of change towards more moderate levels. We shall see clinical examples of this later (especially in Chapter 7).

Summary

A number of methods are available which can help to provide us with a clearer understanding of people with psychological problems. The most commonly used is repertory grid technique, of which there are many variants. There are also less structured possibilities like 'Self Characterisation' and essays. The analysis and interpretation of grids can range from simply 'eyeballing' to quite complex statistical procedures, but at all times is likely to be most fruitful if the clinician or researcher pays heed to the principles of personal construct theory.

Note

1. Slater's Ingrid programme (Slater, 1977) produces a measure of inter-element relationships called 'element distances'. These measures are somewhat different from correlations but they can be used as an index almost analogously to correlations. Norris and Makhlouf-Norris (1976) have suggested the term 'actual self isolation', where in a grid there are no non-self elements closer than a criterion distance from the actual self. One can also produce an index of degree of self isolation by averaging the distances between self and all other elements. As we shall see in later chapters there is evidence that psychiatric patients differ from controls on such measures.

PART TWO

DISORDERS

In Part One, we have seen how Kelly offered an alternative approach to 'diagnosis', one grounded in terms of a person's efforts to make sense of his experience. In Part Two, however, we return to some familiar labels, mainly derived from a psychiatric approach to classification. We hope that this may help you to translate Kelly's general principles into practice. It will become clear, however, that whatever the 'presenting problem', personal construct theory offers both understanding and constructive guidelines to a helping relationship.

3   SCHIZOPHRENIA: WHAT IS LOOSE IN SCHIZOPHRENIC CONSTRUING?

Omer Van den Bergh, Paul De Boeck and Willem Claeys

Introduction

Most general chapters or books on schizophrenia start with stressing the complex and confusing character of this disorder and then proceed with the painstaking effort of classifying all different aspects and/or theories within this vast domain. Fortunately, the title of this book saves us this trouble, because it is obvious that a personal construct (PC) view will be at issue. Nevertheless it is not superfluous to say that this approach has mainly been concerned with only one aspect of this multifaceted disturbance, namely clinical thought disorder.

The first research of this topic, based on Kelly's monumental publication of 1955, remained a one-man job for a good number of years. It was Bannister who conducted a series of studies (Bannister, 1960; 1962; 1963; 1965a) concerned with the schizophrenic's construct system and with the process of becoming thought disordered. In 1966 and 1967 he published together with Fransella, the Grid Test of Schizophrenic Thought Disorder (GTSTD), a diagnostic instrument designed to test whether a patient is thought disordered or not (Bannister and Fransella, 1966; 1967). To some, this instrument may look like the odd sister in the PC family, offspring of a PC-psychologist taking French leave to the differential-psychometric tradition. For it is clear that Kelly's Rep test was certainly not intended to classify people in categories. This GTSTD has nevertheless launched a line of research concerned with typical psychometric questions, as for example its validity and discriminative power (Bannister, Fransella and Agnew, 1971; McPherson, Blackburn, Draffan and McFayden, 1973; Poole, 1976). Although we think that the main contradiction with Kelly's basic philosophy might not be the mere existence of a classical test, but the way it is used and for what purposes, we will not pursue this line of research in the following chapter.

Another frequently mentioned point of criticism in this respect is that thought-disordered (TD) schizophrenics can hardly be approached as a subclassification within the group of schizophrenics, and therefore cannot usefully be contrasted with non-thought-disordered (NTD) schizophrenics (Bonarius, 1980). Thought disorder may be seen in most schizophrenics at particular moments and it is not even specifically present only in schizophrenics (see e.g. Beck, 1963; Harrow and Quinlan, 1977). This point of criticism is valid if one has diagnostic ambitions and uses clinical categories that point to stabilised personality traits or structures. However, if one tries to understand the process of becoming thought disordered, within the general 'Kellyan' assumption that the schizophrenic becomes thought disordered because he tries to stay a 'lay-scientist' anyhow, one can usefully apply the term 'thought disorder' and study the persons that are affected by it. But we think that PC approaches to schizophrenia should not focus too much on only thought disorder.

In this chapter, we will link up with Bannister's original findings and proceed a few steps in the discussion about the schizophrenic's way of construing by formulating a 'divergence hypothesis'. This hypothesis unifies the group of schizophrenics as a whole, but nevertheless allows for the possibility of contrasting TD and NTD construing processes. In the research part, we will present some results in line with this hypothesis and we will finally conclude with some implications for therapy.

The Theory: Construing the Schizophrenic's Way of Construing

The Schizophrenic's Construct System

From Kelly's (1955) fundamental postulate and the construction corollary, it is obvious that the notion of a construct is deeply connected with the notion of anticipation: to construe a person as friendly is basically a prediction that a person will behave in a certain manner in the future. But a construction process is not an isolated activity, it happens in relation with other construing processes to form construct systems (cf. organisation corollary). The relationships between constructs can be viewed as other types of predictions. For example, if in a person's construct system 'friendly' and 'sincere' are closely related, it means that the construction of someone as friendly implies that he is expected to be sincere as well.

When Kelly conceives the schizophrenic's way of construing as 'loose', it is implied that there is something wrong with the way he predicts the world he lives in. De Boeck (1981) analysed Kelly's statements about loose construing and found four characteristics, which will be repeated here. 1. Loose construing means instability in the assignment of elements to construct poles. The allocation of elements to construct poles is varying from one moment to another. 2. In loose construing the application of contructs is extended. This means that the range of convenience is broadened to include elements to which the construct normally does not apply. 3. Loose construing is only approximative. Events are not construed precisely, but as rough approximations. 4. Loosened constructs retain their prior identity. A loosened construct is still a construct in the person's construct system. It remains contrasted with its opposite pole. Only the way it is applied to elements and its relationship with other constructs has changed. Because of the correspondence between construing and predicting, these four characteristics of loose construing are applicable to loose predicting as well: 1. loose construing leads to varying and inconsistent predictions; 2. it leads to predictions concerning events from outside the range of convenience, while irrelevant events can be taken to validate certain predictions; 3. it leads to approximative predictions but 4. the construct will nevertheless still be used as a basis for predictions. De Boeck (1981) shows that each of these aspects can be illustrated with Kelly's own words.

Because predictions can be made from a construct to elements, as well as from a construct to other constructs, loose construing may be observed in both types of prediction. When Bannister started his empirical studies on the basis of Kelly's ideas, he opted for an 'operationalisation' of loose construing in terms of the relationship between constructs: 'It can be argued that the varying predictions of a loose construct are consequent upon the construct having weak relationships with surrounding constructs in the hierarchical system . . . ' (Bannister, 1960, p.1241).

In his first experiment, Bannister asked his subjects to indicate which 9 persons out of a series of 18, all known to the subject, could be allocated to one construct pole. This was repeated for 9 other construct poles, all supplied by the researcher. In a second part, the same procedure was repeated for 18 other known persons as elements. Bannister used four clinical groups (depressives, neurotics, non-thought-disordered (NTD) schizophrenics and thought disordered (TD) schizophrenics) and a control group of normals. From the results he computed four measures: 1. The Intensity of Relationship between constructs: this is the degree to which the constructs are interrelated; 2. The Consistency of Relationship: this is the degree to which the pattern of relationships between constructs in the first grid is replicated in the second. 3. The Coefficient of Variation: this coefficient is intended to measure the variability of the relationships between constructs. 4. The Social Deviation score: this measure expresses the degree of idiosyncrasy in the pattern of relationships between constructs by taking the mean of the group of normals as the norm.

Bannister's most apparent results were that TD schizophrenics and NTD schizophrenics could be differentiated fairly well on the Intensity and Consistency of Relationship measure. On both measures TD patients have a lower score. In a second experiment (Bannister, 1962) some measures were refined, others were added and the procedure was slightly different in that photographs of unknown people were used as elements. Bannister found that the differentiation between NTD and TD schizophrenics had increased on the Intensity and Consistency of Relationship measures. The results showed also a low variability score (Coefficient of Variation) of the schizophrenic group as a whole and a socially deviant pattern of relationships in TD schizophrenics. Moreover, by means of a new measure (Maldistribution score) Bannister was able to show that NTD schizophrenics use predominantly only one pole of the construct dimension, in which they differ from normals and TD schizophrenics. This latter measure is an element measure based on a dichotomous allotment of elements to a construct pole, while other measures are relationship measures. In fact, this measure shows that there may be more in the schizophrenics construct system than can be tapped with the relationship measures. This is also apparent in two later studies, one from Frith and Lillie (1972), the other from Haynes and Phillips (1973). Frith and Lillie (1972) questioned the interpretation of loose construing and hypothesised that lower Intensity and Consistency of Relationship would derive from difficulties in the assignment of elements to constructs. That is to say, TD schizophrenics would not be able to handle large amounts of information and to rank order faces on the basis of a construct. This leads to 'errors' which can be measured more adequately through the 'Element Consistency' score, a test-retest reliability measure per construct. They found that, partialling out the Element Consistency, there was no relationship between Intensity and Consistency of Relationship on the one hand and clinical thought disorder as rated by the psychiatrist on the other hand, while the Element Consistency measure was an equally good predictor of thought disorder as Bannister's measures.

Haynes and Phillips (1973) proposed that TD schizophrenics are simply inconsistent. This is more directly measured by an element measure instead of by a construct-relationship measure. These researchers essentially replicated Frith and Lillie's results: the inconsistency measure discriminated better than Intensity and when partialling out the inconsistency, Intensity did no longer discriminate significantly. Our own research (Van den Bergh, De Boeck and Claeys, 1981) replicated the importance of the Element Consistency measure, although we found the Intensity measure not entirely useless. Also Radley (1974) pointed to the importance of both relationship and element measures. Therefore, Bannister's option to interpret thought disorder as a matter of only weakness in the interrelationship of constructs is seriously challenged: it seems to be just a part of the whole story. Considering the process of becoming thought disordered, more light is shed on this problem.

The Process of Becoming Thought Disordered

How does loose construing develop? If construing is predicting, then the occurrence of events can validate or invalidate a construct or a construct-relation, or can turn out to fall outside the range of convenience of a construct. In what Bannister (1963, p.680) termed 'an advisably oversimple "pilot" hypothesis' he reasoned that 'serial invalidation' could initiate the process, leading to the phenomena associated with the clinical description of thought disorder. If a prediction is invalidated, the person may firstly try to reconstrue the events in terms of the opposite pole, but if invalidation continues, the construction process may oscillate between the two construct poles and finally result in a weakening of the construct relationships (lowered Intensity).

Bannister tested his hypothesis in a series of four experiments of the following general form (see Bannister, 1963; 1965a): normal subjects were asked to rank order an array of photographs on each construct of a list. This was repeated several times and by telling them that they had been very successful or unsuccessful in ranking the photographs according to the experimenter's predetermined plan, validation or invalidation was realised. From the four experiments, Bannister was able to conclude that 1. serial validation strengthens the intercorrelations between constructs, 2. serial invalidation produces changes in the pattern of construct interrelationships, and 3. validation of one constellation of constructs and invalidation of another constellation within the same individual produces respectively an increase and a decrease of interrelationships between constructs.

Although Bannister found in only one of the four studies that the relational Intensity was lowered by the invalidation, he concluded that the finding may be considered the laboratory equivalent of clinical thought disorder, a conclusion that up to now is frequently cited. However, Lawlor and Cochran (1981, p.41) point rightly to the fact that: 'For over a decade, the invalidation hypothesis has rested upon a single unreplicated experiment, following three unsuccessful experiments'.

Probably, serial invalidation does more than only loosening the construct relationships, and this is not surprising. For the serial invalidation can be seen as an operational equivalent of Kelly's definition of anxiety as unconstruable events, and it may be remembered that Kelly has distinguished between two reactions on anxiety, namely loosening and tightening.

So, up to this point Bannister's research endeavours resulted in two problems, the one being the importance of element measures versus construct-relationship measures, the other being the effects of invalidation on the construct system.

A major impetus for the better understanding of these problems was provided by Radley (1974) after an extensive retrospective study of the different research results thus far. According to Radley, both the element measures and the relationship measures are important. On the one hand, subjects may be inconsistent (low Element Consistency) while having a tight relationship between constructs, on the other hand low Intensity scores may be typical for normal but 'cognitively complex' persons (Bieri, 1955), while they may show consistency in the ranking of elements to a particular construct. In this latter respect, he pointed to the possible importance of the Variability of Intensity-score. Bannister (1962) namely, had found that TD and NTD schizophrenics showed an equally low Variability score, that was lower than in normals. According to Radley (1974), the study of Makhlouf-Norris, Jones and Norris (1970) provides a clue for the interpretation of this result. They found the construct system of normals to consist of separate clusters, connected by 'linkage' constructs which make it possible to make independent and even contradictory judgements, while still maintaining coherence through the 'linkage' constructs. In their construct system, Intensity may be low and Variability high. They are more cognitively complex. The low Variability score of schizophrenics means that they are cognitively simple. Because of this cognitive simplicity, schizoid persons are less able to integrate conflicting information very well, through forming superordinate constructs, while precisely conflicting information might be characteristic of their environment (see the double bind hypothesis, Bateson, Jackson, Haley and Weakland, 1956).

According to Radley, a first attempt to deal with this incompatible information, typical for NTD patients, is situated at the level of element allocation to constructs. The person uses only one pole of the construct dimension and tries to neglect the information consistent with the other pole. However, this neglect may not be complete enough, causing a shift to the opposite pole and an attempt to disregard the actual conflicting information. In this way, the schizoid person tries to resolve the invalidating experiences with a minimal change in his construct system. This repeated shifting of elements from one pole to the other may result in 'successive, contrasting impressions of the other, such that a tight system of constructs was applied to events in a relatively inconsistent way' (Radley, 1974, p. 321).

If nevertheless this strategy proves to be insufficient the person may give up and may adopt a new strategy which results in thought disorder. This new strategy consists in that the person uses his constructs only on the basis of tenuous properties that are present in both poles of the construct dimension. According to Radley, this can be called a *dedifferentiation* of the construct. The allocation of elements to constructs becomes more or less a random process. The range of convenience of the construct broadens, which also affects the relationship between constructs, that become looser and more idiosyncratic. This 'solution' is situated both at the level of element allocation to constructs and at the level of construct relationships.

This interpretation is surely provocative, although there are some problems with it. On the one hand, Radley describes the first phase as one in which the person forms 'successive, contrasting impressions of the other . . . ' (p. 321). However, a continuous shifting of the elements from one pole to the other should eliminate a lopsided distribution, while such a distribution is typically found in NTD schizophrenics. On the other hand, continuing the above quote, Radley says: ' . . . such that a tight system of constructs was applied to events in a relatively inconsistent way.' But, it is known that NTD schizophrenics show a relatively high Consistency of Construct relationship and a high Element Consistency (see Van den Bergh *et al.*, 1981, for both remarks.)

According to us, the results of TD and NTD schizophrenics are better interpreted by considering them as two different ways of handling invalidation and one strategy does not necessarily precede the other. Cochran (1976; 1977) reported empirical data supporting the view that invalidation may lead to two different reactions: some people tend to weaken their construct-relations in the face of invalidation, while others tend to strengthen them. Moreover, it was found that lopsidedness of the constructs was an indication for the strengthening reaction. To us, it seems not too far-fetched to suppose that the schizophrenic may experience the completion of a grid type of test as an invalidating situation, when no feedback from the investigator is given. Also in Bateson's double bind hypothesis (Bateson *et al.*, 1956) it is stated that all formal characteristics of a double bind are not necessary anymore in order to experience unavoidable invalidation, once the person has learned to see the world according to the double bind patterns.

For normals, it is known that they tend to intensify their construct relations in case of no feedback, i.e. without comments from the investigator the relational intensity tends to increase from test to retest (Bannister and Mair, 1968). This is in line with the findings of McGuire (1960) (see also Rosen and Wyer, 1972) that cognitions are reorganised in a more coherent way after they have been made explicit. When a belief questionnaire is administered twice, the beliefs show up in a more consistent way during the second administration. McGuire has called this phenomenon the 'Socratic effect.' For schizophrenics, we want to distinguish between two reactions: NTD schizophrenics are expected to react with a strengthening of the relations from test to retest that is even stronger than the usual Socratic effect that is established in normals; TD schizophrenics are expected to show a reversed Socratic effect from test to retest.

This hypothesis is called here the *divergence hypothesis* including that, when retested, TD schizophrenics and NTD schizophrenics diverge from normals in contrasting ways. This two-reactions view looks attractive because it allows for a differentiation within the group of schizophrenics and because it implies that the two groups differ from normals in contrasting ways, so that a general-deficit hypothesis becomes implausible. An additional advantage of looking at the evolution of subsequent grid administrations is that the focus is on the process of construing and less on fixed characteristics of the construction system. The key words are not 'loose' and 'tight', but 'loosening', and 'tightening' with respect to the relationships between constructs.

Although the intensification of interconstruct relations in NTD schizophrenics looks like a tightening reaction, the explanation that we want to give for it implies that constructs are used in a less precise way, because only one or a few aspects are considered whereas others are left out of consideration in order to avoid inconsistencies.

Consider a construct system in which 'bad' means 'unfriendly' and 'rude'. Meeting a friendly rude person would mean an invalidation of the construct 'bad' except when the construing person concentrates on only one aspect, e.g. rudeness. However, doing so leads to an extension of the bad pole of the construct as the allotment conditions are less stringent now. The lopsidedness of constructs might be an indication of this phenomenon, and in fact, NTD schizophrenics turned out to have lopsided constructs (Bannister, 1962). Another aspect of this phenomenon might be that the construction becomes simpler. As only one or a few aspects are concerned, the system tends to become less multidimensional (see also Miller and Chapman, 1968). The relations among constructs to which the focused aspect(s) is (are) relevant may be expected to be intensified as a consequence of the allotment criteria being more simple now. Hence, both TD and NTD schizophrenics have in common that their constructions are loose in the sense of not being as complete as they should be. It is as if schizophrenics leave out at least some of the conditions to use a construct, in order to avoid invalidation. The difference between TD and NTD schizophrenics then reduces to a loosening in a random way by taking into account only one or a few construct aspects on a random-like basis, as contrasted with a loosening by focusing systematically on only one or a few but always the same construct aspects.

The idea of loose construing as being incomplete construing is worked out in De Boeck (1981), where the underlying principle is called 'loss of conjunctivity', i.e. loss of the principle that all of the allotment conditions have to be fulfilled in order for a construct to be considered applicable. Conjunctivity is a notion that is borrowed from the literature on concept learning. Multiple attribute concepts are defined by more than one attribute and by a rule that specifies which attributes have to occur in an element for that element to be classified as an example of the concept in question.

From the concept learning literature (Haygood and Bourne, 1965), the most common rule seems to be conjunctivity, i.e. that all of the attributes have to be present. The opposite rule is disjunctivity i.e. that one of the attributes is sufficient. A rule in between is a compensative rule in accordance to which attributes may compensate for each other. This latter rule might be more in agreement with the new approach that is introduced by Rosch (1973) for natural categories, but also that rule requires that all of the relevant attributes of an element are taken into account. The 'loss of conjunctivity' implies that the conceptual rule becomes less complete, so that no longer all of the attributes are taken into account.

A construct system consists of a network of relations among constructs. Some of the constructs may be considered attributes of other constructs, i.e. conditions that should be considered to allot an element to one of the construct poles. Consider a person to whom 'is a friend' has the following attributes: 'contacts me frequently', 'helps me', and 'is helped by me'. A construction of someone else that is based on only one of these attributes (which are also constructs) would be characteristic of the loss of conjunctivity. De Boeck (1981) has stressed that loss of conjunctivity may account for looseness. Indeed, when only one attribute is considered, the construction is only approximative and it varies on the basis of the attribute in question. Such a construction would also lead to varying predictions depending on whether the other person is considered a friend or not. However, when the loss of conjunctivity is biased in a systematic way by concentrating on one and always the same of the attributes, the result would not be looseness in the sense of varying constructions, but it would be a tightening of the relations with other constructs to which the same attribute is important. A random-like selection of an attribute, on the contrary, would lead to varying constructions and to a loosening of the construct relations.

The Specificity of Schizophrenic Thought Disorder

Clinicians, working with schizophrenic patients, will all have their stories on the fluctuations of TD according to differences in moments, subjects of talk or partners in the conversation. One of the authors (O.V.d.B.) had the opportunity to observe many instances of these fluctuations. A frequently occurring situation is one in which the schizophrenic is able to discuss coherently about politics (and it can be assured that this is a complicated matter in Belgium), actuality and so on, while touching the topic of the patient's family obviously makes him confused.

Similar examples can be found in reports of ex-patients about their psychotic episodes (see Green, 1964; Sechehaye, 1950).

Laing and Esterson (1964) analysed conversations in the Lawson family and found that Agnes' thought disorders were highly selective and occurred only when certain topics were at issue.

Also other authors (Haley, 1959a; Lidz, 1973) studying schizophrenia from the viewpoint of interpersonal relations acknowledge the variability of the occurrence of thought disorder within the same patient.

In PC-research, the hypothesis was set up that thought disorder would be more pronounced when handling psychological constructs in the interpersonal domain because invalidation may have occurred more in contact with people.

This hypothesis is especially important because it challenges theories of schizophrenic thought disorder as a generalised inability to handle large amounts of information (Frith and Lillie, 1972), or as a general inconsistency (Haynes and Phillips, 1973).

In a pioneering study by Bannister and Salmon (1966) photographs of people and names of objects were rank-ordered on respectively psychological and physical constructs. However, the incomparability of these two tasks prevented drawing firm conclusions from this study. McPherson and Buckley (1970) used the same series of photographs of people to be rank-ordered on psychological and physical constructs and found evidence in favour of the specificity hypothesis. A number of subsequent tests have been carried out, each with some methodological improvements, while still favouring an interpretation in line with the specificity hypothesis. For example, Heather (1976) tested the hypothesis with photographs of unknown people and names of known people as well. McPherson, Armstrong and Heather (1975) carried out some major improvements, such as equating the level of difficulty, the test-retest reliability and the level of intensity and construct consistency scores for the physical and psychological constructs.

It is not our aim to review these studies and discuss the methodological problems associated with this subject. The importance of the specificity subject for our purposes lies herein that, if our divergence hypothesis proves right, as well as its interpretation in the context of the invalidation hypothesis, this divergence should be specific too. This means that the differences between TD and NTD disorder should be more pronounced when construing people psychologically. In fact, such a result may be considered a kind of validity test.

Research: Testing the Divergence Hypothesis

We will report here on two studies with TD schizophrenics, NTD schizophrenics, and normals. Both studies are intended to replicate the major conclusions from the personal construct oriented research on thought disorder, and at the same time to test the divergence hypothesis. A first major conclusion that has to be replicated is that the relations among constructs have a lower Intensity in TD schizophrenics than in other subjects, and that the same is true for element-construct relations. It might even be argued that the latter phenomenon is stronger than the former. A second conclusion we want to replicate is that the loosening and hence the thought disorder is somewhat specific to the interpersonal domain. The divergence hypothesis must be considered in addition to this and as a specification of the difference between TD and NTD schizophrenics.

In the first study, the focus is on the difference between TD schizophrenics and NTD schizophrenics and normals with respect to interconstruct relatedness (The Intensity measure) and on the stability of element-construct relatedness (the Element Consistency measure). Furthermore, the divergence hypothesis is considered, using a Maldistribution score for lopsidedness of the constructs and by studying the evolution of the interconstruct relatedness (Intensity) during subsequent grid administrations.

In the second study, the focus is on the specificity of thought disorder to psychological construing. Intensity and Element Consistency are considered. Furthermore, the divergence hypothesis is combined with the specificity hypothesis, leading to the expectation that the divergence is specific to psychological construing of persons.

Study One

The first study is reported by Van den Bergh *et al.* (1981). Therefore, only a short description of the method is given here. Subjects were 32 normals and 32 young schizophrenics admitted to a psychiatric hospital (none of them was chronic). In the treatment units, the patients were divided in hierarchically ordered groups reflecting different recovery levels. A patient normally starts at the lowest level and according to the progress she/he makes in terms of a behaviour rating system, she/he goes up to the next level (see Cosijns, Peuskens and Tilmans, 1977). For this study, four subgroups were formed. The first two subgroups were TD and NTD schizophrenics from the lowest recovery level. The third and fourth subgroups were from the middle and from the highest recovery levels, respectively; none of them was thought-disordered, so that all of these subjects were considered NTD schizophrenics. Thought disorder was assessed by the independent clinical judgment of both the ward psychiatrist and the therapist, using the Mayer-Gross, Slater and Roth (1954) description.

Four types of grids were administered, each with eight elements and six constructs: (1) the Grid Test of Schizophrenic Thought Disorder with supplied elements and supplied constructs (Bannister and Fransella, 1966); (2) a grid test with the supplied elements from (1) but with elicited constructs; (3) a grid test with elicited elements but with the supplied constructs from (1); and (4) a grid test with elicited elements and with elicited constructs. The subjects were required to rank-order the elements of each type on each of the constructs. Furthermore, for two constructs of each type also binary judgments were asked (construct pole applicable or not). All four variants of the grid were administered twice, once in the test phase and once in the immediately following retest phase (only a short rest pause was provided). Within each phase the order of the four types was varied so as to have each type of grid equally often in each position.

Among the measures that are used in the study, the most important ones are Intensity, Construct Consistency (stability of interconstruct relations), Element Consistency, and Maldistribution (on the basis of the binary judgments). It was found that TD schizophrenics were differentiated from NTD schizophrenics and normals with respect to the first three of these measures in a significant way. As usually, TD schizophrenics obtained lower scores on Intensity, Construct Consistency, and Element Consistency (for more details, see Van den Bergh *et al.*, 1981).

It is important to notice that TD schizophrenics were differentiated from the other groups much better with respect to Element

Consistency than with respect to Intensity. The element-construct relations, as reflected in the Element Consistency measure, seem to be impaired more than the construct-construct relations that are reflected in the Intensity measure. Moreover, the difference with respect to Intensity disappeared in an analysis of covariance with Element Consistency as a covariable. The same was true when Element Consistency was used as a convariable of Construct Consistency. The finding that Element Consistency is more crucial in differentiating TD schizophrenics from other subjects may stem from the grid test procedure in which element-construct relations are tapped in a direct way by rank-ordering elements with respect to constructs, whereas construct-construct relations are derived from the rank orders. If one would be interested in a direct assessment of interconstruct relations, one should ask the subjects what the implications are, that constructs have to each other.

In line with the divergence hypothesis, the NTD schizophrenics turned out to exceed normals and TD schizophrenics with respect to the Maldistribution score, indicating that the constructs of NTD schizophrenics are more lopsided. Furthermore, analysis of variance revealed an interaction effect with respect to the Intensity measure. From test to retest TD schizophrenics showed a decreasing Intensity, whereas NTD schizophrenics and normals showed an increasing Intensity.

As four grids were administered to each subject, a further exploration of the evolution in the interconstruct relatedness was made possible. A new analysis of variance was carried out with group as a between-subjects factor and with order (first two grids vs. last two grids) and test/retest as within-subjects factors. Again a significant interaction effect was found which shows that within the test phase TD schizophrenics strongly weaken their interconstruct relations, whereas NTD schizophrenics, especially those from the lowest recovery level, strongly intensify their interconstruct relations (see Table 3.1). Within the second half of the procedure, i.e. within the retest phase, the Intensity did not change from the first two to the last two grids. The results from table 3.1 clearly support the divergence hypothesis.

An additional finding is that the intensification as well as the weakening of interconstruct relations in schizophrenics is accompanied by a decresasing differentiation of the interconstruct relations. The variability of the relations decreased from test to retest in

Table 3.1: Intensity Scores of First and Last Two Grids of the Test Phase, as a Function of Subjects Group

	TD schizophrenics	NTD schizophrenics			Normals
		level 1	level 2	level 3	
first two grids	30.19	34.87	36.63	27.74	33.46
last two grids	21.80	44.78	38.89	28.64	36.17

The Intensity scores are mean squared rho's x 100; they have to be multiplied by 30 to be comparable to the scores from the Bannister and Fransella (1966) test.

the schizophrenic subgroups, whereas it increased in the group of normals (the interaction was significant, see Van den Bergh *et al.*, 1981).

Although in NTD schizophrenics as well as in normals the Intensity increased from test to retest, the differentiation of the interconstruct relations decreased in the former subjects and increased in the latter subjects. This finding is in line with the explanation given earlier for the intensification of interconstruct relatedness in NTD schizophrenics, i.e. that the construing becomes simpler by being oriented to only one or a few aspects of the elements.

With respect to the three subgroups of NTD schizophrenics, it should be noticed that in Table 3.1 especially the NTD subjects from level 1 contrast with TD subjects, whereas those of level 2 and 3 are more like normals in their evolution from the first two grids to the last two grids. Aggregating the data from all NTD schizophrenics, as is usually done in personal constructs research on schizophrenia, would have concealed the construing processes we now have established in the level 1 subjects.

Study Two

The second study concerns the specificity of thought disorder. In former studies either persons and objects served as elements and the constructs were psychological and physical, respectively (Bannister and Salmon, 1966), or only persons had to be construed with psychological and with physical constructs (Heather, 1976; Mc Pherson *et al.*, 1975). In none of the studies were all four combinations of persons and objects and of psychological and physical con structs used. In the present study, persons, i.e. photographs of faces, and objects, i.e. photographs of chairs, are combined with psychological constructs as well as with physical constructs. In order to exclude alternative explanations for the specificity phenomenon, the constructs were chosen so as to make equivalent: (a) the intensity of the inter-construct relations in all four combinations, at least for normals; and (b) the degree of difficulty of the tasks. Ths degree of difficulty was operationally defined as interpersonal agreement (via Kendall W-coefficients of element rank orders from different subjects) and also by making use of subjective ratings of difficulty.

In a first preliminary investigation 24 constructs were judged by 14 normals on their being psychological vs. physical and on their applicability to both persons and chairs. In a second preliminary investigation 8 persons and 8 chairs had to be rank ordered on the 24 constructs by 16 normal subjects.

On the basis of the two preliminary investigations a selection of constructs was made, resulting in a set of three psychological constructs: 'friendly', 'gracious', and 'calm', and a set of three physical constructs: 'heavy', 'ugly', and 'robust'. All of the selected constructs were considered applicable to persons as well as to chairs, and the first set was considered rather psychological, whereas the second set was considered rather physical. The degree of difficulty (Kendall W's as well as subjective ratings) and the inter-construct intensity were about equal in the four combinations of elements and constructs.

Then, the four resulting grids were administered twice to three groups of subjects: 10 TD schizophrenics, 10 NTD schizophrenics, and 10 normals. The three groups were matched with respect to age, sex, and education, and the two schizophrenic groups were from the lowest recovery level. The order position of the four grids was varied so that each type of grid was placed equally often in each order position.

Because of the high variance within the two schizophrenic groups in comparison with the normals, the subject with the highest variance within each schizophrenic group (i.e. with the highest variance with respect to the scores that are derived from the 4×2 grids) was left out of the data analyses. Analyses of variance of the Intensity measure and of the Element Consistency measure were conducted with one between-subjects factor (the three groups) and with two within-subjects factors, type of elements and type of constructs. None of the analyses revealed a significant interaction of element type or construct type with the group, so that on this initial test no evidence was found in support of the specificity hypothesis.

However, an important difference with the typical design of the studies in which the specificity hypothesis was supported (Heather, 1976; McPherson *et al.*, 1975) is that in those studies only persons were used as elements and that Element Consistency was not considered. Therefore another analysis of variance was planned only for Intensity and without the data from the grids with objects as elements. Furthermore, in order to test the specificity hypothesis in the most direct way, the between-subjects level was reduced to two levels: TD schizophrenics vs NTD schizophrenics and normals. The analysis now revealed a group × construct type interaction ($F(1,26)=3.84$, $p < 0.10$). The interaction is shown in Table 3.2.

Table 3.2: Intensity of Interconstruct Relations for Psychological and Physical Constructs Used for Persons as Elements by TD Schizophrenics, and by NTD Schizophrenics and Normals[a]

Construct type	TD schizophrenics	NTD schizophrenics and normals
Psychological	23.65	30.65
Physical	32.51	29.34

[a] The intensity scores are mean squared rho's × 100; they have to be multiplied by 30 to be comparable to the scores from the Bannister and Fransella (1966) test.

When data were considered that are similar to the data from previous studies, the specificity hypothesis received some, but not very strong support. With respect to psychological constructs used for persons, TD schizophrenics obtained a lower Intensity score than others ($t(26)=1.80$, $p < 0.05$, one-tailed), and their Intensity measure for psychological constructs was lower than that for physical constructs ($t(8)=2.42$, $p < 0.05$, one-tailed).

The specificity hypothesis is confirmed here in its absolute version. TD schizophrenics are not inferior with respect to physical constructs but only with respect to psychological constructs, whereas NTD schizophrenics and normals do not show any difference between both types of constructs.

The specificity of the thought disorder being replicated, the question arised whether also the divergence of test-retest differences was specific to psychological constructs used for persons. Therefore, an analysis of variance was used with group (the three groups), construct type and test/retest as factors with the Intensity score from the grids with persons as a dependent variable. The expected interaction between the three factors was not significant, but the results were in line with the divergence hypothesis (see Table 3.3). The Intensity scores of TD schizophrenics decreased from test to retest when psychological constructs were used, whereas the same scores of normals and NTD schizophrenics increased either to some extent (in normals) or to a rather large extent (in NTD schizophrenics). The differences concerning physical constructs were much smaller. When only psychological constructs were considered, the interaction of group × test-retest turned out to be significant ($F(2,25)=4.65, p <0.05$).

Table 3.3: Test-retest Intensity Score Differences in Grids with Persons and with Psychological and Physical Constructs used by TD Schizophrenics, NTD Schizophrenics, and Normals

Construct type	TD schizophrenics	NTD schizophrenics	Normals
Psychological	−6.25	15.89	3.48
Physical	1.13	2.13	−1.32

TD schizophrenics seemed to weaken their psychological construct relations while construing persons, whereas NTD schizophrenics intensified the relations, clearly more than normals do. Moreover, the loosening of psychological constructs by TD schizophrenics was specific to the construing of persons, as the comparable retest-test difference for chairs is −0.27 (for physical constructs and chairs it is 4.19).

In summary, study one and study two are in line with the classical findings (1) that TD schizophrenics have less intense interconstruct relations and also less stability in their element-construct relations than NTD schizophrenics and normals, and (2) that the lower intensity of TD schizophrenics is specific to the psychological construing of persons. The more crucial findings, however, concern the divergence hypothesis stating that TD and NTD schizophrenics diverge in the evolution of their subsequent interconstruct relational intensity after an initial construing phase.

The divergence of TD and NTD schizophrenics was theoretically underpinned earlier by an interpretation of loose construing as 'incomplete construing' (the 'loss of conjunctivity'). Incomplete construing would lead to an intensification of construct relatedness when the incompleteness has a systematic bias in favour of one or a few aspects of the elements, whereas it would lead to a weakening of construct relatedness when the incompleteness has a random-like basis.

An explanation of schizophrenic construing as incomplete construing is in agreement with Schilder's hypothesis of 'abortive thought' (Schilder, 1951) stating that schizophrenics stop the microgenetic thought process too early (see also: Flavell and Draguns, 1957). It is argued by De Boeck (1981) that links may also be seen with Bleuler's theory that a central and fundamental symptom of schizophrenia is the breaking of associative threads between ideas (Bleuler, 1911), with Von Domarus' (1964) 'paralogical reasoning', with the 'overinclusion hypothesis' from Payne (1961) and Cameron (1964), and with the 'loss of set' formulation from Shakow (1963). Other theories may offer hypotheses on which aspects are or are not left out of consideration in the incomplete construing process. According to Chapman and Chapman's (1973) theory of excessive normal bias in schizophrenia, those aspects which are most salient to normals would be taken into consideration; and according to Salzinger's (1971) immediacy hypothesis one might expect that the most immediate aspects (close in time and space, intense, or unconditioned) remain, whereas the less immediate aspects are dropped from the construing process. It may be noted in passing that the immediacy hypothesis seems to have some relevance to grid data, as is shown by De Boeck *et al.*, (1981).

Implications for Therapy

Our current knowledge about the aetiology of schizophrenia requires humbleness in formulating therapeutic proposals. Within the PC-approach of schizophrenic construing a major therapeutic attempt was realised by Bannister, Adams-Webber, Penn and Radley (1975) for which the present ideas may have some relevance. We will limit ourselves in this section mainly to this.

Bannister's (1963; 1965a) testing of the serial invalidation hypothesis showed in all four experiments that validation led to a tightening of construct relationships. Given his interpretation of loose construing as a loose relationship between constructs, it is a logical step to attempt to tighten up the schizophrenic's construct system through a validation procedure. In a thorough investigation of each experimental subject, Bannister *et al.* (1975) tried to find clusters of relatively related constructs within the generally loose construct system. The authors write in this respect:

> It was hoped to discern the nature of his vague expectations and then repeatedly engineer situations in which these expectations would be fulfilled. Thereby the links between the constructs which had generated the expectations would gradually be strengthened and other constructs which were part of the same loose constellation might be drawn in, so that eventually the whole subsystem (. . .) might be strengthened and elaborated. (p. 171)

Generally speaking, the experiment's results were inconclusive, the reason for which might be tied to some practical and theoretical considerations. According to these authors, one rather theoretical point might be that the constructs get different, idiosyncratic meanings before they become loosely related. In our view, constructs get indeed different, idiosyncratic meanings because of the loss of conjunctivity: a verbal label is applied after the construction process had taken into account only some, but not all of the essential and necessary aspects.

In some patients, there is a systematic bias with respect to the type of aspects that are taken into account, leading to a relatively invariant and simple construct system that is tightly related. For example, this type of patient may describe the hospital as a concentration camp, only because he is not allowed to go anywhere anytime and he may feel himself tortured, only because he should do things he does not like to do according to the treatment programme. It is obvious that almost any situation can be construed in such a way that the bias is confirmed. In other patients the construing process is similarly functioning, but the lack of systematic bias makes their construct system loosely related. Therefore, their utterances are more fragmented and incoherent.

This means that according to us, the therapeutic focus should not lie in the tightening of the construct relationships, but in the re-instatement of conjunctivity, in the sense of completion of the construction process without overlooking too many aspects of the events that are construed. In 'biased' patients, this may result in a loosening of construct relationships, since the bias toward one or a few of the aspects would be removed so that again all of the relevant aspects can be considered. In 'unbiased' patients it might result in a strengthening of the relationships since the basis of the construction would become more stable instead of random-like. It is to be expected that for both types a reinstatement of conjunctivity leads to an increase in the differentiation of the construct system by the fact that more aspects of the events will underlie the construction process.

It is clear that a direct strengthening strategy through validation of the existing relationships does not guarantee that the basic problem is touched.

Therefore, it seems more advisable to offer an environment that allows for new but stable relationships between elements and constructs and between different constructs to be formed on a more complete basis, than to start with strengthening whatever construct relation the patient has.

This being put forward at a theoretical level, the problem arises how to realise this aim in practice. Bannister *et al.* (1975) stress the difference between their approach and operant programmes such as token economies, because in this latter treatment, emphasis lies on the motivational-emotional value of the reward. However, token economies may offer important possibilities from the point of view presented here. For there is evidence to suggest that token economy programmes may be effective in the treatment of schizophrenic patients because of other factors than the reward (Baker, Hall, Hutchinson and Bridge, 1977). One of these reasons might be that a coherent environment is offered in which a clear set of rules allows for predictivity on a conjunctive basis. The hierarchical ordering of groups with respect to the number of criteria that are to be fulfilled in order to receive the back-up reinforcer is a successive approximation of this conjunctivity principle. For example, at low levels of complexity, tokens are given immediately upon the simple presence in the occupational therapy room. At higher levels, the patient has to be present for a certain duration and has to produce a certain amount and quality of work before receiving his tokens.

Also, at the lowest level, the back-up reinforcer can be obtained at the end of each day. At the highest level, the back-up reinforcer can be obtained at the end of the week (a free weekend) provided that each day a minimum number of tokens is received.

Thus, the predictivity rule at lower levels is a rather simple if –
then relation; at higher levels the rule is mostly an if . . . and
if . . . and if . . . (. . .) then relation.

Another important feature of such a programme might be the
gradual increase of social reinforcers as compared to tangible
rewards. This is important not only because external rewards can be
detrimental to the development of intrinsically motivated behaviour (Levine and Fasnacht, 1974) but also in view of the specificity of thought disorder. For token economy programmes are a
coherent environment for the team members too. Therefore, their
reactions in response to the patients' behaviour are also more
predictable, because the set of rules specifies what behaviour
should be reinforced by the team members. It is obvious that in this
way, coherence and predictability may be more important than
reward and it can be expected that any ward organisation that
provides the same amount of structure will be equally effective with
respect to the treatment of thought disorder.

However, it may be expected that 'biased' patients should be
more difficult to treat than 'unbiased' patients in such a programme,
because the fact that they have a tight theory of the world that is
protected by a loose application rule, makes them less apt to change
their way of construing.

Of course, the treatment of the schizophrenic patient does not
stop with ward organisation. Probably, such a structured environment provides only opportunity to regain cognitive coherence at
subordinate construct levels. The development of higher order
constructs around the self and important others that allow for a
better integration and differentiation of the personal construct
system is also required. An interesting diagnostic approach in this
direction might be found in Space and Cromwell (1977). However,
therapeutic success in this respect will be dependent on progress in
all different domains of schizophrenia research. In the PC
approach, much importance is attached to the occurrence of unconstruable events, but it is not specified whether such events are
unconstruable because of the structure of the events or because of
the structure of the construct system, or because of both. It may be
mentioned in passing that research as to the pathogenetic effect of
double bind situations points to an overstatement of its importance
(Sluzki and Ransom, 1976). Probably, one should not under-
estimate the person-side of the matter. But neither is it specified

whether the structure of the construct system has become too simple because of rearing influences or because of biological factors or because of the combined influence of both (see Shean, 1978, for an introductory review). It seems to us that the PC approach is ideally suited to the integration of developments in different domains into a comprehensive and detailed description of the process of schizophrenia . Therefore, it is hoped that PC-theory of schizophrenia will keep and expand contacts with these domains.

Acknowledgement

The authors wish to thank Dr J. Peuskens, supervisor in the University Psychiatric Centre, Kortenberg, Belgium (Medical Director Professor Dr Pierloot).

4 PERSONAL CONSTRUCTS IN DEPRESSION: RESEARCH AND CLINICAL IMPLICATIONS

Robert Neimeyer

Elsie S. was a 52-year old woman who sought psychotherapeutic help from an 'experimental' treatment programme incorporating personal construct concepts and methods, after 15 years of relatively unproductive psychoanalytic sessions with various therapists. During her intake interview, she reported a number of painful symptoms, including insomnia, appetite disturbance, and loss of energy to pursue her responsibilities at home or in her part-time work as a bank teller. She described feeling chronically 'down', and spent at least part of each day crying in response to apparently minor disruptions of her routine. Gradually, she had withdrawn from many of the activities and hobbies she once enjoyed, as she became increasingly critical of her ability to meet the high demands she placed on herself in connection with her gardening, craftwork, painting, and the like. Elsie also felt more and more 'introverted' around people, and by then had 'zero interest' in sexual relations with her generally sympathetic husband of 30 years. The future seemed to offer only a 'downhill' course, leading toward further ageing and isolation, so she seldom contemplated it in detail. At her worst moments, Elsie found herself vaguely wishing she were dead, but she had no actual plans to take her own life.

In the diagnostic terms employed by most mental health workers, Elsie was 'depressed'. Specifically, both clinical interviews and psychological test data indicated that she was suffering from moderate, non-psychotic, unipolar depression of a chronic nature. The terms by which Elsie described herself were more vivid. On her Repgrid she construed herself as 'numb and tearful' rather than 'feeling good,' as 'closed up' rather than 'vulnerable', and as 'self-absorbed' rather than 'giving'. Both through her formal grid responses and in her informal conversation, Elsie conveyed the sense of living out a diminished, restricted existence which she was powerless to change.

In its general outlines, at least, Elsie's case is not unique. Studies in the United States and Europe indicate that approximately 10 to

82

20 per cent of the adult population will experience at least one episode of major depression at some point in their lives (American Psychiatric Association, 1980). When one considers that these figures do not include the substantial numbers of persons who experience depressive symptoms, but who receive other primary diagnoses, and that depression is often implicated in high-risk suicide attempts, the condition may be 'the most frequently seen, and perhaps the most lethal, of the psychiatric disorders' (Rush, 1982, p. 1).

In the present chapter, I will attempt to outline a personal construct model of depression, and consider the research that presently exists for each of its propositions. In addition, I will formulate some general assessment and treatment implications that seem consonant with this model and its research base. This latter effort will be admittedly speculative, since most personal construct research to date has been more concerned with a conceptualisation of the disorder than with its treatment. But by deriving some therapeutic hypotheses from existing research and theory, I hope to encourage subsequent clinical investigators to evaluate and refine these preliminary conjectures.

The Personal Construct Model

By analogising human behaviour to scientific inquiry, construct theory highlights our need as persons to build informal theories which enable us to interpret, organise, and anticipate a widening range of experience. In the course of human development, this takes the form of our accommodating our construction systems to a lifelong series of 'novel' events, events which are only inadequately construed in the light of our existing system (Mancuso, 1977). In Kelly's own terms, this process represents an ongoing 'dilation' of our awareness, a 'broadening of the perceptual field in order to reorganise it on a more comprehensive level' (Kelly, 1955, p. 476).

Almost by definition, this dilation entails a certain degree of *anxiety*, 'the recognition that the events with which one is confronted lie outside the range of convenience of one's construct system' (Kelly, 1955, p. 495). Of course, if the novel event being construed is only minimally discrepant with the person's existing system, the individual may experience nothing more than a mild arousal that motivates her to elaborate her construing in order to interpret the experience meaningfully (cf. Mancuso and Adams-Webber, 1982). But if the novel event is too discrepant, the anxiety it generates can be substantial. Thus, for a woman who has interrupted her career in order to raise a family, the decision to return to work may pose an interesting elaborative challenge, while for a more traditional wife and mother with little work experience outside the home, the same decision can be a source of considerable anxiety. This illustrates that the anxiety is not a function of external events in themselves, but is instead a function of the degree to which the individual's construct system is structured to anticipate them.

When confronted with events that are not easily assimilated into the existing construct framework, the individual can respond in one of three ways. As Kelly (1955, p. 847) explains:

> If . . . dilation presents the person with a situation he cannot handle, he can do one of three things. He can live with his anxiety for a time; he can crawl back into his shell for a time; or he can immediately start doing something about his constructs. If he crawls back into his shell he is using *constriction*, a device that enables him to postpone the revision of his constructs. The procedure is also a concession that his constructs are impermeable, that, while they fit the sorts of things he had previously found them useful for, they are not applicable to his newest venture.

At times, all of us use constriction to reduce the number of incompatible events with which we have to deal; it can serve as a temporary respite from the relentless process of reconstructing our outlooks. But such necessary constriction becomes depressive at the point that 'spontaneous elaboration is sharply curtailed' by a person in an 'effort to cut his field down to manageable size' (Kelly, 1955, p. 845). Like Elsie, the depressed individual typically shows 'withdrawal tendencies on all fronts' (Kelly, 1955, p. 1116), placing novel events psychologically out of bounds in order to minimise the risk of further invalidating the existing construct system. Ironically, this constrictive stance is often adopted after considerable invalidation (particularly at the level of the person's self-concept or 'core role structure') has already been sustained. Thus, the depressed person may continue to feel vulnerable and self-critical, but refuse to experiment with the new behaviours or self-constructions that might lead to the development of a more satisfying identity or way of life.

Most personal construct research on depressed individuals has been descriptive, focusing on those distinctive features of their construing that give rise to the depressive predicament. The picture that emerges from this research highlights the negative or ambivalent self-construing characteristic of the disorder, and attendant disruptions in the individual's self-image. As depression deepens, the individual's construct system becomes increasingly tailored to extracting negative, rather than positive information from ongoing experience. Similarly, the depression-prone person develops a 'set' to interpret events in highly polarised 'all-or-nothing' fashion, and to form global undiscriminating emotional judgements. Finally, such an individual tends to view him or herself as essentially different from others, a tendency that is not reducible to their proneness to see themselves in negative terms. I will first review research bearing on each of these features before examining the implications of this research for psychotherapy for the disorder. Readers interested in a fuller discussion of research on depression and suicide from a personal construct standpoint may wish to consult R. A. Neimeyer (1984; 1985a).

Negative Self-construing

At least since the seminal writings of Freud (1955), self-devaluation has been considered one of the cardinal features of depression. In Freud's theory of melancholia, this tendency toward self-criticism was seen as a reflection of 'anger-turned-inward' toward an introjected, but disappointing love object. Thus, the melancholic may have unconsciously identified with a loved one, establishing a representation of the other as an 'ego-ideal'. Upon losing the other through rejection or death, the melancholic may then turn the ensuing anger or rage upon the self, which contains the only remaining representation of the lost object. While this complicated psychodynamic sequence is often rejected as implausible by authors outside the psychoanalytic camp (e.g. Hollon and Beck, 1979), self-devaluation itself is none the less observed in about 80 per cent of depressives (Beck, 1973), and is included in nearly all instruments designed to diagnose the disorder (Glazer, Clarkin, and Hunt, 1981).

From a personal construct standpoint, this implies that depressed individuals, relative to others, will construe themselves under more negative poles of their personal constructs, a finding that has been confirmed in several repertory grid studies using both psychologically 'healthy' and non-depressed psychiatric comparison groups (e.g. Ross, 1985; Space and Cromwell, 1980; Sperlinger, 1976). In addition, a tendency toward negative self-construing has been found to correlate with severity of vegetative and affective symptoms (sleep disturbance, feeling 'blue' or sad) within a group of carefully diagnosed depressed subjects (Neimeyer, Klein, Gurman and Griest, 1983).

While these general trends seem to hold across several studies, recent work also suggests that the relationship between negative self-construing and depression may be more complex than most mental health workers assume. Both Space and Cromwell (1980) and Space, Dingemans and Cromwell, (1983), for example, discovered that even severely depressed hospitalised patients rarely construed themselves in consistently negative terms, though they were prone to higher levels of self-devaluation than controls. Instead, these patients displayed a tendency toward what these researchers termed *mixed self-valence*, the tendency on the grid to evaluate themselves both positively and negatively on different constructs within the same construct subsystem. Clinically, this could be registered as an ambivalent or equivocal self-evaluation within a given domain: Elsie, for instance, viewed herself as 'loyal' and 'dependable' as a close friend, but also as 'insecure' and 'cold' within the same relationship. Space and Cromwell (1980) conjectured that the instability of such mixed self-valence could predispose the individual to *slot movement*, the sweeping reconstruing of oneself in positive or negative terms in response to relatively minor changes in circumstances. Thus, the depressive may unwittingly cognitively structure his experience to maximise his susceptibility to unpredictable mood shifts. Support for this hypothesis has been provided by Ross (1985), who asked depressed and non-depressed persons to perform daily ratings of themselves on a sample of personal construct dimensions over a two-week period. As predicted, the former showed greater tendency toward slot change on a day-to-day basis.

A second set of findings suggests that while depressives do not simply construe all events in negative terms, they do become cognitively 'primed' to attend selectively to negative, rather than

positive, information. Dingemans, Space and Cromwell (1983) discovered that subjects with more vegetative symptoms (fatigue)
were more likely than less symptomatic subjects to provide a
negative description on the emergent pole of the construct; it
became the way in which most acquaintances were seen as alike,
with only a few acquaintances being seen as positive exceptions to
this general rule. Similarly, Sheehan (1981) found that when
depressed patients completed a grid rating the way they felt significant others viewed them, they placed nearly two-thirds of their
self-elements under the negative construct pole. What emerges
from these studies is the implication that as depression increases,
one develops a construct system that is increasingly tailored to
encoding, storing, and retrieving negative information about the
self and others. This formulation adds detail to the general cognitive
model of the disorder outlined by Beck, Rush, Shaw and Emery
(1979), and contributes to the conceptualisation of the depressive
self-schema outlined in a later section.

Conceptual Differentiation

One of the most influential concepts introduced by personal
construct researchers is the notion of 'cognitive complexity',
defined as 'the degree of differentiation in an individual's construct
system, i.e. the relative number of different dimensions of
judgement used by a person' (Tripodi and Bieri, 1964; p. 122). The
idea that some construct systems may be 'complex' (composed
of a large number of relatively unrelated construct dimensions)
while others are 'simple' (contain only tightly related constructs that
are used virtually identically to interpret experience) has formed
the basis for a large body of personal construct literature in
personality, social, and developmental psychology (Adams-
Webber, 1979b).

In psychopathology research, both extremely differentiated and
undifferentiated systems can be viewed as problematic (cf. Landfield, 1980a). On the one hand, the overly differentiated individual
may tend to construe events, other persons, and even the self in
fragmented terms, depriving experience of a sense of coherence or
meaning. On the other hand, the massively undifferentiated person
may construe things so globally that much subtle information about
the social environment is lost. These extremes in construct system
structure have been associated with schizophrenic thought disorder

(Bannister; 1960; see also Chapter 3) and obsessive-compulsive disorder (Makhlouf-Norris, Jones and Norris, 1970; see also Chapter 5), respectively.

One could argue, as have Ashworth, Blackburn and McPherson (1982), that the constrictive process operative in depression should produce an increasingly undifferentiated conceptual structure for construing social experience. These investigators did find some equivocal support for this position: relative to manics, schizophrenics, and alcoholics, depressives employed construct systems whose first three factors accounted for a larger degree of variance. Currently symptomatic depressives, however, could not be distinguished from either recovered depressives or non-psychiatric controls, suggesting that the above findings may reflect the conceptual fragmentation of the other three pathological groups rather than the cognitive simplicity of depressives *per se*. Further doubt is cast on the interpretation of these results by the consistently negative findings of other researchers (Dingemans *et al.*, 1983; McPherson *et al.*, 1973; Space and Cromwell, 1980; Sperlinger, 1976). To date, there is no evidence that depressives employ less differentiated general construct systems than normals.

But on a more specific level of analysis, the structure of the depressive's construct system may indeed display unique features. This possibility is suggested by Silverman's (1977) finding that although depressed subjects could not be distinguished from normal controls in the gross structure of their interpersonal construing, they did indeed appear more monolithic in the use of their mood-related constructs. This implies that while the depressed client may be able to make fairly fine perceptual discriminations in many areas of her experience, she may be prone to much more global, inflexible construing when she confronts emotionally charged issues.

A second distinctive feature of the depressed individual's cognitive structure may be the relative absence of intra-system *conflict* it displays. As suggested by Kelly's (1955) fragmentation corollary (see also Landfield, 1982), our construct systems are seldom logically water-tight. Ordinarily, they are 'loosely' enough fashioned that they permit some degree of implicative inconsistency, as when we construe someone who is 'unsympathetic' as 'unable to face reality', and believe that this inability to face reality leads to 'unhappiness', but paradoxically construe unsympathetic people as generally happy. Sheehan (1981) employed an ingenious grid measure of this kind of cognitive inconsistency, and found that depressives tended to have *less* of such conflict than controls. She interpreted this as consonant with a constriction argument: depressed persons may employ a construct system that minimises the perception of inconsistency. Unfortunately, Carroll (1983) was unable to replicate the finding on a similar sample, casting some doubt on the generality of this phenomenon.

Depressive Self-schema

One of the most interesting specific structural characteristics of depressive construing concerns the nature of the individual's 'core role structure' or self-schema. In keeping with the structural emphasis of personal construct theory, the 'self' is not considered simply a unitary object or concept that can be placed within the construct system (Bannister, 1983). Instead, it might more accurately be considered a network of self-perceptions, with various aspects of ourselves being viewed as more or less linked up with one another (cf. Mair, 1977b). In the limiting case a person might construe himself in invariant terms in a variety of social settings or relationships: in the home or on the job, with friends or with superiors, such a person sees himself as open, honest, intelligent, etc. On the opposite extreme, another person may see herself as having a very different personality in different contexts: at work she is fastidious, but at home is sloppy; with friends she is talkative, with superiors, quiet. Thus, an individual's self-schema may vary in its degree of differentiation or consistency.

Sheehan (1981) examined the possibility that members of a depressed group (most of whom were hospitalised) would display less complex, more 'intense' self-schemas than normal controls. She assessed the coherence of their self-structure by administering a *multiple perception of self* grid, in which subjects rated themselves from the viewpoint of significant others in their lives. Evidence appeared to support her hypothesis: depressives showed less differentiated core-role structures than controls. Recent research by Neimeyer *et al.*, (1983), however, produced different findings. Using a methodology similar to Sheehan's, these authors found no relationship between level of depression in a moderately symptomatic client group and coherence of the core-role structure.

These apparently conflicting findings might none the less be integrated from the standpoint of a personal construct model of the disorder (see R.A. Neimeyer, 1984, 1985a). Specifically, it would be predicted that normal, non-depressed individuals typically construe themselves in predominantly favourable terms across a number of social roles. This evaluative consistency would be reflected in a relatively undifferentiated but positive self-schema; the individual tends to apply to himself the positive poles of his self-referent constructs in virtually all contexts. With the onset of depression, however, negative self-evaluations begin to be assimilated into the person's core-role structure. This produces some loss of organisation in the self-schema (differentiation), producing at moderate levels of depression the pattern of 'mixed self-valence' noted by Space and Cromwell (1980). Gradually, as depression deepens, a consistent self-structure may again crystallise, but along negative rather than positive lines.

Support for this hypothesised curvilinear relationship between core-role differentiation and intensity of depression comes from two sources. First, research within experimental psychopathology (e.g. Kuiper and Derry, 1981) suggests that whereas moderate depressives are able to recall readily material that is either negatively or positively valenced, severe depressives show superior recall only for negatively valenced material. Since memory for an event is a function of whether or not the individual has available appropriate cognitive schemata with which to 'encode' it, this implies that the self-schemas of moderate depressives are more evaluatively differentiated, whereas those of severely depressed individuals are more negative, but also more consistent (see R.A. Neimeyer, 1984, for discussion).

Research by Neimeyer, Heath and Strauss (1985) provides additional support for this model. Partitioning a group of carefully diagnosed depressives into four groups on the basis of their severity, they discovered that the most depressed subjects (quartiles 3 and 4) displayed less differentiated self-schemas than the moderately depressed group (quartile 2). The least depressed group was intermediate in differentiation, and could not be reliably distinguished from the other groups.

It is important to emphasise that although the research to date has examined the relationship between core-role differentiation and depression only in cross-sectional designs (i.e. using different subject groups), the most important clinical implications may be longitudinal. For example, a given individual who is becoming increasingly depressed may undergo subtle but significant disruptions in her self-image, as outlined above. This interpretation of these findings suggests that different clinical strategies might prove useful at various points in the development of the disorder, a topic to which I shall return in a later section.

Polarised Construing

One particular form of cognitive rigidity that theorists have associated with psychopathology in general and with depression in particular is 'dichotomous thinking', or 'the tendency to place all experiences in one of two opposite categories; for example, flawless or defective, immaculate or filthy, saint or sinner' (Beck *et al.*, 1979). For Elsie, this took the form of seeing herself as either the 'ideal mother' or as a 'complete failure as a parent', with no in-between. In personal construct terms, this represents a tendency to use constructs as binary categories into which events are roughly classed, rather than as graded dimensions on which events are placed (cf. Kelly, 1955, pp. 141–5). This tendency to construe reality in simple and extreme terms appears to represent a developmentally less mature mode of thinking, one that precedes the acquisition of more flexible dimensional construing (Applebee, 1976).

Neimeyer *et al.*, (1983) were able to demonstrate that within a group of depressed individuals, symptom severity correlated with the tendency to evaluate the self in extreme, absolutistic terms. This finding was conceptually replicated by Dingemans *et al.* (1983), who discovered that this trend toward dichotomous thinking discriminated both depressives and schizophrenics from normal controls. Therefore, while polarised construing does not appear to be *uniquely* associated with depression, it does seem to be operative in the disorder, especially in more severe cases. Moreover, given the connection between chronic dichotomous thinking and serious suicide ideation (Neuringer and Lettieri, 1971), this feature of depressive construing is an especially important target for therapeutic intervention.

Self-other Distance

Holland (1977) has argued that most theories of personality and psychopathology tend to underemphasise the social dimension of our behaviour, instead restricting their scope to the examination of intrapsychic events. This criticism might be levelled even more strongly at cognitive theories, which by definition focus on the internal processes and structures by which individuals impute meaning to their experience. Yet construct theorists have taken at least a first step in the direction of including interpersonal as well as intrapersonal processes in their study of depression, by exploring the degree to which distressed persons construe themselves as isolated from or unidentified with significant other people.

Based on extensive clinical contact with several severely depressed clients, Rowe (1978) first described the tendency of such individuals to operate on the basis of 'propositions that enclose', that emphasise their separateness from both relatives and potential friends. Empirical support for this view was subsequently provided by Space and Cromwell (1980), who discovered that depressives indicated much less perceived similarity (or identification) between self and others (parents, spouses) in repertory grid ratings than did either other psychiatric patients or non-disturbed control subjects. This finding was all the more significant, because this trend toward greater self-other distance held even after the effects of negative self-construing were statistically partialled out. These findings appear reliable, since they have been replicated by Space *et al.* (1983).

Related research by Adams-Webber and Rodney (1983) demonstrates the hazard of assuming a simple causal relationship between cognitive set and emotional response. These investigators asked non-depressed subjects to complete a repertory grid under normal conditions, and then to retake it under instructional sets designed to induce both elated and depressed mood. They found that in the depressed affect condition, respondents rated themselves as less identified with others, despite the fact that both self and others were rated more negatively than in the baseline condition. Conversely, under the elation set, subjects viewed themselves as more identified with others. These preliminary findings point up the potential usefulness of mood induction techniques in precipitating changes in construct system structure, a strategy which will be discussed more fully below.

Clinical Implications

Research in psychopathology represents both basic and applied science, leading on the one hand to the development of empirically validated models of disorders and on the other to the refinement of the methods by which they are assessed and treated. The studies reviewed above aim almost exclusively at the former goal, leaving their clinical implications largely unarticulated. For this reason, I would like to extrapolate cautiously from this growing literature in order to formulate a few diagnostic and treatment recommendations.

Assessment

As in most areas of personal construct research, the vast majority of studies discussed in this chapter rely primarily or exclusively upon adaptations of Kelly's (1955) Role Construct Repertory Grid or Repgrid. Perhaps the most obvious question raised by this methodological commitment concerns the clinical utility of the grid in assessing depressed clients. What information can it provide that cannot be derived from more straightforward questionnaires or clinical interviews? Are there indications or contraindications to its use with depressives?

For the most part, the advantages and disadvantages of employing grid technique with depressives are similar to those encountered in most other clinical applications. For example, the grid embodies the strengths of both projective tests (e.g. elucidation of the client's subjective world) and objective questionnaires (e.g. quantitative rigour permitting the sensitive assessment of treatment efficacy). It integrates the study of both cognitive *content* (in the form of elicited constructs provided by the client) and cognitive *structure* (reflected in derived scores of system differentiation, etc.). It is an enormously flexible technique, one that can be tailored to assess the client's relation to significant others, or his or her own self-image. Above all, it is congruent with the humanistic aspirations of construct theory, permitting the assessor 'to survey the pathways along which the subject is free to move' rather than merely 'to classify him as a clinical type' (Kelly, 1955, p. 203). Of course, the general drawbacks of grid technique also apply: there are few developed norms for grid scores, making interpretation of their results more difficult, and they are oriented more toward the measurement of extant psychological states, rather than the temporally extended process of construing and reconstruing (see Fransella and Bannister, 1977; Neimeyer and Neimeyer, 1981b and Button, Chapter 2, for further discussion).

Apart from these general considerations, the specific use of grid technique with depressives has some distinctive advantages and disadvantages. Among the former is its ability to tap structural features of depressive cognition (such as globality or polarisation) that figure prominently in conceptualisations such as Beck's (1976), but which are left unaddressed by other assessment techniques (Arnkoff and Glass, 1982). In the clinical setting, of course, grid results can be interpreted highly idiographically to help pinpoint particular areas of the individual's construing requiring intervention. Sheehan (1981), for instance, notes that extreme ideal self ratings by a client may indicate the need to moderate the client's excessive standards, since these may represent perfectionistic ideals that are virtually impossible to attain. Such close examination of a client's grid responses often discloses material that would take much longer to emerge in unstructured interviews. For example, prior to her therapy Elsie completed a grid in which the elements were aspects of herself in various social roles (see Neimeyer, *et al.*, 1983, for details concerning grid format). Looking over her responses, I noticed that whereas she construed herself in predominantly positive terms in relating to 'people she liked,' she construed herself highly negatively (as angry, closed, etc.) in the role of 'close friend'. This primed me to raise concerns about her experience of herself in superficial as opposed to intimate relationships early in the therapy.

The administration of grids to this client group should be done thoughtfully, however. Obviously, for the severely depressed client experiencing psychomotor retardation and difficulties concentrating, completing a paper-and-pencil grid requiring hundreds of specific ratings can become a gruelling test of endurance. For this reason, it is sometimes useful to administer the grid in structured interview form (Kelly, 1955; Neimeyer and Neimeyer, 1981b) possibly even breaking it down into two phases, construct elicitation and element placement. The timing of grid administration should also be considered. In his own therapy with a distraught client, for example, Kelly postponed grid testing until the sixth session, after he had established the general outlines of the client's problems and provided some provisional assistance with an unexpected crisis (discussed in Neimeyer, 1980).

At a theoretical level, it bears emphasising that the grid's structural and content emphasis, while useful, also renders it less sensitive to the cognitive *processes* that are implicated in depression. Thus, the development of constriction *per se* has yet to be studied, despite its centrality in the personal construct model. This implies that the clinician will have to remain alert to such processes as the client's gradual withdrawal from previous interests and relationships, tendencies that will be only indirectly hinted at by grid results.

Finally, it should be remembered that any comprehensive assessment of the depressed client should draw upon other measures that complement the strengths of the repertory grid. For example, such symptomatic and behavioural rating scales as the Beck Depression Inventory (Beck *et al.*, 1979) and the Pleasant Events Schedule (Lewinsohn and Libet, 1972) are useful, since they help operationalise the criteria (mood and behaviour change) by which therapy will be judged successful. Other assessment techniques employed within construct theory can also prove valuable adjuncts to formal grid testing. For example, assigning the self-characterisation (Kelly, 1955) as homework can serve diagnostic and therapeutic ends: it gives a clinically rich portrayal of the depressed client's self-image, and at the same time invites her to view herself in a more sympathetic and detached manner than she may be accustomed to doing. Similarly, the use of daily grid ratings by the client (Ross, 1985) can serve as a self-monitoring tool that can be made integral to certain therapeutic interventions. This and other applications of assessment methods in the context of treatment will be discussed in the following section.

Treatment

Ultimately, the clinical utility of any psychological theory must reside in its ability to (a) explain the mechanisms by which existing treatments produce their effects, and (b) generate new and more-effective forms of intervention. Although personal construct theory's contribution at this level to the treatment of depression is at only a rudimentary stage, some implications for various types of therapy are beginning to take shape. For convenience, I will cluster my remarks under five headings, bearing on hospitalisation, pharmacotherapy, behavioural procedures, cognitive procedures, and group therapy.

Hospitalisation. Discussion of the effects of inpatient treatment are curiously scarce among psychological theories of depression, despite the fact that depressives may account for as much as 75 per cent of all psychiatric hospitalisations (Secunda, Katz, Friedman and Schuyler, 1973). Kelly (1955, pp. 845–6) acknowledged that brief institutional treatment could sometimes have its place. Specifically, he believed that it could represent a short-term expedient for helping a severely anxious client constrict his perceptual field, 'as he finds that he is no longer compelled to face that for which he had no adequate structure.' Thus, if timed properly, it can help forestall further invalidation of the client's construct system by substituting a simpler, more predictable environment for the more threatening, unpredictable life-situation currently being confronted by the client. Providing such a refuge may be especially important when the client's construct system shows signs of increasing loss of structure, as when he or she is undergoing a transition from one stable core-role structure to another. As both Kelly (1961) and Landfield (1976) have argued, such increasing disorganisation may provide a cognitive context for the suicidal act.

Unfortunately, hospitalisation is at best a means of arresting further invalidation, and at worst may simply exaggerate the client's helplessness when she confronts a suddenly dilated field of problematic events at discharge. The extent of reconstruction that occurs over the course of brief institutionalisation is suggested by the findings of Hewstone, Hooper and Miller (1981). These investigators discovered that patients' identification with others improved during their hospital stay, a change that seemed to correlate with their improved mood. No change was evident, however, in a number of other features of their construct systems (e.g. negative self-construing, system differentiation). Interestingly, pretreatment assessment of a client's constructions may help predict his or her likelihood of benefiting from in-patient treatment. Sperlinger (1976), for example, has reported that depressives who employ constructs suggesting high 'self-sufficiency' (e.g. competent, independent) tend to improve during hospitalisation, while those who use few self-sufficiency constructs do not. Future studies in this area would be of greater value if they were to isolate or at least clearly describe the specific interventions administered during in-patient treatment, so that the effects attributable to various forms of therapy (e.g. medication, behaviour therapy) can be distinguished from those resulting from simple custodial hospitalisation *per se*.

Pharmacotherapy. Traditionally, pharmacotherapy has been considered the treatment of choice for most depressives (Winokur, 1981). Despite some significant side effects of these medications, it is generally acknowledged that drug therapy using the tricyclic antidepressants, monoamine oxidase inhibitors, or (for bipolar disorder) lithium carbonate can be helpful in minimising many of the disabling vegetative symptoms of acute depression. The question posed to personal construct researchers concerns the nature and extent of conceptual change accompanying successful drug treatment.

The controlled evaluation of drug therapy conducted by Sheehan (1981) offers some tentative answers to this question. Monitoring shifts in the construing of unipolar depressives, she found a clear decrease in self-ideal self distance occurring over 6 to 8 weeks of unspecified drug therapy. No such change was evident in untreated controls. Similarly, Sheehan found that the treated depressives increased in the number of high forcefulness and social interaction constructs they employed, and showed correspondingly less reliance over time on constructs connoting low forcefulness and emotional arousal. The construct content of controls remained stable over the same interval. In contrast, no changes in several aspects of construct system *structure* were evident in response to pharmacotherapy. These findings suggest that drug therapy may produce some incipient changes in the content of construing, but has little effect on the system at deeper structural levels. As such, it may be useful in making the severely depressed person more amenable to treatment, but should not be expected to carry the full weight of therapeutic reconstruction.

Behavioural Interventions. It is a common misperception that personal construct therapy is a highly intellectualised or verbal affair (cf. Rogers, 1956). Yet Kelly (1955, pp. 995–6) clearly recognised that 'sometimes it is more feasible to try to produce personality readjustments by attacking the symptoms than by going directly after the basically faulty structures.' In the case of the severely constricted, withdrawn client, Kelly suggested that this could take the form of prescribed occupational, recreational or social activities assigned to the client as between-session homework (pp. 997–8). For example, he might suggest that the constricted homemaker take a part-time job, or do some spring cleaning before the next therapy session. What distinguishes this approach from a straightforward behavioural intervention is Kelly's emphasis on using activity scheduling as a vehicle for 'controlled elaboration' of the construct system. For example, after the above assignment, Kelly would spend time considering with the client the 'similarities and contrasts . . . between what she finds herself doing and thinking while on the job and what happens in her household' (1955, p. 997). Thus, in addition to dilating her field of experience, the exercise could help her construe herself and her activity in less restrictive terms.

The systematic use of activity scheduling is a major technique employed by Lewinsohn and his colleagues (e.g. Lewinsohn, Munoz, Youngren and Zeiss, 1978) in their behaviour therapy for depression. By first monitoring the client's activity level and then assigning selected activities, the therapist seeks to provide the client with experiences of accomplishment or pleasure, and thereby improve his or her mood. Directive strategies of this kind may be especially helpful when the client appears disorganised, alternating between one set of behaviours or self-perceptions and the next.

Activity monitoring can also be used in conjuction with more cognitive/reconstructive strategies. Extending Ross's (1985) method, a therapist might ask the client to perform daily self-ratings on a set of personally significant construct dimensions, and to keep an accompanying log of events that seemed to 'trigger' any dramatic slot-movement from one side of these scales to the other. Therapeutic discussion might then focus on the nature of the precipitating events and the interpretation the client placed on them. Enactment techniques such as fixed role therapy can be especially useful at this point in helping the client approach the problem situation differently (see Adams-Webber, 1981, for general discussion, and Bonarius, 1970, for specific application to depression). Since these interventions begin to address both 'external' behavioural and 'internal' cognitive change, more attention will be given to the latter in the next section.

Cognitive Interventions. One of the more revolutionary recent developments in psychotherapy for depression has been the emergence of cognitive therapy (Beck *et al.*, 1979), an approach whose efficacy in treating unipolar depression has become well established (Weissman, 1984). Cognitive therapists assume that depressives commit certain predictable errors in processing information (e.g. by overgeneralising on the basis of failure experiences, engaging in black-or-white thinking) and thus maintain the apparent validity of a cognitive 'triad' consisting of a negative view of the self, the world, and the future. Therapy consists of a set of cognitive and behavioural strategies to help the client first recognise the way that his mood relates to the interpretations he places on events, and then test those interpretations for their validity. As Sheehan (1981) and R.A. Neimeyer (1984) note, there is much in Beck's approach that is compatible with a personal construct perspective, although the former tends to be somewhat more limited in the range of disorders it addresses and more focused on the role of logic and rationality in mental health (c.f. R.A. Neimeyer, 1985a).

From a personal construct standpoint, the therapeutic challenge facing the therapist working with a depressed individual is to reactivate the client's movement through the 'experience cycle' (R.A. Neimeyer, 1985a). For Kelly (1955), experience consisted of more than simply the events people confront. Rather, it described the process of framing an *anticipation* of an event, *investing* oneself in the outcome, *encountering* the event, recognising the *confirmation or disconfirmation* of one's anticipation, and finally, *revising* one's construct system in light of the outcome. Since this revised system then provides a point of departure for new anticipations or predictions, the continuous movement through this cycle describes the process of psychological growth. The depressed individual often has so seriously constricted his range of activities that he is arrested in his movement through the cycle, preventing himself from encountering the events that could invalidate or enlarge upon his rather rigid and negative constructions.

Ultimately, then, the goal of therapy is to help the client encounter a richer, more dilated field of experience, and to use this experience to elaborate a more adequate view of the self and others. Mood induction techniques like those employed by Adams-Webber and Rodney (1983) may be useful in setting the stage for this behavioural experimentation. This could take the form of encouraging the client to imagine herself in some detail in a more positive life role ('Try to picture exactly what it would be like if you were having a pleasant and intimate relationship with your husband,' or 'Let's fantasise for a moment about how you'd feel about yourself if you were able to find that executive job you've been looking for'). This may help the client experience in imagination an alternative to her existing constructions, and thus may instil a more hopeful view of herself and others. Elaborating on the above examples, the client might then be encouraged to behave on the assumption that an intimate conversation with her husband *is* possible, or that suitable professional work *can* be found. This may help counter the self-fulfilling prophecy that such goals are unattainable, and hence, not worth striving for. Of course, in keeping with Kelly's (1955, p. 998) caveat about real-life behaviour change, more difficult behavioural experiments (e.g. opening a personal conversation with a reserved spouse, seeking a job interview) should be discussed and enacted in the safety of the therapy room before being implemented in the client's actual life.

The therapeutic efficacy of such techniques has been investigated by Neimeyer *et al.* (1985), who have studied the reconstruction resulting from a group adaptation of cognitive therapy for unipolar depressives. Based substantially on the work of Beck *et al.* (1979), the treatment programme included behavioural interventions (e.g. activity scheduling), cognitive interventions (e.g. developing rational responses to dysfunctional thoughts), and personal construct techniques (e.g. assessing personal belief systems through the laddering technique). Offered weekly to six randomly constituted groups of clients, the therapy proved superior to a wait list control condition in reducing both depressive symptomatology and suicide ideation. More important in light of the model advanced above, treated subjects, relative to controls, showed decreases in both negative construing of themselves in the future and 'as they really were,' and in polarised construing of themselves across a variety of social roles. These results provide evidence that an amalgam of personal contruct and cognitive interventions can produce not only symptomatic remission of depression, but substantial revision at the level of 'core role' structure. Further cross-fertilisation of the two approaches seems to hold considerable promise for effecting specific changes in those aspects of construing that seem most clearly linked to depression-proneness.

Group Therapy. A final implication of the personal construct model of depression concerns the potential utility of group psychotherapy (see Chapter 15), a format that is gaining increasing credibility in the treatment of the disorder (R.A. Neimeyer, 1985b). The usefulness of an explicitly interpersonal treatment has been suggested by Space and Cromwell (1980), who viewed it as one means of increasing the depressive's identification with other people. Additionally, Sheehan (1981) has observed that as a client's interpersonal milieu changes, this provides new 'elements' in the form of people to be construed, so that group therapy necessarily entails a dilation of the client's field of social experience. Thus, group treatment may not only serve to reduce the client's perceived distance from others, but also foster experimentation with new forms of interpersonal construing.

The only group therapy study focused on depression from a personal construct viewpoint (Neimeyer *et al.*, 1985) produced mixed evidence on these putative benefits. While substantial change in both depressive symptoms and construct system structure occurred over the course of this brief, cognitively oriented therapy, group members did not show a significant decrease in self-reported 'detachment' from others in general. Whether this negative finding reflects the relative insensitivity of the non-grid measure of detachment used, or the failure of the highly structured treatment to produce increased identification must be answered by further research.

Unanswered Questions

In the above review I have attempted to glean from the burgeoning empirical literature on personal constructs in depression, a tentative model of the disorder, and have tried to examine a few of its implications for clinical assessment and treatment. In so doing, I have tried to point up the compatibility of a personal construct approach with some existing theories (particularly cognitive-behavioural formulations), since it is my belief that the most humane and effective treatment for depression will follow from a comprehensive model that integrates aspects of them all. Clearly, much of this conceptual work remains to be done. Just as clearly, there are a number of pressing questions that confront clinical researchers in this area.

At a theoretical level, the explanatory status of many of the processes and styles of construing in depression highlighted in this review remains obscure. For example, does the globality of affective construing among depressives detected by Silverman (1977) represent a cognitive style that predisposes certain individuals to become depressed, or a kind of conceptual rigidity that develops only with the depressive syndrome itself? Does therapeutic reduction of polarised thinking (e.g. Neimeyer *et al.*, 1985) simply help ameliorate an acute depressive episode, or does it also serve a preventive function, reducing the risk of future mood disturbance? Elsewhere (R.A. Neimeyer, 1984), I have discussed such questions in light of the larger issue of whether these processes are *symptom-*

linked (i.e. covary with level of depression) or *vulnerability-linked* (i.e. place currently non-depressed individuals at greater risk for developing the disorder). Answering questions of this type will necessarily entail longitudinal, prospective studies of a kind that have not yet been attempted.

At a clinical level, the most serious question facing personal construct researchers concerns the specification and evaluation of treatment strategies. Most research to date has examined only the impact of broad, non-specific interventions (e.g. hospitalisation, psychotherapy), and then only on a few cognitive or symptomatic outcome variables. Clearly, if clinically relevant knowledge is to be produced, investigators must begin to study the impact of particular interventions (e.g. fixed role therapy, building mastery through activity scheduling) on several aspects of construing (e.g. negativity and differentiation of the self-schema, self-other distance). Only after the efficacy of such procedures is established can a comprehensive treatment programme for depression be assembled on rational grounds.

In conclusion, the growing concern of construct theorists with the phenomenon of depression has begun to clarify the personal dimensions of the disorder. I hope that the continuation of this work will permit us not only to understand, but also to help change the painful and constricted world in which the depressed individual lives.

Acknowledgement

This work was supported in part by funding to the Dept. of Psychology's Center for Applied Psychological Research granted through the Centers of Excellence Program of the State of Tennessee. Reprints may be obtained from Robert A. Neimeyer, PhD, Dept of Psychology, Memphis State University, Memphis, TN. USA 38152.

5 NEUROTIC DISORDERS: THE CURSE OF CERTAINTY

David Winter

Theory

The traditional psychiatric view of the neurotic individual is of a person beleaguered by anxiety, whose symptoms either represent direct expressions of this anxiety or defensive manoeuvres adopted in an attempt to control it. Kelly's description of neurosis was not dissimilar to this, for he also regarded the neurotic as someone who 'is always fighting off anxiety', and who consequently 'casts about frantically for new ways of construing the events of his world' (p. 895). It will be recalled that, in personal construct theory terms, anxiety is the experience that events are largely unconstruable, that they lie mostly outside the range of convenience of one's construct system. Construing could therefore be considered always to be directed towards the reduction of anxiety, although Kelly regarded this as a negative statement of his theory's view of motivation, of the individual's quest for predictability and certainty. Anxiety was also by no means seen by Kelly as necessarily a sign of pathology but rather, in limited degrees, as an essential prerequisite for adventure and reconstruction, 'a harbinger of change' (p. 836). Thus, the normal person 'keeps opening himself up to moderate amounts of confusion in connection with his continuous revision of his construct system. He avoids collapse into a total chaos of anxiety by relying upon superordinate and permeable aspects of his system' (p. 896). In this passage, Kelly draws on his Modulation and Fragmentation Corollaries, which together imply that a person can tolerate a certain degree of incompatibility in their construing provided that their superordinate constructs are sufficiently permeable to accommodate these inconsistent constructions. Neurotics are unable to rely on permeable superordinate constructs in this way

As well as offering a general formulation of neurosis, personal construct theory provides some indication of the processes which may be reflected in particular neurotic symptoms. Thus, free-floating anxiety and depersonalisation may be viewed as direct manifestations of a person's awareness of an inability to predict their world. Free-floating anxiety is not, however, a particularly meaningful concept in construct theory terms for, in a sense, all anxiety could be considered as essentially free-floating: in the words of W.H. Auden (1976), 'The fears we know are of not knowing'. By developing phobic, obsessional or hysterical symptoms the neurotic could therefore be seen as attempting to provide some 'structure "at any cost" ' (Tschudi, 1977, p. 338) in an otherwise unpredictable, anxiety-provoking world. Thus, in the case of the phobic, anxiety in the face of largely unconstruable events is replaced by fear of a concrete object, while the obsessive-compulsive client finds a certain haven of predictability and structure within the narrow confines of their obsessional concerns. In Kelly's view, the obsessional's construct system 'is characteristically impermeable; he needs a separate pigeonhole for each new experience and he calculates his anticipation of events with minute pseudomathematical schemes' (p. 89). Phobic avoidance reactions and the rituals of the obsessional can also be considered to represent clear behavioural expressions of a constrictive process, the drawing in of the outer boundaries of the perceptual field to minimise apparent incompatibilities in the construct system. Similar considerations apply to the neurotic depressive, but as the predicament of such clients has been a concern of the last chapter, it will not be discussed here. Constriction can also be regarded as serving to maintain the client's symptoms, in that continuation of the phobic avoidance or obsessional routines prevents invalidation of predictions that cessation of this behaviour is likely to have catastrophic consequences. At the same time, evidence of such dangers may be collected assiduously, and constructions of the safety provided by maintenance of the phobic or ritualistic behaviour are validated. The client who presents with hysterical conversion symptoms may also resist testing out their predictions, in this case those concerning their purported ill-health. Kelly viewed such a client's symptoms as an expression of 'preemptive' dualistic construing in an individual whose construct system may otherwise be loosely structured. Their physical complaints may preclude a psychological construction of their situation and involve preverbal, dependency constructs, which the individual uses 'to build a relationship with his doctor or anyone else who enjoys having people dependent upon him' (p. 869).

If the neurotic's symptoms do serve the function of structuring their world, the loss of these symptoms may be an anxiety-provoking prospect. For example, the phobic may have highly elaborated constructions of their phobic object, and of the self as a fearful person, whereas the implications of seeing the self as un-afraid may be relatively few. It would follow from Kelly's Choice Corollary that such an individual may construe the self as phobic because by doing so they may anticipate greater possibilities for the elaboration of their construct system (possibilities which now include the opportunity to join various phobic societies) than if they were to face the world without fear. Such considerations can pro-vide some explanation of the so-called 'neurotic paradox' of be-haviour which is 'at one and the same time self-perpetuating and self-defeating' (Mowrer, 1950). Other explanations are also pos-sible. If a central aspect of a person's core-role structure is con-struing the self as fearful, the loss of phobic symptoms may be resisted not only because such a comprehensive change in core structures would be threatening, but because it could be accom-panied by guilt in Kelly's sense of 'dislodgement of the self from one's core role structure' (p. 533). Further, as will be seen below, seemingly paradoxical neurotic symptoms may be comprehensible in terms of implicative dilemmas in which the symptoms carry particular positive implications for the client.

Personal Construct Theory and Other Theoretical Perspectives

The major alternative approaches to the explanation and treatment of neurotic disorder are the biological, the psychodynamic, and the behavioural. Biological models have emphasised high arousal level, which in some disorders has been regarded as a major aetiological factor (Lader and Matthews, 1968). Similarly, Eysenck (1960) con-siders neuroticism to be a manifestation of a labile autonomic nervous system, with the particular symptoms developed by a neurotic client being related to their personality type in that both symptoms and personality reflect the client's degree of cortical arousal. In common with Eysenck, the personal construct theorist would not view the neurotic's 'choice' of symptoms as divorced from other areas of their life, but here any similarity between the two approaches ends. While personal construct theory would cer-tainly not disregard a client's level of arousal, or any other feature of their biological state, this would be considered to be just one other construable aspect of their world. Of relevance here is attribution theory, developed from the demonstration by Schachter and Singer (1962) that an individual labels their state of physiological arousal in a way which is consistent with their expectancies regarding their situation. For example, there is some experimental evidence (Gochman and Keating, 1980) in support of the view that in phobic anxieties a high arousal level resulting from some life stress may be wrongly attributed to contact with the phobic object.

Attributions, expectancies, and such other cognitive factors as self-statements, irrational beliefs, and failures in information processing are also increasingly being incorporated in behavioural formulations of neurotic disorders, which traditionally had relied on classical or operant conditioning paradigms. Kelly was fairly dismissive of conditioning models of neurosis, as is evident from his discussion of the difficulties faced by learning theory in attempting to explain Mowrer's (1950) 'neurotic paradox'. Thus, he states:

> 'From the standpoint of the psychology of personal constructs. . . there is no neurotic paradox. Or, to be more correct, the paradox is the jam certain learning theorists get themselves into rather than the jam their clients get themselves into . . . Within the client's own limited construction system he may be faced with a dilemma but not with a paradox.' (Kelly, 1969a, pp. 84–5).

Many behaviour therapists also now recognise the inadequacy of traditional learning theory formulations of neurotic symptoms, and particularly the lack of evidence for a classical conditioning component in their aetiology. Similarly, there is a growing awareness of the importance of cognitive processes in behavioural treatments of the neuroses. The importance of expectancies in such treatments has been indicated (Marcia, Rubin and Efran, 1969), while Bandura (1977) has suggested that enhancement of perceived self-efficacy is an active ingredient in behaviour therapy. Repeated disconfirmation of expectations has been proposed to constitute the most effective method of weakening avoidance behaviour (Seligman and Johnston, 1973) and obsessional rituals (Meyer, Levy and Schnurer, 1974), while Rachman (1983) has outlined a 'therapy by disconfirmation' for agoraphobia, which he suggests may also be applicable to other disorders. In terms of personal construct theory, these approaches could be regarded as directed towards the invalidation of constructions underlying neurotic symptoms, and as counteracting the neurotic's characteristic avoidance of such invalidation. However, although cognitive and Kellian formulations of neurotic disorders are not inconsistent, personal construct theory does, as Neimeyer and Neimeyer (1981b) point out, plug the gaps in cognitive approaches which Sarason (1979) referred to as the 'three lacunae of cognitive therapy'. Specifically, it is able to address the client's cognitive history, the different levels of accessibility of their cognitions, and interactions between these cognitions.

Such issues are also, of course, central to psychoanalytic perspectives, which would accord a central defensive role in neurotic disorders to the repression of unacceptable impulses and the displacement of the associated anxiety in such a way that these impulses may receive symbolic expression. Several aspects of this classical analytical view of neurosis, such as Freud's 'hydraulic' model, are at variance with construct theory formulations. Kelly regarded the analyst's interpretations of the symbolic significance of some aspect of a client's experience as being more likely to be indicative of the construing of the analyst than that of the client. Therefore, as Tschudi (1977) points out, analytical interpretations may involve 'hostility' on the part of the therapist in the way that Kelly defined this term. Nevertheless, such interpretations may indeed have some validity and utility as explanations of the client's predicament, if only because psychoanalytic constructs are now so prevalent in Western society. Further, although personal construct theory would not, like traditional analytical approaches, attribute an overriding importance to the client's early development, and would not employ similar models of developmental stages and fixation, it would accept that childhood experiences may be relevant to the development of neurotic symptoms in that the neurotic's construing may have some basis in the constructions of their parents.

In other areas, there is greater correspondence between the psychoanalytic and personal construct theory views of neurotic disorder and its treatment. Both approaches, although conceptualising these areas rather differently, can accommodate the phenomena of transference and of resistance to therapeutic change. Both can also explain the possible emergence of other forms of psychological distress if therapy is solely directed towards symptom removal, and the payoffs, or secondary gains, of the client's symptoms. Personal construct theory does not employ a concept of the unconscious but, as we have seen in Chapter 1, it does indicate various ways in which a client's construing may be at a low level of cognitive awareness, and which may be relevant to neurotic symptomatology. Thus, Kelly (p. 474) gives a case example, which would not be altogether out of place in psychoanalytic text, in which 'suspended' constructions concerning sibling rivalry are shown to underlie a client's phobia of water. Numerous other examples are provided by Ryle (1975) in support of his contention that the defence mechanisms employed by the neurotic 'can be reformulated in terms of the predominance of certain restricted constructions of events, and of certain rigidly maintained plans for action, resulting in the exclusion of alternative interpretations and plans' (Ryle, 1978, p. 589).

There is, then, some degree of congruence between the personal construct theory explanation of neurotic disorder and those derived from alternative theoretical frameworks. A major difference, however, is that the personal construct theorist would not regard the neurotic as a passive victim of biological processes, unfortunate reinforcement contingencies, or the ebb and flow of libidinal forces. Rather, neurotic symptoms, just like the behaviour of a normal individual, would be considered to reflect the client's active search for meaning in their experiences. This view will now be further elaborated by consideration of research investigating the constructions underlying neurotic disorder.

Research

Structure of the Construct System

Most reviews of research on construing in psychological disorder take as their starting point Bannister's investigations of the construct systems of thought disordered schizophrenics. This will be no exception because these studies (Bannister, 1960, 1962; Bannister and Fransella, 1967; Bannister *et al.*, 1971) included control groups of neurotic clients and thus provided the first, albeit incidental, experimental evidence of the structure of the neurotic's construing. Bannister (1962, p. 834) took the view that

> the essence of neurotic construing is a tendency to have over-tight construct relationships . . . which imply a gross restriction in the number of ways in which a neurotic can view any given situation. This would mean that all situations tend to be seen as more or less exact replications of situations previously experienced and behaviour becomes consequently rigid and stereotyped.

The resulting hypothesis that neurotics would show stronger inter-relationships between constructs (higher 'Intensity') and greater stability in the pattern of these relationships (higher 'Consistency') than normal subjects was not confirmed at a statistically significant level. However, the mean Intensity score obtained by neurotics was higher than those of all other groups in each of the four studies. while they obtained the highest mean Consistency score in two of the studies. In one of the studies, neurotics also exhibited significantly greater uniformity than normal subjects in the strength of relationships between different constructs. suggesting that their construct systems showed little in the way of sub-system differentiation.

While the evidence of tight construing in neurotics which can be gleaned from these studies is suggestive rather than strong. various considerations should perhaps be borne in mind in interpreting their results. For example. Bannister and Fransella (1971) observe. as will be discussed further below. that some of the neurotic clients in their sample obtained scores indicative of very loose construing. It would follow that, in view of the high mean scores of the neurotic sample, some of the neurotic subjects must have obtained scores indicative of very tight construing. The heterogeneity of the neurotic samples in these investigations is also reflected in the high standard deviations of their grid scores. In addition. as the clients studied were in-patients. it is perhaps notable that on the whole neurotics had tended to maintain highly structured construct systems despite having undergone the potentially invalidating experience of admission to psychiatric hospital. which might in itself have been expected to lead to loosened construing (Bannister. 1963). Finally, the grids used in this research employed supplied constructs, and so may not have been tapping the structure of the clients' *personal* construct systems.

Studies specifically designed to elucidate the construing of neurotics. and conducted on predominantly out-patient populations using grids with elicited constructs, have provided somewhat firmer indications of structural abnormalities in the neurotic's construct system. Thus, neurotic disorder has been associated with high levels of construct interrelatedness (Caine. Wijesinghe and Winter 1981: Ryle and Breen, 1972c), and with a high degree of logical consistency in construct relationships (Winter. 1983a). If neurotics are characterised by tightly knit construct systems. they might also be expected to show less differentiated construing than normal subjects on 'cognitive complexity-simplicity' measures (Bieri, 1955), and some indirect evidence in support of this prediction has been provided by the demonstration that a person under stress becomes less cognitively complex (Miller, 1968). Although other studies have failed to find an association between neuroticism and cognitive simplicity, none of them were carried out on homogeneous samples of untreated neurotics (Frazer, 1980; Robertson and Molloy, 1982; Space, 1976). In another small, atypical sample, Leitner (1981b) provided some evidence that clients diagnosed as neurotics or 'personality disorders' showed the literal relationships between their constructions of feelings, values and behaviours which would be expected of individuals whose constructs are highly interrelated. A further area of investigation has been the way in which neurotics and anxious subjects use construct scales. In neurotic out-patients, an association has been demonstrated between neuroticism and the making of polarised judgements (Margolius, 1980; Ryle, 1981; Ryle and Breen, 1972c), although findings with non-client populations are more equivocal (Bonarius, 1977a; Chetwynd, 1977). 'Lopsided' construing, the tendency to use only one pole of a construct scale, has also been related to manifest anxiety (Chetwynd, 1977; Fransella and Bannister, 1977).

The profusion of different (although not independent) structural indices of construing does not lend itself to a ready integration of the results of studies which have used these various measures in attempting to elucidate the predicament of the neurotic. Nevertheless, the evidence presented above generally supports the view that such an individual tends to operate with a tightly organised construct system, to construe events in a polarised manner, and to be intolerant of fragmented, inferentially incompatible constructions. This would not be inconsistent with Kelly's suggestion that the neurotic's superordinate constructs do not have the permeability which would allow them to cope with a certain degree of uncertainty and confusion, their only available response to which may be constriction of the construct system. The lack of differentiation evident in the neurotic's construing would also be indicative of a tendency towards 'constellatory' constructions: for example, construing of the self as 'lacking in confidence' might also imply that it is perceived as 'stupid', 'socially inept', and characterised by a host of other negative attributes. Evidence of the specific difficulties which are likely to be faced by the individual whose construct system is structured in this way is presented in other chapters. It will be seen, for example, that such an individual is likely to be particularly hampered in their anticipation of the construing and behaviour of others, and thus in interpersonal relationships (Chapter 10). The tight structure of their construing may also belie 'potential chaos' (Adams-Webber, 1970) in that, faced with invalidating evidence, few alternative constructions would be available. To quote Adams-Webber (1979b, p.60), 'in such a tightly organised system, even a few minor revisions of his initial impressions of an event may have sweeping implications throughout his system as a whole'.

Nevertheless, as in the case of every other individual, the ways in which the neurotic characteristically construes reality can be considered to represent strategies directed towards the optimal anticipation of events. Their undifferentiated construing may thus serve the purpose of increasing the predictability of their world. However, a more precise indication of the strategic functions served, and the problems posed, by the neurotic's construing requires a consideration of the content of the construct system as well as its structure.

Construing of Self and Others

A considerable body of evidence, much of it from research employing semantic differential ratings of the self and the ideal self, attests to the low self-esteem of neurotic clients (Bond and Lader, 1976). In their repertory grid study, Ryle and Breen (1972c) demonstrated that neurotics not only tend to construe themselves as dissimilar to their ideal selves, but also as different from other people. They conclude that the neurotic is 'someone who sees himself as unlike others in general and unlike his parents in particular, who is dissatisfied with himself, who tends to extreme judgements and operates with a less complex construct system than do normals, and who tends to construe others in ways which depart from consensual values in respect of certain attributes' (p 488). Essentially similar findings have been obtained by Space (1976) and by Caine *et al.* (1981), who demonstrated that the negative self-construction of the neurotic is associated with a correspondingly positive construal of other people. Ryle (1981) has also extended his earlier work, finding that neurotics construe not only themselves, but also relationships in which they and their significant others are involved, more unfavourably than do normal subjects. Margolius (1980), in addition to providing further evidence of the extreme but unfavourable construing of the self in neurotics, demonstrated an association between neurotic disorder and high levels of logical consistency in constructs salient to various aspects of the self. These results would suggest that the neurotic's tendency to construe events in a polarised fashion and to be intolerant of ambiguity is particularly pronounced in their construing of the self, which tends to be seen as 'all bad' and contrasted with other people, who are seen as 'all good'. This is consistent with the view expressed by Makhlouf-Norris and Norris (1973, p. 287) that 'in neurotic patients the need for self-certainty is such that they construe the self in a way which predicts undesirable outcomes which are certain to be validated, rather than predict desirable outcomes which would be open to invalidation'. Such arguments provide a further illustration that the apparent self-destructiveness of the neurotic is only paradoxical if human behaviour is seen as being directed towards manifestly hedonistic ends rather than towards making sense of one's world.

The difficulties in social relationships which are likely to be experienced by the neurotic as a result of their tendency to perceive the self as different from others are indicated by the finding that the more an individual construes their social world in this way, the less easy it is for other people to anticipate their construing (Adams-Webber, 1973). It has also been shown consistently that normal subjects tend to perceive similarities between themselves and others approximately 62 per cent of the time and dissimilarities 38 per cent of the time, this being the ratio in which differences between self and others would be highly salient (Adams-Webber, 1979b). As neurotics do not organise their judgments in this manner, it is likely that, while in a general, blanket sense perceiving more dissimilarity between the self and others, they may display a less subtle sensitivity to such dissimilarities. However, such aspects of the neurotic's construing, and their relationship to interpersonal difficulties, require further investigation.

The Complaint

In complaining of a particular symptom, the client may be considered, in a sense, to be actively choosing one aspect of their experience on which to focus their psychological distress. It might be expected, therefore, that the neurotic's choice of symptom would be likely to reflect the characteristic ways in which they construe their world. Some support for this argument has been provided by demonstrations that clients who tend to construe others in objective terms (giving constructs such as 'old-young' or 'male-female' in a construct elicitation procedure) are likely to report somatic symptoms, in contrast to the 'psychic' symptoms of clients whose construing indicates more concern with the psychological characteristics of others (McPherson and Gray, 1976; Smail, 1970). McPherson and Gray regard psychic and somatic symptoms as particular constructions placed on the sensations accompanying the high state of arousal experienced by the anxious individual. In the 'objective construer', such constructions are likely to emphasise physical sensations; in the 'psychological construer', emotional responses. Smail's study also indicated that those neurotic clients whose construing shows a predominant awareness of their internal rather than external reality tend to report psychic rather than somatic symptoms. Similar conclusions have been reached by researchers using the 'locus of control' dimension (Emmelkamp and Cohen-Kettenis, 1975; Johnson and Sarason, 1978), and by Caine *et al.* (1981), who report that their 'data suggest a broad differentiation between patients who emphasise interpersonal difficulties and those who present complaints with an external locus (e.g. phobic or somatic)' (p. 110).

An individual's predominant constructions of their world would be expected to derive from the most tightly organised section of their construct system. If these are the constructions which are reflected in their symptom choice, it would follow that the constructs which they apply to their symptoms should show a high level of interrelationship with other constructs within their system. As we have seen, such conclusions might also follow from the notion that choice of a particular symptom serves to increase the predictability of the individual's world and to provide a 'way of life' (Fransella, 1972), the loss of which would be resisted if no viable, well-defined, alternative constructions are available. As Hayden (1979) has shown, a person will only adopt a more favourable, new self-construction if it carries more implications for them than the old. An indication that such considerations may be relevant to the predicament of the neurotic client is provided by Winter's (1983a) demonstration that constructs describing their symptoms show a 'tighter' organisation, and also greater logical consistency in terms of interrelationships with other constructs, than is apparent elsewhere in their construct system. An alternative interpretation of these findings would be that it is in those areas of their life in which their construing is most rigid and intolerant of ambiguity that the neurotic is most likely to experience difficulties which come to be presented as symptoms.

A further indication that the symptom with which a client presents may be serving some purpose for them can be obtained by consideration of its personal meaning for the client, its implications in terms of other constructs. Several single case studies (e.g. Tschudi, 1977; Winter, 1982; Wright, 1970) have adopted such an approach and have demonstrated that a symptom may have positive implications or 'payoffs' for the client. The neurotic's symptoms might therefore be expected to be doubly resistant to change if they not only reflect an area of particularly tight and rigid construing, but are also associated with certain positive self-constructions. Some of the clearest indications of the way in which inflexible construct structure and idiosyncratic construct content may interact to maintain neurotic behaviour are provided in the work of Ryle. Having demonstrated that he was able blindly to differentiate the repertory grids of neurotics from those of normal subjects (Ryle and Breen, 1971), much of his subsequent work has been directed towards delineating more precisely the differences between these two groups. His more recent formulations of the constructions which underlie neurotic difficulties are in terms of 'dilemmas, traps and snags' (Ryle, 1979a). Dilemmas are defined as false dichotomies or associations, such as the tendency of Ryle and Breen's (1972c) neurotic students to construe cold people as likely to succeed academically, and warm people as passive and likely to need psychiatric help. It might not be surprising if individuals holding such constructions were repeatedly to fail examinations, to experience difficulties in self-assertion, or indeed to complain of any psychological symptom, for in so doing they would receive the payoff of at least being able to construe themselves as warm. In a study comparing neurotic clients and normal controls, however, Ryle (1981) failed to provide evidence of a greater frequency of dilemmas in the former group, but as the dilemmas considered were formulated in terms of supplied constructs, they might not have been of personal relevance to the subjects.

Specific Complaints: (a) *Obsessive-Compulsive Disorders.* As mentioned above, some of the neurotic clients in the standardisation sample for the Bannister-Fransella Grid Test were found to construe very 'loosely'. Bannister and Fransella (1971) report that, unexpectedly, these clients were mostly diagnosed as suffering from obsessive-compulsive neurosis. Although Makhlouf-Norris and her colleagues (1970, 1973) failed to demonstrate any significant difference between obsessive-compulsive clients and non-psychiatric patients in the strength or consistency of their construct relationships, they did find that the groups differed in terms of the subsystem organisation of their construct systems. Specifically, while the construct systems of control subjects were characteristically 'articulated', consisting of more than one cluster of constructs, but with linkages between clusters, this tended not to be the case with the obsessionals. The interpretation of these results linked them to the additional findings that obsessional clients characteristically construed the self as dissimilar to the ideal self (Makhlouf-Norris and Jones, 1971), and rated it more highly on constellatory constructs (defined as those which were most central to their principal dimension of construing) than did normal subjects. In effect, therefore, not only was the obsessional's construct system unidimensional but the opposite poles of this dimension were defined by the self and ideal self. Complex constructions of other people would not be possible with such a system and, nearly everyone being construed more positively than the self, the obsessional 'is not only bad but he is the worst person he knows' (Makhlouf-Norris and Norris, 1973, p. 286). By engaging in compulsive, ritualistic behaviour, the obsessional is thought to avoid testing this prediction of their unlimited badness. Makhlouf-Norris and Norris conclude that these features of the obsessional's construing serve not only to reduce uncertainty regarding the self but to maintain a conception of the ideal self as highly virtuous.

The apparent differences in the findings of Bannister and Fransella and Makhlouf-Norris *et al* have been explained by Fransella (1974) as being due to the two studies tapping different areas of the obsessional's construct system. As the repertory grid used by Makhlouf-Norris employed elicited elements and constructs, it would have been more likely to indicate features of the construct subsystem concerning the self and symptoms than would the Bannister-Fransella Grid Test. Fransella points out that an individual's construct system need not have a uniform structure and that the obsessional's 'non-articulated' construing of the self and their obsessive concerns may represent an island of tight structure in an otherwise loose system. To quote Bannister and Fransella (1971, pp. 172-3), 'it was as if the obsessional person was living in the only world that was meaningful to him — outside the area of his obsessions all was vagueness and confusion.' As Fransella points out, this 'vagueness and confusion' is likely to be experienced by the obsessional as anxiety when they are faced with events unrelated to the self and symptoms, while any invalidation of predictions within this one realm of tight construing will pose a considerable threat to the system. She suggests that the obsessional's situation represents the outcome of a process of constriction of the construct system in the face of invalidation of the rigid, brittle predictions of a person whose construing was initially tightly structured. That the resultant non-articulated system may be particularly vulnerable to invalidation is indicated by Bannister's (1963) demonstration that loosening following invalidation is more likely if the invalidated constructs form a discrete cluster unrelated to any which are being validated. The non-articulated system is also one in which, as in a client described by Rigdon and Epting (1983), superordinate constructs are likely to be impermeable, and which would therefore not facilitate resolution of inconsistent experiences. An explanation may thus be provided for the obsessional's tendency to avoid ambiguity and to exhibit difficulties in integrating experiences and in reaching decisions (Beech and Liddell, 1974; Hamilton, 1957; Milner, Beech and Walker, 1971; Reed, 1969a, 1969b).

A more recent study by Millar (1980), however, casts some doubt on these conclusions. Using a grid with elicited elements and constructs, he failed to replicate the finding of a greater frequency of non-articulated construct systems in obsessionals than in normal controls, and while the cognitive complexity of obsessionals was lower than that of normals, it was comparable to that of the mixed neurotic sample studied by Ryle and Breen (1972c). In addition, obsessionals exhibited a more extreme and negative view of the self, and a greater tendency to see the self as dissimilar to others, than did both normals and Ryle and Breen's neurotics. Therefore, while there is some consistency in the research findings that obsessional neurotics construe themselves in a highly unfavourable light and as alienated from other people, the evidence that such constructions are particularly characteristic of obsessionals is not strong. The design of the Makhlouf-Norris study, comparing obsessionals with normal controls, could not reveal aspects of construing specific to obsessional disorders as opposed to neurotic disorders in general. Although Millar's investigations did attempt to differentiate obsessionals from other neurotics, he admits that his in-patient obsessive-compulsive clients and Ryle and Breen's out-patient neurotics may not be comparable groups, and that differences observed between their construct systems may merely reflect different degrees of severity of neurotic disorder. A study is now required which compares the construing of obsessive-compulsive neurotics with that of a matched sample of neurotics not presenting with obsessional symptoms.

Specific Complaints: (b) *Agoraphobia.* The predicament of the agoraphobic has also received specific attention from the personal construct theory viewpoint. Single case studies have indicated how a consideration of the relationships of a construct concerning a phobic symptom with other constructs in an individual's system may reveal the extent to which the client dissociates the phobia from other areas of their life, and the specific implications for them of the phobia and its loss (Wright, 1970; Bannister, 1965b). Frazer (1980) found that agoraphobics construed themselves less favourably and identified less with males, including their fathers, than did non-agoraphobic neurotics and normal subjects. Other aspects of their construing appeared to be reflections of neurotic disorder in general in that they did not reveal significant differences between the two neurotic groups, although differentiating both groups from normal subjects. Thus, as in previous research, both neurotic groups were found to construe themselves as more dissimilar to other people, and to have somewhat less articulated construct systems, than did normal controls. On the basis of these findings and responses to a questionnaire concerning subjects' perceptions of their parents, Frazer interprets the agoraphobic's situation as resulting from a family background in which strict rules were imposed, particularly concerning the expression of emotions. He suggests that, as a result of this parental inflexibility, the child is rarely in a position to experience invalidation of their construing, and consequently unpredictable events later in life are extremely anxiety-provoking. However, caution should be exercised in drawing conclusions on the basis of Frazer's study in that, as his agoraphobic subjects were all receiving behavioural treatment and his neurotic controls were undergoing psychotherapy, it is unlikely that the construing of either clinical sample was in its pristine neurotic state. He remarks that it is unlikely that behaviour therapy would have affected the phobics' responses to the test battery but, as will be seen below, this is a questionable assumption.

The construing of agoraphobics has also been examined in relation to that of their spouses. Thus, Hafner (1977a, 1977b) found evidence of complementary patterns of self-esteem and the expression of hostility in severely disabled agoraphobic women and their husbands. Increase in self-esteem and symptomatic improvement of the phobics during therapy corresponded with changes in the reverse direction in their husbands, who recovered when the phobics relapsed. Hafner therefore concluded that these husbands were resisting their wives' therapeutic improvement, and that denial of hostility by the husbands was a major factor in this regard. The concept of denial, with its implication that there is a correct way of construing the world, does not rest easily within a personal construct theory framework. Nevertheless, as Ryle (1975) has pointed out, such concepts may be reformulated in construct theory terms (e.g. as low cognitive awareness of constructions of negative qualities and interpersonal conflict) and operationally defined with repertory grid measures. In a study using a repertory grid with supplied elements and constructs, the latter mostly selected from constructs previously elicited from a large agoraphobic sample, Winter (1983b) has also investigated self-esteem and construal of interpersonal conflict in agoraphobics and their spouses. Similarly to Hafner's study, high self-esteem in the spouses of agoraphobics was found to be associated with high symptom levels in the phobics, and these spouses showed significantly higher self-esteem than did normal subjects. Agoraphobics and their spouses also perceived less selfishness and anger, and agoraphobics less jealousy, than did non-agoraphobic neurotics and normal subjects. This 'lopsided' construing suggested a tendency to 'submergence' of construct poles concerning conflict and lack of tenderness. In other words, the agoraphobics and their spouses in this study tended to perceive significant others as uniformly good and virtuous, and this was more pronounced in the more disabled phobics. However, one area where this was not the case was marital infidelity. Agoraphobics showed a greater tendency than other neurotics to associate the ability to go out with a likelihood of infidelity. Apart from this, though, they and their spouses idealised the ability to go out and imagined that after the phobic's treatment they would be more similar to their ideal selves than they were even before the commencement of the phobic symptoms. This would appear to be an example of Fransella's (1972) 'if only' syndrome, in which symptomatic improvement may be resisted because both partners are able to maintain an idealistic fantasy of life without phobic symptoms only as long as the client remains agoraphobic. The agoraphobics and their spouses had very similar construct systems, and the finding that the greater the correlation between the grids of phobic and spouse the fewer hours per week the phobic spent out of the house suggested that such similarity in construing reflected a collusive pattern of interaction which served to exacerbate the phobic symptoms.

That aspects of the construct systems of phobic and spouse may be of prognostic significance was also demonstrated in this study by considering the clients' responses to behaviour therapy. Thus, a more positive therapeutic outcome was observed in those cases where phobic and spouse initially differentiated more between people in terms of interpersonal conflict and lack of tenderness, but for whom infidelity was a less salient construct. An additional finding, corroborating those with other client groups, was that therapeutic improvement was more pronounced in phobics whose construct systems were initially less unidimensional, and therefore possibly more flexible. Such flexibility of the construct system would be expected to facilitate reconstruction, and changes in construing were indeed found to accompany therapy. Both phobics and spouses came to construe the client more favourably, while therapeutic improvement was also associated with a reduced likelihood of seeing infidelity as an implication of confidence, independence, and the ability to go out. The phobics came to discriminate more between other people in terms of constructs concerning tenderness, while ability to go out became a less salient construct for them. In the more improved phobics, going out became less idealised while confidence came to carry more positive implications. Symptom loss in the phobics was also associated with an increase in the flexibility of their spouses' construing.

Winter suggests that these findings indicate that the agoraphobic's construct system is ill-equipped to deal with situations of interpersonal conflict, which by virtue of their unpredictability are likely to generate anxiety. This, and the fact that anxiety is one of their more superordinate constructs, would explain the observation by Goldstein (1982, p. 185) that such clients 'go to great lengths to avoid such feelings as anger and frustration', misapprehend the causal antecedents of emotional distress, and 'label almost every state of arousal as anxiety or fear'. The phobic strategy to avoid the anxiety associated with conflict may involve constriction of the construct system, and a delimiting of the individual's interpersonal world to a spouse whose construing is similar to their own. If the superordinate constructs of this shared 'family construct system' (see Chapter 16) are 'weak, anxious, invalid' versus 'strong, confident care-giver', a complementary pattern of phobia and counter-phobia, as described in numerous case studies (e.g. Holmes, 1982), is likely to be maintained. The relationship between phobic and spouse is also likely to be one of validation of constructions, just as Frazer (1980) suggested was the case in the phobic's relationship with their parents.

Treatment Allocation and Response

The way in which neurotics construe their world may be expected not only to determine the type of symptom with which they present but also their expectations of therapy, the clinician's decisions regarding their treatment allocation, and the form of therapy to which they are most likely to respond. Some indication that this is indeed the case was provided by Caine *et al.* (1981, 1982). They demonstrated that neurotic clients whose construing was oriented towards external reality, who construed their situation in terms of lack of self-sufficiency but a high degree of structure, and whose symptom constructs were superordinate showed expectancies favourable to a directive, structured, symptom-centred treatment such as behaviour therapy. They were also more likely to be selected for, and to show improvement in, behaviour therapy. By contrast, internally oriented clients, who construed themselves and their symptoms in terms of inactive, deficient social interaction, and whose symptom constructs carried few implications in terms of other constructs tended to favour an introspective, interpersonally focused form of therapy such as group psychotherapy. Again, this was the treatment to which they were most frequently allocated, and which was most likely to eventuate in a positive outcome. Clients allocated to therapy groups were also more likely to show conflict in their self-construing, as indicated by a high discrepancy between their use of a self construct and a self element, and more likely to improve if they initially construed themselves in an extreme and unfavourable light, perhaps indicating greater motivation to change. In addition, less improvement during group psychotherapy was shown by clients whose constructs were organised in a tight, undifferentiated fashion, while the reverse was true for behaviour therapy (Winter, 1983a).

If neurotic disorders are associated with particular patterns of construing, reconstruction in these areas should be apparent in those clients who improve over the course of therapy. Ryle has provided evidence, largely in the form of single case studies, of the occurrence during focused psychotherapy of predictable changes in the neurotic's construing (Ryle, 1975, 1979b, 1980; Ryle and Lunghi, 1969). In one of these studies there was some, albeit slight, indication that clinical ratings of improvement were associated with change in those aspects of construing which Ryle and Breen (1972c) had found to characterise neurotics. Similar findings have been obtained in other investigations of neurotic populations, where it has been demonstrated that clients over the course of therapy come to construe the self as more similar to the ideal self and to other people. Such changes have been related to independent indices of therapeutic outcome (Caine *et al.*, 1981; Fielding, 1975; Koch, 1983a) and, in group psychotherapy, to aspects of the therapeutic process (Caplan *et al.*, 1975; Fielding, 1983; Fransella and Joyston-Bechal, 1971; Koch, 1983b).

However, demonstrations of reconstruction in neurotics are not confined to insight-oriented psychotherapy. Caine *et al.* (1981) found comparable changes in construing over the course of therapy in their group psychotherapy and behaviour therapy clients, while the neurotic depressives studied by Hewstone *et al.* (1981) came to see themselves as significantly more similar to other people during short-term hospitalisation, which was accompanied by a reduction in depressed mood. The additional finding of this latter investigation that general changes in construing were not significantly greater in the depressives than in a non-psychiatric control group highlights the need for caution in drawing conclusions from the many uncontrolled repertory grid studies of reconstruing during therapy. A major shortcoming of these studies is that they are unable to separate changes arising from therapy from those which may result from the serial grid assessments themselves. One such artefact of repeated grid administration is a tightening of construct relationships, which might mask the expected tendency for the neurotic's construing to become more differentiated during successful therapy. In considering the fact that only modest changes in construing during therapy have been observed in some studies, it is also of relevance that reconstruction is less likely to be demonstrated on general grid indices of 'neurotic construing' than on individualised grid measures (Caine *et al.*, 1981; Koch, 1983a;

Winter and Trippett, 1977). In the Caine *et al.* study, the individually predicted changes were part of a general reduction in the polarisation of the neurotic's construing. However, it was only in the specific areas of content of the individualised predictions, which largely concerned dilemmas and construing of the self and significant others, that decreased polarisation of construing was associated with therapeutic change on other measures. These findings are, of course, quite consistent with the idiographic emphasis of personal construct theory, and they have led to the development of guidelines for individualised prediction of therapeutic changes in the neurotic's construing on the basis of pretreatment repertory grid assessment (Winter, 1979, 1982). It is perhaps by such individually tailored monitoring of therapeutic reconstruction that the validity and utility of personal construct theory formulations of the predicament of neurotic clients can most clearly be demonstrated.

Summary of Research Findings

Although the research findings on construing in neurotic disorder are not unequivocal, they do indicate a characteristic pattern of tight, polarised construing and intolerance of ambiguity. This is particularly apparent in the construct subsystems concerning the symptoms and the self, which is typically perceived unfavourably and as different from others. Similar features of construing have been found to characterise depressives to a somewhat greater degree, but, as Button (1983a) has indicated, apparently different psychological disorders may indeed reflect similar vulnerabilities to invalidation, strategies directed towards its avoidance, and failures to anticipate others. As such, the general therapeutic aims in different disorders may be similar. With the individual neurotic client, however, it would appear that a personal construct theory formulation of their difficulties may render apparently self-defeating behaviour explicable both to clinician and client, and may facilitate the planning of an appropriate therapeutic strategy. Such applications of the construct theory model will now be illustrated in relation to each of the general aspects of the neurotic's construing which have been highlighted by the research results.

Applications

Structure of the Construct System

'I may not be able to hold the castle but at least I can hold the keep' (description by an obsessional neurotic of his difficulties).

Sidney had always considered himself a responsible, law-abiding family man. As he was returning from work one day, a police car screeched to a halt beside him, and he found himself pinned to the ground with such force that his arm was broken. It later transpired that the incident was a case of mistaken identity, but following it Sidney has been so crippled by phobic anxiety that he is unable to leave his home. His description of the occurrences of that day is notable for its lack of condemnation of the police officers concerned. Rather, its predominant tone is one of incomprehension, and he remarks that, as the groundsman at a police sports centre, he had always regarded police officers as his friends. At repertory grid assessment, he was unable to think of anyone he disliked. This assessment revealed a very unidimensional construct system, the first principal component of which accounted for 83 per cent of the variance and contrasted 'courteous', 'principled', 'homely' people, who 'wouldn't tolerate anything wrong' with people who are 'quick-tempered'.

It might be predicted that, in common with many other neurotic clients, a positive therapeutic change for Sidney would involve a loosening of the tight structure of his construct system and the development of permeable constructs which could allow some resolution of his inconsistent and confusing experiences. Thus, a construct such as 'over-diligent' might allow him to subsume both the positive qualities he had always attributed to the police, and the behaviour of the police officers who accosted him. An increase in the permeability of his construct system might also allow negative evaluations of others to enter his awareness, and the construal of his autonomic responses in terms of such emotions as anger rather than anxiety.

As will be discussed in Chapter 14, Kelly outlined various ways in which a therapist may induce loosening of the client's construing. Interestingly, the techniques which he considered can achieve this aim have been much employed by clinicians of other theoretical orientations with neurotic clients, although for reasons which have been conceptualised very differently. The therapist who is loosening a neurotic client's system should tread carefully, however, because the process may admit to the client's perceptual field material which their tight constructions had previously excluded and which, by virtue of its unpredictability, may occasion intense anxiety. As we have seen, considerable anxiety and threat may also be generated by any invalidation attempted by the therapist of the neurotic's predictions because their tight, brittle construct system may be particularly susceptible to structural collapse following invalidation. An untimely intervention may lead our obsessional client to lose his keep as well as his castle!

It may be, then, that the therapist will at times need to control the neurotic's anxiety level and to curb a loosening process which appears too rapid or extensive. Support and reassurance may serve this purpose, but a more fundamental protection against anxiety and uncertainty, facilitating the client's experimentation and revision of their constructions, is provided by permeable superordinate constructs and by the development of linkages between discrete construct clusters. The therapist may, therefore, attempt to increase the permeability of a neurotic's constructs, extending their range of convenience, by demonstrating their applicability to new elements. With more permeable superordinate constructs, the client's ability to tolerate inferentially incompatible construct sub-systems will increase, and as a consequence elaboration of the construct system will be facilitated and previously suspended constructions may return to the client's awareness. The end-result of a personal construct psychotherapist's interventions may therefore include what a psychoanalyst might term making conscious the unconscious.

Construing of Self and Others

'Altogether, I see myself as being weak, insipid, ineffectual, boring and totally unattractive either to my wife as a husband, or to others as an acquaintance or friend. Not a very nice picture'. (The conclusion of the autobiographical sketch completed by Simon at the commencement of personal construct psychotherapy.)

It may be self-evident that a major aim of psychological therapy is modification of the client's self-constructions. The research findings on neurotic clients would suggest that in this group, as in Simon, a positive treatment outcome would generally involve construing the self less extremely and negatively and as more similar to other people. The experiments in which a therapist encourages the neurotic client to engage may often be designed to produce evidence which will validate a more favourable self-perception and, as Bandura (1977) has indicated, it is possible to view many behavioural techniques in these terms. In common with the behaviour therapists, Kelly was by no means averse to 'action rather than words' in therapy. Thus, in answering his question 'What if a person thinks he is neurotic — or even is neurotic — does he have to act that way, or continue to live that way?', he concluded that 'the key to therapy might be in getting the client to get on with a new way of life without waiting to acquire insight' (Kelly, 1969b, p. 59). Here he is suggesting that many neurotic clients are, in a sense, trapped in their 'autobiographies', but also that therapeutic procedures designed to free them from these traps and to modify their self-constructions are more likely to succeed if threat and guilt can be minimised by disengaging their 'core' constructs from this process. This was one reason for the emphasis which Kelly placed on the therapeutic use of enactment methods such as fixed role therapy, which may demonstrate to the client their possibilities of choice and that the self, and its construal by others, is not immutable. Such changes may also be facilitated by asking the client to write self-characterisations from different role perspectives, or to view the self metaphorically as if it were a 'community of selves' (Mair, 1977b), each with its allotted role. All these methods may be especially useful with neurotic clients because of their potential to replace impermeable self-constructions, which had previously limited movement, by more permeable constructs which can encompass apparent inconsistencies in the self.

Mair also provides a reminder that any change in self-construing necessarily involves change in the client's construing of others inasmuch as the self can be considered to be one pole of a self-other construct. It will be recalled that many of the studies indicating reduction in polarisation of self and others during therapy have focused on group psychotherapy, which may therefore be of particular value with neurotic clients. By discussing similarities and differences between each other, and between themselves and people outside the group, group members would be expected to increase the permeability of their role constructs and, finding their constellatory or preemptive constructions of each other wanting, to develop more 'propositional' modes of construing. Experimentation in the interpersonal laboratory of the group may be allowed to proceed 'informally' or may be facilitated by the use of group enactment procedures or Landfield and Rivers' (1975) method of 'rotating dyads' (see Chapters 8 and 15). This latter approach has been found to facilitate group members' ability to construe the construction processes of others and thus, in terms of Kelly's

Sociality Corollary, their ability to form role relationships. It may, therefore, be appropriate for neurotic clients who, by virtue of their tight construing, experience difficulty in empathising accurately with others.

The Complaint

Repertory grid assessment of Arthur, who had presented with severe obsessive-compulsive symptoms, revealed a non-articulated construct system and a dilemma involving the construct 'feeling-unfeeling'. Thus, for him being feeling was highly associated with being obsessional, unstable, introverted, and worried, all of which were part of his one major cluster of constructs. While behaviour therapy served to reduce the intensity of his obsessional symptoms, he became increasingly anxious and depressed, and accordingly was eventually transferred to a psychotherapy group. No significant reconstruing was evident in a grid completed at the termination of behaviour therapy, but a further grid assessment at the time of leaving the psychotherapy group demonstrated reversal of the correlations of 'feeling-unfeeling' with constructs relating to his symptoms, and a reduction of the former construct to impermeability in that it was no longer significantly correlated with any other construct. This apparent resolution of his dilemma was also accompanied by his construct system becoming articulated.

The personal construct psychotherapist, viewing constructs as if they were bipolar, will not only be concerned with the personal meaning of the neurotic's presenting complaints but also with the implications of their loss. For example, construct elicitation with Peter, who presented with social anxieties and difficulties in self assertion, indicated that he contrasted being 'assertive' with being 'calmly logical'. As in Arthur's case, such considerations may elucidate the purpose which the symptoms serve for the client and therefore the likely obstacles and resistances to therapeutic change. Although his own therapeutic approach has a basis in object relations theory, the framework outlined by Ryle (1979a) may be of value to the personal construct psychotherapist in conceptualising the limiting constructions of the world underlying a neurotic's complaints. As Ryle has demonstrated, the formulations thus provided are easily comprehensible to the client and can be used both to focus and to monitor brief psychotherapy. Such therapeutic ventures may even on occasion involve exploration of the client's early life for, as Ryle and Lunghi (1969) have suggested, the construct relationships underlying a dilemma may represent generalisations from significant past relationships. For example, it may have been that Arthur's dilemma of being either obsessional or unfeeling derived from his childhood experience of an obsessional, caring father and a disorganised, unfeeling mother. An active attempt to delimit the range of convenience of the obsessional-unfeeling construction to these particular people, and ideally to these particular people at that particular time, might have served to reduce the construct to impermeability more rapidly than did Arthur's three years of therapy. He would then have been free to experiment with alternative constructions of himself and others, including the possibility of being at the same time unobsessional and humane. To use Tschudi's (1977) terminology, Arthur's obsessional symptoms constituted a 'loaded question', an oblique way of obtaining some conception of his own virtuousness, and appropriate aims of therapy could therefore have been the provision of ways to achieve this objective apart from via the symptom, or alternatively a devaluing of the objective.

It would follow from Fransella's (1972) view of the symptom as a 'way of life' that therapeutic approaches which purely focus on the symptom are unlikely to be effective as the client, in a sense, knows too much about the symptom already. If an equally meaningful alternative way of life is not elaborated during therapy, the client's predicament might be similar to that of a phobic described by Bannister and Fransella (1971, p. 192): 'The young man had a phobia for telephones and travelling. About a year of systematic desensitisation treatment enabled him to travel and use the telephone. He commented on the utter pointlessness of such an achievement since he had no-one to ring up and no-one to travel to'. Nevertheless, a symptom-oriented treatment approach, by demonstrating the client's ability to confront previously avoided situations and invalidating predictions that the consequences of so doing are likely to be catastrophic, may set off what Yalom (1970) has termed an adaptive spiral, involving considerable reconstruing by the client and significant others. This may indeed facilitate elaboration of a construction of the self without symptoms.

Treatment Allocation and Response

Sylvia presented with agoraphobic symptoms, and principal component analysis of her pre-treatment repertory grid revealed the loadings of elements on its second principal component which are indicated in Figure 5.1. She failed to respond to behaviour therapy, but subsequently lost her phobic symptoms when her husband was imprisoned for incest.

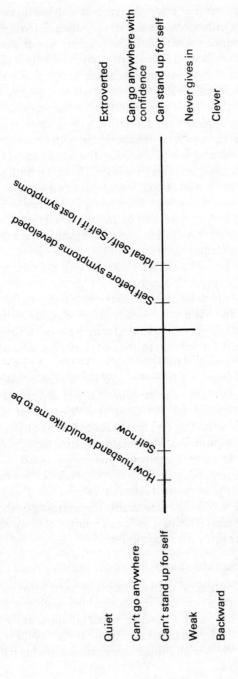

Figure 5.1: Loadings of Elements on the Second Principal Component of an Agoraphobic's Repertory Grid

It will now be apparent that in treating neurotic clients the personal construct psychotherapist may adopt a variety of treatment strategies, including some which have been developed within alternative theoretical frameworks. As Karst (1980) has pointed out, such technical eclecticism is coupled with a clear therapeutic rationale in that treatment choice will be based on assessment of the client's construct system and directed towards effecting specific changes in construing. More generally, the research reviewed above would suggest that the therapist would do well to allocate the client to a form of treatment which is close to the focus of convenience of their construct system, taking into account such considerations as the client's constructions of the self and of their symptoms, and the extent to which their construing is dominated by awareness of their 'inner' or 'outer' reality. In reaching such a decision, the therapist may find it useful, in addition to a clinical interview, to employ more formal assessment procedures such as a repertory grid, self-characterisation, or the Claybury Selection Battery, developed by Caine *et al.* (1982) for use in the treatment selection procedure. The clinician's major concern here will be the selection of a form of therapy which, being meaningful to the client, is likely to mobilise their expectancies of change and hence their reconstruing.

It may be argued that no radical change can be produced if the client is allocated to a treatment which matches their expectations because such an approach would only serve to validate existing constructions and maintain the status quo. However, no change at all is possible if the client is not available to be worked with, and the client whose symptoms are highly salient but who is allocated to a form of treatment which does not concern itself with their symptoms is likely to drop out of what they may feel to be a meaningless therapeutic exercise. In this connection, it should be emphasised that the initial choice of treatment may be made with a view to 'holding' the client in therapy but that there may be switching of therapeutic approaches if some reconstruction is achieved. If a client's constructs are highly impermeable, the therapist might feel that they would be unable to anticipate the behaviour of other members of a psychotherapy group, which would therefore be too anxiety-provoking to be considered as an initial treatment option. However, if more permeable constructs can be developed in the individual therapy situation, subsequent group psychotherapy may then be appropriate to allow some experimentation with these new constructions prior to their use in the 'real world'. There may also be a further reason for switching of treatment methods in the case of the client who, like Arthur in the example discussed previously, is initially in a dilemma as a result of an association between the symptom and a 'payoff construct'. If, as in this case, constructs relating to the client's symptoms occupy a superordinate position in their construct system, a symptom-oriented approach such as behaviour therapy may be considered appropriate and may indeed serve to reduce the intensity of the symptoms. However, in the absence of any other change in the client's construing, a reduction in symptom severity would lead the client to shift their self-concept towards the undesirable pole of the payoff construct, in Arthur's case unfeeling. For treatment gains to be maintained, it may then be necessary for therapy to change its focus to the exploration and attempted resolution of this dilemma, and the client may well be more amenable to such an approach if the amelioration of their symptom has resulted in a reduction in its implications for them and its centrality to their self-concept (Winter, 1981, 1982).

Whatever resolution of a client's dilemmas occurs during therapy, however, treatment gains are unlikely to be maintained if these constructions are at the same time being validated by the client's family. The case of Sylvia, and the research findings on construing in agoraphobia, highlight the importance of considering, and possibly attempting to modify, not only the neurotic's personal construct system but also the system of constructs which operates in their broader social network. The fact that the vast majority of clients diagnosed as agoraphobic are female also indicates that common patterns of construing in a cultural or political context, in this case the constellatory constructs which define sex role stereotypes in Western society, may influence the way in which neurotic difficulties are presented. The further possibility that such constellatory social constructions play an aetiological role in neurotic disorders of course carries considerable implications for preventative work. In general, the clinician who adopts a Kellian approach to the prevention and treatment of neurotic complaints will, in common with the Eastern philosopher and the theoretical physicist (Zukav, 1980), convey the message that the certainty provided by constellatory constructions, and by taking a unidimensional view of a multidimensional world, is an illusion for which the indivudiual or society trades adventure and freedom. As Barnes (1983, p. 42) remarks, 'To mimic the beautitudes it can be said both of psychotherapists and of their patients that blessed are the confused for they will find their way, cursed are the certain for that's the way they'll stay'. In finding their way, the neurotic, like any other individual, will need at times to be confused, without becoming lost; at times certain, without clinging to certainty.

Acknowledgment

I am indebted to John Gosling for his comments on an earlier draft of this chapter.

6   SUICIDE

Charles Stefan and Judith Von

Each of us gives his life for something . . . to seek to die well is the object of the full life, and those who fail to live well never succeed in finding anything worth dying for. Thus life and death can be made to fit together, each the validation of the other.

George A. Kelly (1961)

Suicide tantalises us with its inherent but debatable paradox. How is it that individuals engage in an act which runs counter to our most fundamental truth, i.e. the basic belief that all human beings are impelled towards self preservation? Our religions, systems of ethics and resulting social codes are all based upon this assumption. Bakan (1967) summarises this issue. He writes,

> Then, living, in the social sense, maintains life. When one drives a car on the highway, one assumes that the other driver will continue to stay alive until his car has passed. Thus, there is a very important sense in which living is a social obligation. And suicide must either actually, or at least symbolically, be a defection in social obligation (pp. 117–18).

An analysis of suicide should be comprehensive enough to describe conditions under which any man (including ourselves) would consider suicide as an alternative to life. In meeting this prescription, we are led into treating suicide as an act that occupies a place of universality within the historical and behavioural repertoire of man. In so doing we avoid the inherent limitations of a theory that would force us to view all suicides as pathological.

In this chapter we will argue that it is advantageous to consider suicide as a simple human act. Our conceptualisation of suicide will draw its roots then from Kelly's view of human behaviour. From the Kellian position, suicide must be considered as preserving, extending or defining a person's system. The crucial question being, what suicide is expected to accomplish for the individual at the moment it's being considered.

As clinicians, what are our gains and losses if we allow ourselves to be guided by Kelly's prescriptions when dealing with suicidal behaviour? It will be a loss if Personal Construct Theory (PCT) is merely another pot in which to boil the same bones. If it offers a mere translation of the same events into another language, it is redundant and what follows from its viewpoint would not qualify it for serious consideration. It will be a gain, if from PCT we are able to clarify what we already know, extend the body of knowledge and are pointed toward further questions regarding the suicidal crisis. In order to be able to judge whether or not PCT accomplishes this, a review of existing conceptualisations of suicide is necessary.

Theoretical Conceptualisations of Suicide

The following review is by no means exhaustive. Rather, it is an attempt to highlight major conceptualisations of suicide, drawing from diverse yet representative areas of study. Numerous motivations have been offered to account for the suicidal act. Mintz (1968) has presented the following summary: hostile impulses directed towards an introjected loved one; aggression turned inward; retaliation; attempts to force affection; attempts at restitution; efforts to rid oneself of unacceptable impulses; desire for reincarnation or reunion with a lost loved one; and the desire to escape from physical pain or distress.

Psychoanalytic theories have focused on internal, unconscious motives. Specifically, that suicide was the result of hostile or aggressive impulses directed toward an introjected and ambivalently perceived love object. In his classic work, *Man Against Himself*, Menninger (1938) states that suicide involves (1) the wish to kill, (2) the wish to be killed and (3) the wish to die.

Sociological theories have focused on man's role in society in an effort to account for suicidal behaviour. Durkheim's well-known work, *Le Suicide* (1897) has provided the prototype for later sociological theorising. Briefly summarised, Durkheim posited three types of suicide; egoistic (the result of too few ties to society), altruistic (a response to societal demands) and anomic (suicide resulting from a sudden change in one's relation to society).

More recently, theorists have focused on the cognitive attributes of the suicidal individual, such as 'hopelessness' (Beck, 1963; Beck and Rush, 1978), dichotomous thinking (Neuringer, 1961), impaired problem solving ability (Levenson and Neuringer, 1971), and rigidity of thought (Neuringer, 1964, 1974).

Linehan (1981) presents a model of suicidal behaviour based on social-behavioural formulations of personality. The model results from an eclectic combining of sociological, biological, psycho-dynamic, cognitive and learning formulations of suicide. Emphasis within this approach is given to maintaining a balance between cognitive, motor and physiological/affective systems. Linehan argues that negative stressors in any one area adversely affect the total organism, thus enhancing suicidal risk.

Conceptions of Suicide From Personal Construct Theory

Kelly (1961) relied on the metaphor 'The present is a bridge between the past and the future', to illuminate a major theme within personal construct theory.

The metaphor is interpreted as casting the individual in an active role of a pilgrim who makes choices. Each choice is a bridge or link between where he has been and what he has done, with where he is about to go and what he will become. Man does not simply leave his past behind, rather he uses it by reflecting on it and at times re-creating it in his future. Clearly this is an image of man standing in 'the midst of personal risk and personal choice' (Mair, 1983).

The relationship of this metaphor to questions about suicide is apt. It brings together at once, the basic time factors that need consideration if an understanding of suicide is to emerge. In using the metaphor as an introduction to Kellian thinking regarding suicide, we have pushed it ironically to the extreme range of its applicability. Yet in using the metaphor we are acutely aware of treading near the edges of our own ability to draw out its exhaustive meaning. Kelly equated the activity implied in the metaphor to 'the essence of life'.

The metaphor's relevance to suicide is two-fold. To begin, suicide is an act of life, an act embodying choice among alternatives under-taken at a moment of crisis within life itself. The choice to suicide arises out of personal consideration of reflected past and antici-pated future. To the extent that suicide involves and is traceable to an individual's biography, we are left with residuals which can be investigated (e.g. personal accounts from attemptors, notes from successful suicides.)

To the extent that suicide is involved with the future as it is anticipated by the suicidal person, we are faced with an imponder-able problem. Left with our own private constructions of death and our related anticipations, we are stripped of fitting methods of investigation. Indeed we are at our methodological limits, left at a point requiring what Mair (1983) neatly described as a 'psychology of the edge'.

As a theory, PCT has both a focus of convenience with regard to suicide and a range of convenience where its limits or edges are found. Within its area of focus, it will straightforwardly offer up conceptions to clarify the nature of suicide. Within its broader range of convenience (as a psychology with edges) it should point towards promise of extension by generating further questions. To arrive at an understanding of suicide, a careful reading of Kelly's two volumes and essays is necessary, as there is no one chapter or section devoted to suicide. Keep in mind that Kelly rested his thoughts about human activity on an assumptive base which when summarised became the fundamental postulate of Personal Construct Theory. It states 'a person's processes are psychologically channelised by the way in which he anticipates events' (Kelly, 1955, p. 46): the key phrase being 'psychologically channelized'. What follows is a theory regarding how the composite attitudes, expectations, and constructions of a person channel or direct his activities. Thus if we are to find an indication of what constitutes suicide it will be found in terms descriptive of an individual's psychological processes. Further, since processes are channelised it will be necessary to define suicide as a psychological act, i.e. a cessation or giving up of psychological life or any aspect of it. To give up any attempts at gaining meaning or failing to go beyond what man already knows (i.e. the reconstructive process) is Kelly's definition of suicide.

In summary, to give up the reconstructive process in degrees is to give up on life in degrees. To abandon the psychological process totally is suicide. Any physical act culminating in death is merely the behavioural statement signifying the premature end of a psychological process. 'In reaching terminal conclusions, moral or psychological, man commits the ultimate suicide of his race.' (Kelly, 1969c, p. 13).

Kelly's Formula For the Analysis of Suicide

PCT is an exclusively psychological theory. It addresses man's efforts in developing effective ways to meet the circumstances he expects to occur. It accounts for man's choice of direction and his disposition to reflect upon the effect of his actions. At his peak effectiveness, man's constructions are the result of considerations of outer and inner events, past experience and future expectations. Continuously operating amid pairs of opposites, man makes choices to maximise his freedom and simultaneously insure a degree of personal certainty. If living means choosing to remain psychologically engaged, then by contrast, suicide is an abdication of that process.

Kelly (1961) provided a brief but seminal application of PCT to a suicide case history involving a 23-year-old college student (referred to as A.S.) who made a suicide attempt by ingesting 75 barbiturate capsules. A.S.'s attempt followed a family conflict wherein his parents rejected the woman he loved and planned to marry. He was found unconscious in his hotel room and was brought to the emergency room of a large general hospital, where he was interviewed and the resultant anemnesis was the base Kelly used for his analysis.

Kelly began by providing a definition of his theory. He focused his analysis of the case by contrasting the conceptions of what he saw as relevant and irrelevant to suicide. Like Hillman (1976), Schneidman (1968) and Bakan (1967), Kelly drew the act away and out of the domain of mental illness. Once pathology was dismissed as inadequate, the inner world of the individual took on major importance. Namely, what was it the person thought he would accomplish when he engaged in the suicidal act? Once divested from a view of the suicidal individual as a victim of circumstance or pathology, Kelly by necessity had to treat biographical details in a unique manner. He viewed biography as containing evidence of how the individual used past events and as the record of the experiments he performed to develop personal meaning. According to Kelly (1961, p. 257) biography is to be treated as the 'grounds he [A.S.] used for the meanings he invented and as the outcomes against which, over the years, he must have so often checked his anticipations.' The person's experiments and interpretations are the important aspect. Obviously this is much different from the traditional view where biography is exclusively used as the data base for the observer to apply his categories to another's behaviour or as a record of antecedent causal events which preordain suicide.

From the Kellian perspective, an analysis of the suicidal event must go beyond biography. Be reminded, the 'present is a bridge linking past with future'. Biography is but half the equation of human behaviour; the other half is anticipation. For a complete analysis, what the person anticipates needs to be considered. Biography provides the medium in which anticipation is rooted and from which it springs. Anticipation (what the individual expects to happen, what events he readies himself to face or avoid) provides the grounds for behaviour. In as much as the past determines what is to be anticipated, anticipation supplies purpose and meaning to behaviour. In order to understand what the individual is trying to accomplish when he suicides, both personal past and anticipated future must be considered.

PCT however, goes beyond anticipation by viewing suicide as an act of anticipated validation. That is, the ability to project into the future that one's actions will be confirmed or disconfirmed. By employing the notion of validation we are forced to consider the act's meaning as residing within the individual's personal construct system. An analysis which seeks clues to personal intention and meaning is much different than an analysis that applies simple dogmatic statements such as 'He attempted suicide because he was depressed or psychotic.' It is also different from saying a suicide occurred because of hopelessness or pessimism. An understanding of an individual's suicide can only be had if we are willing to view it as a personally validating act. Indeed we may conclude after analysis that it was a cry for help, an opportunity for vengeance, a relief from boredom, the only sensible thing the enactor sees to do, but we cannot begin here.

By introducing suicide as a validating act, Kelly unties another knot. There is a tendency within other formulations to attribute some degree of illogicality to the enactor's motives. Once spoken the attribution is treated as fact. Ignored are the central issues which channel the individual's behaviour in the direction of suicide. By invoking the notion of validation, the act is lifted out of the realm of illogicality and at the same time the clinician's task is set. This task is to determine what the suicidal act was designed to accomplish or avoid. Thus the knot produced by the clinician's premature conclusions is circumvented.

In his analysis of A.S., Kelly proposed a dualistic categorisation, 'dedicated acts' and 'mere suicides'.

Suicide As a Dedicated Act

Utilising the lives and deaths of Socrates and Jesus, Kelly (1961) exemplified suicide as a dedicated act. In a brief discussion of their lives, he interjected the following notions. The individual finds himself presented with a choice that reduces to life or death. If continuing to live requires turning one's back on one's core system (that which provides structure and determines direction), then the resultant situation may be more costly than suicide. This is especially true if death via suicide promises confirmation of those core issues. The anticipated confirmation stems from the possibility that others may extend the meaning found in the suicidal person's life. In this way, suicide becomes a sensible and dedicated act. As Kelly (1961, p. 260) writes, 'the act is designed to validate one's life, to extend its essential meaning rather than to terminate it.'

It has been said that all acts of suicide involve the social fabric. Our definition of the social fabric will flow from Kelly's sociality corollary. What is inferred in this corollary is that individuals do not live their lives in vacuums. Instead, there exists a social interrelatedness that goes beyond simple barter or exchange. It is a dependency on interconnectedness recognised and described by Jung (1959) as sychronicity and by Kelly (1955) as an 'ultimate internal bond.' Mair (1970) comments, ' . . . I am convinced of the irretrievably interpersonal nature of each person's system for organising and making sense of the world around him.' Thus, the interrelatedness of individuals becomes the *sine qua non* in developing and maintaining personal construct systems. In dedicated acts of suicide the social fabric (or interrelatedness) is not broken. If the individual opts to live in a set of circumstances calling for a recantation, not only is his system (that which he lived for) destroyed, but the systems of others are also negatively, perhaps irrevocably affected. Continuing to live offers a poor choice, tantamount to psychological suicide. If suicide is chosen, the destruction of one's system is not experienced. The social fabric remains intact and one's personal meaning is provided extension through others who may apply the inherent implications in their own lives. Kelly (1961, p. 258) referred to this type of interpersonal anticipation as 'sublime anticipation.' In so doing he created an overview of mutually dependent human activity in which men are bonded to each other for the validation of their truths. This process constitutes social progress. Whereas some may self destruct for reasons tied to the shortcomings of their systems, the possibility exists that some may seek death to reaffirm and insure a continuance of the meanings that had guided their lives. Thus if something is worth living for, it is worth dying for and death becomes but one side of the coin of human enterprise, life the other, each side totally dependent on the other for meaning.

As a Mere Suicide

'Mere' suicide result from a personal system that is flawed. The individual finds himself in circumstances wherein his constructions allow for neither extension nor clarification. It is not that circumstances do not provide opportunity (they never do), but rather that the person is unable to consider alternatives. In effect, the person is caught in his own trap. Rowe (1983) recognised this condition within depressives and referred to it as 'created prisons'. Addressing the same phenomenon, Ryle (1975) termed it self-created 'frames and cages'.

Kelly (1961, p. 260) viewed 'mere suicides' as resulting from 'two limiting conditions' of personal construction which he labelled realism and indeterminacy. 'The first is when the course of events seems so obvious that there is no point in waiting around for the outcome. The score is so lopsided there is no reason to stay to see the end of the game.' From this deterministic attitude, the person anticipates utter boredom, constancy and repetition. His conclusions point toward a predictably determined future.

The latter condition, indeterminacy, occurs when 'everything seems so unpredictable that the only definite thing one can do is to abandon the scene altogether' (Kelly, 1961, p. 260). Here the suicidal attempt is made impulsively in a context of anxiety and is seen as the only way to inject sensibility into an already chaotic system. Reliable bearings to guide and to generate anticipations have been lost. Further, behaviour, the means of understanding the world, is rendered ineffective.

Those who behave suicidally from either pole of limited construction are validating their point of view. The determined outlook seeks definition via suicide for a system that does not promise extension, where all future outcomes are expected to end with the same results. For those experiencing chaos, suicide promises certainty to a system which is already beyond extension. Further experimentation simply is expected to add to the overwhelming confusion. The only certainty left is simply death.

In summary, by creating the dualistic categories (mere suicide and dedicated acts) Kelly provided a way out of the trap of having to view suicide as necessarily pathological. Primarily the distinction pivots around: (a) choice, (b) commonality, (c) social progress. The choice, in dedicated acts, is to preserve one's system, in mere suicides the choice is to abandon it. In dedicated acts, the purpose of the act projects its meaning to others. In mere suicide, the assignment of meaning is clouded by the idiosyncratic nature of the act. That is, an outsider viewing the act sees alternatives, which the enactor does not. Dedicated acts leave the social fabric intact, thus maintaining social progress. Mere suicides destroy the social order by adversely affecting significant others.

Personal Construct Investigations of the Suicidal Event

The study of suicide is the study of a strategic process undertaken to accomplish a personal end. The following is a review of investigations into suicide from the vantage point of PCT. Stemming from our view of suicide as a process, we have chosen to group and thus view these studies as pertaining to the time course inherent in the suicidal act. That is, suicide past — the organised patterns a person brings to bear; suicide present — the crisis event; and suicide future — the person's expectations regarding the results of his actions.

The Organisation of Construct Patterns

Studies of the construct organisation of the individual have formed the backbone of PCT in general and of suicide in particular. Landfield (1976) examined the 'instigating context' of suicidal behaviour. By instigating context he referred to the 'imminence of construct system breakdown' and stated specifically that suicide 'will be found in the context of disorganisation and constriction of one's personal construct system.' In order to test his hypothesis, Landfield employed a modified version of the Repertory Grid Test from which he developed three indices of measurement. Two were assumed indicative of constriction; the third, disorganisation. An individual was considered to be operating from a constricted system when (a) he could not apply his constructs to the individuals in his grid, (b) he could not decide which end of his constructs applied to those individuals and (c) the constructs he developed were judged as overly 'concrete'. The individual's system was considered disorganised when the degree of interrelatedness between constructs with constructs, and elements with elements were analysed and considered functionally independent of each other. Employing the grid with different populations (e.g. attemptors, ideators, long-term therapy clients, etc.), Landfield found that attemptors showed significantly more concreteness and system disorganisation, thus confirming his hypothesis.

Ryle (1967) undertook a broad investigation into the meaning and consequences of the suicidal act. Specifically he sought to examine the belief that suicidal individuals are often ambivalently and symbiotically bound to a significant but pathological individual. Further, Ryle sought to demonstrate the application of repertory grid technology to the study of dyadic relationships. In so doing, he established a precedent for employing grid methodology in the study of suicide. Ryle presented a case history involving a 19-year-old woman who made a suicide attempt in the context of preventing her boyfriend from leaving her. During the course of therapy with the suicidal woman, he administered Repertory Grid tests to both her and her boyfriend on two occasions. He offered an interpretation of the grid results consistent with PCT (i.e. the young woman considered self destruction less painful than the task of revising her construct system). It is felt that he could have elaborated the dynamics of the act more fully. Missing are themes of hostility, threat, guilt and core role invalidations.

Lester (1968) discussed suicidal behaviour from the vantage point of PCT. Specifically, he suggested that the Kellian notion of hostility may account for findings indicating that suicidal individuals are rigid in thought and are prone to extorting and distorting evidence. Lester (1971) attempted to demonstrate that suicide attemptors differed in 'cognitive complexity' from non-suicidals. He gave the Situational Resources Grid to both groups and compared their results on four developed indices of cognitive complexity. He failed to find significant differences between groups. It should be noted that Lester's definition of cognitive complexity differs from both Bieri's (1966) and Adams-Webber's (1979b). In addition, Bannister and Fransella (1982, p. 111) caution against considering 'cognitive complexity' the simple equivalent of a trait dimension. They argue that subsystems within the total construct system, may have more or less degrees of simplicity vs. complexity when compared to one another.

R.A. Neimeyer (1984) provides an exhaustive review of the depression and suicide literature from the PCT perspective. Integrating his own and others' findings, Neimeyer presents evidence which suggests that similar cognitive factors may be present in depression and suicide. He cites the following as areas where these similarities occur: (a) constriction of events; (b) system disorganisation; (c) anticipatory failure; (d) negative self construing; (e) polarisation of dichotomous construction; and (f) interpersonal isolation. Neimeyer argues the need for future research to determine if these factors are symptom or vulnerability linked.

The Crisis Event

It is difficult, if not impossible, to focus solely on the crisis event, in that it encompasses both personal past and anticipated future. Yet that period of time wherein the decision to suicide emerges is of special importance. It is characterised by those factors inherent to transition. Landfield (1976) recognised system disorganisation as part of the crisis and termed it an 'instigating context.' Stefan and Linder (in press) in elaborating Kelly's two limiting conditions for suicide present a description of the suicidal crisis in PCT terms. Suicide is viewed as a choice undertaken either to prevent total chaos (ultimate indeterminancy) of one's core constructions or as a choice taken to prevent a fatalistic (ultimate realism) outcome. The general strategies employed by field-determined individuals (those who derive meaning from the thrust of outer events) and by construct-determined individuals (those who derive meaning from creating inner-based constructs) are explored within the context of the C-P-C cycle (Kelly, 1955 and Chapter 1 this book).

What Result the Suicide Attemptor is Expecting

Rowe (1983), and Stefan and Linder (in press) have argued that the individual experiencing chaos reaches for certainty or clarity. The individual experiencing fatalism seeks some way to extend or escape this entrapment. Landfield (1976) describes the suicidal attempt as a 'bid for clarity'. In doing so he is offering a description of what the person expects will result.

Parker's (1981) investigation sought to distinguish what personal meaning a group of high intentioned suicide attemptors versus low intentioned attemptors would assign to their suicidal behaviour. She developed a grid of 11 interpersonal conflict situations and 9 supplied constructs. The grid was given to parasuicidal subjects who were matched for age and the suicide method employed. The Beck Suicide Intent Scale was used to determine levels of intentionality. Results indicated that these groups differed in the following way. Low intentioned individuals viewed overdosing as a way to escape tension, analogous to getting drunk or crying. This group was optimistic about talking as a means of conflict resolution.

Moderate-to-high intentioned individuals construed overdosing as related to death and not analogous to getting drunk or crying. They were pessimistic about the effects of talking, viewing it as an opportunity to assign blame and avert the real problem.

This study assumes that suicidal intention is personally defined, an assumption in keeping with PCT. It also supports the contention that suicide is undertaken as an experiment in one's social environment either to provoke a change or find an avenue of escape. Parker's investigation is important in that it offers a finer grained analysis of what suicidal individuals are attempting to accomplish by their behaviour.

We have referred to Kelly's analysis of the case of A.S., in which he elucidates two limiting conditions of suicide: realism and indeterminacy. The following case histories are offered both as illustrative examples of these conditions and as a vehicle from which to offer treatment strategies.

Clinical Examples

Suicide Within a Context of Realism (i.e. believing that the world and oneself are determined)

Lena quit school upon turning sixteen. Having been mislabelled a slow learner, Lena was assigned to special classes. As a result of this class assignment and a mild speech impediment, Lena became the brunt of her peers' teasing. Her only friend was a boy, also from special classes who eventually quit school with her. In spite of her parents' wishes, Lena married him. Her marriage quickly turned sour as she and her husband strongly disagreed over her role. In addition, relations between her husband and parents worsened to the degree where he forbade any contact between them. This included their seven-year-old daughter. Then, against her husband's wishes, Lena obtained a job as a cashier. She was soon fired, however, when her employer terminated all cashiers because a theft had occurred and he was unable to determine the culprit. Having lost her job, Lena turned to religious activities as a way to fill in the gaps: however, her husband soon demanded that she stop.

Cut off from all outlets, Lena decided that a suicide gesture (via overdose) would bring her family together and force her husband to make amends. She anticipated that all would meet at her hospital bed. Indeed it worked, but the effect was only temporary. Her husband again became oppositional and forbade family contact. In addition, sexual relations had become painful due to a physical problem for which Lena was being treated. Severe quarrels ensued, to which her daughter reacted by her own attempt at suicide. Her daughter's action became the grounds for a strong experience of guilt for Lena. In addition, she reported loathing her husband and his sexual advances. She seriously contemplated shooting him — 'below the belt.' However, she anticipated the devastating consequences to her family — they would have a murderer for a mother and daughter and she would be capitally punished or imprisoned for life. With these as the results, she concluded her life would be over. She chose to kill herself. She took a gun to her heart, but instead shot herself through the pectoral muscle.

Analysis and Evaluation. During a series of interviews, it became evident that Lena relied primarily on the negative descriptions that were applicable to her past experiences (school, lost job, etc.). She concluded she was unable to deal with the events which emerged. This self construction cast her in a passive posture simply waiting for events to occur. Indeed her first attempt cast her into a passive role of 'patient'. Her daughter's suicide attempt was interpreted by her as evidence that she was an unfit mother and, dislodged from her core role of mother, she saw no channel of movement open to her. The future life she anticipated would trap her. She chose death as a way out of a failed life, hence our assignment of her to the fatalistic pole.

Suicide Within a Context of Indeterminacy (i.e. believing that the world and oneself are chaotic)

Patti, an excellent college student and athlete, experienced the disintegration of her system when she began questioning her sexual identity. She was not dating and had no close friends. Her sexual experience was limited to a series of teenaged experimental encounters with an older cousin.

Patti interpreted her social isolation and athletic prowess as evidence of homosexuality. This interpretation was strengthened by her realisation that she was associating exclusively with females. Patti began hearing voices telling her that she was a boy, a misfit and would be better off dead. In response, she tried to jump from a bridge but was prevented and briefly hospitalised. During her hospitalisation, Patti was visited by a female teammate with whom a complex and dependent friendship developed. Patti interpreted this friendship as homosexual, an interpretation that was not held in common. Her friend became attracted to a young man and began dating. As their dating intensified, Patti spent increasingly more time alone. In a spate of vengeance, Patti shot herself in the stomach with a small calibre rifle. Because of the resultant pain she sought aid and was rehospitalised.

During a series of interviews, Patti described her intended vengeance as wanting to hurt her friend by removing herself as a source of validation on which she believed her friend was dependent. Of central importance was Patti's expectation that her suicide would create a state of chaos for her friend while ending her own experience with it.

Analysis and Evaluation. Interviews with Patti revealed that she had prematurely concluded she was homosexual. Once the pre-emptive label was applied, all events became evidence to her that her conclusion was valid. After being dislodged from the friendship she believed provided an arena for experimentation, Patti chose suicide to prevent an utter loss of certainty. Viewed in contrast, for Patti the anticipated future represented threat and anxiety: for Lena there was nothing left in which to engage.

It might be argued that these cases simply exemplify suicide in a context of depression or psychosis respectively. This may be a valid diagnostic view. Yet it has serious limitations, in that it conveys little understanding of the individual's choice to suicide. In addition, the diagnostic view lacks predictive utility. It is well known that not all depressed or psychotic individuals suicide. If suicidology is to be advanced, we must be able to differentiate those who will from those who will not. We would argue that the potential for suicide increases once core constructions of self are centrally implicated in the experiences associated with realism and indeterminacy. The self statement, if uttered, would be 'I am totally controlled, with no freedom of movement' or 'I am incapable of ever making sense of anything, not even myself.' Once such self determinations are made, the realm of despair is entered.

Assessment

A variety of useful clinical techniques and instruments exist for assessing a suicidal individual. The range includes structured interviews, factorial scales on the MMPI, projective tests and specialised scales which focus on issues of intent, lethality, risk/rescue factors, and others which predict the potential for future attempts. As a group, they are useful in both research and clinical applications. They are most useful in providing support for clinical judgments and bringing related issues into focus.

When specific questions arise regarding why an individual entertained the choice, what the context was interpreted as being, and what was expected to result, the existing pool of tests is limited. While helpful in initiating an investigation, they lack utility in drawing out the personal meaning assigned to surrounding events and the act itself. Once they help fill in the gaps from the outside point of view, the clinician is still left with the suicidal individual and the question remains: What does he do with thim? What do they do with each other? More specifically, what therapeutic directon should be taken?

There is presently no structured assessment device useful in determining whether or not an individual chose suicide in a context of realism or indeterminacy. Clinical experience in applying this dimension to suicidal cases suggests that it is a useful reference axis because it brings together at once a view of suicide as the coincident of inner and outer experience as subsumed by the individual's point of view and from which treatment implications follow.

Regarding interviews, we propose that they be conducted in a manner consistent with PCT. That is, the individual is to be viewed as an expert regarding himself, and he is to be maintained in that role. Further, the credulous approach is to be fostered. Broadly translating Perry's (1978) work, we argue that there is no place for a preemptive motivational analysis which leads to attributions of hostility, manipulation or psychopathy.

In summary, the interview should be conducted toward the end of allowing the personal perspective to emerge, the ultimate goal being an understanding of the act which subsumes the individual's description, assigned meanings and anticipations. From this understanding, directions for treatment should result.

Treatment Implications

We have argued that suicide is a behavioural statement signifying that the individual is either blocked from or has lost sight of the course of action he set for himself. At this point he considers death more desirable than the anticipated futility or utter senselessness. Our purpose is to describe a therapeutic approach which focuses on that actual experience of being blocked or lost.

It has become clear from listening to survivors that the attempt itself has had an impact on the total scope of their lives. New problems emerge as a result of engaging in suicidal behaviour. The act places the individual in a state of delicate transition wherein new constructions are quickly developed and old constructs changed. Concern regarding the ability to control suicidal urges is often expressed. Indeed, intimate others often begin to relate as if the individual will always be prone to suicide.

There is a tendency for the suicidal person to operate in one of two extreme ways. The first is to do nothing, avoid or deny the issue, perhaps hoping 'it' will go away. The authors reviewed the Suicide Intent Scale responses of 76 newly hospitalised suicide attemptors; 83 per cent indicated they did not intend death. One possible interpretation is that these attemptors were distancing themselves from the act, trying to manage impressions by denying they were suicidal.

Many suicidal persons give up attempts at self direction and experimentation. They allow themselves to be treated as having a specifiable condition, which lies outside the realm of their influence. They begin relying on medication to lift and lower their spirits. They become fearful and suspicious of strong emotion; regarding it as a harbinger of lost self control. Borrowing the language of their doctors, they discuss their 'manic-depressive illness' and place their hopes on a 'cure' which they believe will result from adjustments in medications. When extreme positions such as these are taken, problematic anticipations arise.

Other individuals merely await their next 'predetermined' attempt. The authors worked with a suicidal woman whose single attempt set the stage for repeated hospitalisations. Each hospitalisation was triggered by her anticipated loss of control. All ordinary experience was translated into an opportunity to lose control: all objects were seen as potential implements of self destruction. She believed there was nothing she could do to prevent her suicidal behaviour; an opinion shared by her family.

Equally as serious are those individuals who become inarticulate in therapy. Unable to discuss their concerns and feelings, they resort to gesturing and crying.

The preceding examples are not rare. They illustrate passive anticipatory strategies which once set in motion, affect future behaviour. In order to deal therapeutically with these strategies, some general principles designed to maximise effectiveness will be offered. First and foremost, fears of the therapist notwithstanding, the attempt must be discussed openly and frankly. Therapy should be timed to begin as soon after the attempt as possible. Regardless of what the therapist may or may not do, the client will begin to reconstrue immediately following his attempt. Although the individual's premature conclusions (regarding his attempt) are to be circumvented, those held by intimate others cannot be ignored. These individuals control and create the social context for the attemptor. They can also offer a source of support and hence should be brought into therapy to the extent possible.

While the primary goal of therapy is to prevent future attempts, a concurrent goal is to foster reconstruction. Stefan and Linder (in press) have used the term 'encoding' to refer to the process of binding the suicide attempt into the construct system of the attemptor. A central outcome of the process is that the attempt becomes viewed as a strategy that was employed to deal with circumstances that have passed and are no longer relevant. The task of encoding can be viewed as an attempt to transfer one system of communication (behaviour) to another (words). If the attemptor has difficulty articulating, various techniques can be applied. He can be asked to describe a picture that he would paint depicting his feelings and then to compare and contrast that with a picture of the most comfortable period in his life. He can be encouraged to write a series of characterisations describing himself at different points in time. These exercises are undertaken to produce themes, thus providing therapeutic communication and direction. Therapy must address the preemptive conclusions reached by those who decide that they are controlled by alien forces. The person should be encouraged to rely on his own senses and to avoid short-circuiting his behaviour by preemptively concluding. Small psychosocial experiments aimed at shifting control from the condition to the person are suggested. Encouraging the person to engage in propositional ('as – if') thinking is often helpful, as are efforts to view suicide as a multi-determined act. However, simple rephrasings of the original problematic conclusion should be avoided. The strategy is to inspire progress towards personal movement, not confirmation of negative circumstances. Rather than viewing suicide as an event outside his control, an interpretation is offered to the client that suicide may have been his means of communicating or his attempt to influence the direction of his life.

For attemptors who view themselves as unable to anticipate (i.e. those who expect chaos) therapy begins by offering a *temporary* belief which stresses personal capability and shifts blame onto stressful circumstances. They are cast into the psychological role of self-expert (i.e. as a person capable of self understanding and direction). These individuals are threatened by anticipations of overwhelming self-destructive urges. This anxiety is enhanced by their inability to reach conclusions — preemptive or otherwise. The basis of this anxiety is their lack of confidence in their own capability to direct their life and future reliably. Useful techniques rely on tacit displays of faith in the client's ability to demonstrate a general competence, which in turn enhances self confidence. In a hospital situation, this can be accomplished by gradually increasing freedom of self determination in *all* areas.

The goal of therapy is to have the client suspend his use of the control issue to the point where it becomes irrelevant. The issue of anticipation couched as 'control' is very difficult to address in therapeutic discussion. Those convinced they do not possess it, manage to prove they do not in numerous ways (almost always 'hostilely'). Treatment strategies should revolve around encouraging the individual to engage in ordinary life activities to gain evidence that he has control over his suicidal feelings. This must be done quickly for the individual will find his own preemptive conclusion in an attempt to allay his anxiety (or he will attempt suicide). If he preempts, he will resist efforts to experiment with alternative propositional conclusions.

What we are describing are therapeutic directions to be taken after an attempt has been made or after the person has identified himself as suicidal. We have stated that the purpose of therapy is to prevent further attempts. We believe that future attempts occur as a result of how the client construes the situation. It is an infrequent and rare occurrence to witness an individual reattempting suicide shortly after an attempt has been made. Those who do are usually in the throes of psychosis and have made the initial attempt within that context. Re-occurrences of suicidal thought and action typically emerge during periods of transition, that is, when adaptive solutions are needed to meet new circumstances. What is frequently observed is that the individual casts about in an effort to understand his self-destructive behaviour. Restating the therapeutic task, the client is assisted in arriving at an understanding which addresses his concerns, avoids pejorative labels, and allows the attempt to be construed as bound in time (i.e. as a strategy no longer necessary). Failure to reach this goal increases the probability that suicide will re-emerge as a strategy. The high frequency of attempts observed at time of discharge is interpreted as evidence of the failure of therapy to deal with these issues.

Once the client begins considering alternative hypotheses regarding core self constructions and developing personal goals, other therapeutic techniques may be implemented. It is useful to see the application of these techniques relative to the chaos-determinism axis.

For the client inclined towards a deterministic outlook, therapeutic interventions should be directed towards loosening the individual's structure to the point where new constructions may be employed on a propositional basis. Psychosocial experiments are suggested as a medium for testing new hypotheses and introspecting about results. Therapy is designed to expand the person's system to the point where new constructions are admitted which will allow personal freedom of movement and control.

For the individual anticipating chaos, therapy centres on tightening procedures, thus bringing the person into contact with elements of the environment. The individual needs to be exposed to alternative perspectives and steps should be taken to maximise the client's problem-solving ability. Bannister and Kelly have addressed the process of tightening and loosening in therapy. The reader is referred to their work for further discussion.

Group Therapy

We have argued that the opportunity to engage in psychosocial experimentation is a strong facilitator of movement. Group therapy in particular, provides such experimentation. For those who have difficulty describing circumstances and private experiences, the words used by others become starting points for their own descriptions. In addition, pre-emptive concluding (the bane of suicidal individuals) is effectively thwarted by group therapy. Suicide must be viewed as a multi-determined event because of the variety of motives offered by group members.

The mere presence of others who have been through a suicidal experience creates an atmosphere of security. This is particularly true for the person who is preoccupied with what others think of him for having done something so 'silly, dumb, crazy, etc.' The final point to be made is that an opportunity for confirmation as well as disconfirmation is readily available in group sessions. Strongly influenced by Mair's (1977a) arguments for employing metaphors, the authors have utilised structured exercises within a group format. Groups composed primarily of suicidal individuals are asked to describe in detail, their 'ideal house'. They are encouraged not to consider circumstantial restraints and to construct the house as an environment wherein they will thrive. As much detail as possible is sought (e.g. location, surroundings, size, style, occupants, visitors, interactions, etc.) This exercise provides a medium for more central problems to emerge. Yet the individual maintains a sense of security as critiques are directed toward the house and not the person. The therapist's role is that of facilitator, one who will aid the client in reconstruing his circumstances. The exercise's relevance to the issue of suicide is that the creation of a positive environment is a future oriented goal and as such, it sets into motion issues of anticipation. The 'Ideal House' offers a meaningful goal with recognisable components that can be broken down into attainable mini-goals. It provides steps that can be taken in the present, thus fostering hope. Finally, the exercise provides individualised material for the development of psychosocial experiments.

Unfortunately, the technique is not applicable to all. The individual who rigidly holds to his pre-emptive conclusion often will not engage in therapeutic exercises. For psychotic individuals, the image provides too much structure as they are unable to contain their descriptions to an ideal house. However for many individuals, this brief exercise provides a direct, fast focus on relevant issues. In summary, the purpose of the group process is to provide hope through triggering the person's anticipations. We agree with Bannister and Kelly that therapy is conducted to enable the individual to meet life's next series of surprises effectively. Nowhere in clinical work is this theme more poignant than when working with suicidal individuals.

Conclusion

The established tradition within suicidology seeks to uncover a universal path to suicide and is based on theoretical considerations which view the suicidal event as stemming from unconscious drives or circumstances outside the range of human influence.

PCT views suicide as resulting from the interpretations the individual has developed regarding the circumstances in which he finds himself. Hence, as a theory, PCT offers ways to account for why a particular individual's theory led to suicide. Kelly offered a description of three basic ways circumstances are typically interpreted. However, he does not limit us to just these three views. The first is of suicide as a dedicated act. A second interpretation is suicide as a reaction to the boredom experienced after one rigidly concludes that they have experienced all that will ever be new. The final path to a suicidal crisis is described as occurring in a context of personal confusion, experienced when they lose sight of their ability to determine and maintain a reliable personal construct system. All three involve an experience of being blocked from the reconstructive process.

7 EATING DISORDERS: A QUEST FOR CONTROL

Eric Button

We have seen how the process of construction can apply to many contexts. Throughout this book we have been particularly concerned with the context of people, particularly as this relates to people's behaviour in a social context. Construing of people, however, does not have to be restricted to behaviour. Many of our impressions and anticipations of people relate to 'physical' characteristics such as 'well-dressed-scruffy', 'blond-brunette' or 'thin-fat'. That is not to suggest that 'physical' construction is unrelated to more 'psychological' construction. Far from being unrelated, our construction of people's physical characteristics may act as a basis for anticipation of people's behaviour. For instance, we might infer that a man who is six-feet odd and almost as broad is 'not a person to tamper with'. We don't have to look far to see evidence of this kind of construction. It is as if people enact their hopes and expectations by the images they present to others. In this way we can view the physical representations as evidence supportive of our personal and shared theory of people. White coats for doctors, interview suits for interviewees and the unshaven look for cowboy film stars all communicate something about how the 'actor' wants and expects to be seen. This seems to be an essentially social process rather than just an idiosyncratic individual act. The 'observer' typically is expecting the actor to conform to his expectations. Queens who don't look like queens, doctors who don't act like doctors and comedians who don't look funny don't exactly go down well. It does not seem adequate, therefore, just to dismiss such physicalistic construing as somehow inferior or misguided. Rather it may be more fruitful to examine how the perception of physical characteristics may be used by people as a way of expressing their choices and of defining or extending their view of the world.

One inescapable way in which we communicate to others is through our bodies. This starts from the moment we are born with expressions like 'bonny baby', 'bouncing boy' and 'a tiny little thing' conveying a lot about our hopes for this new person. One particular facet of our bodies of which we will doubtless become aware is whether we are too fat, too thin or just right. The predominant

153

societal construction in affluent societies is of the desirability of being slim, thin and certainly not fat. The negative stereotype of obesity is well established (e.g. Maddox, Back and Liederman, 1968) and is quite clearly evident from an early age in children (Staffieri, 1967). There is also evidence that this is a sex-related goal with females more likely to engage in dieting behaviour (Nylander, 1971) and more prone to develop a psychological disorder surrounding weight concern (e.g. Button and Whitehouse, 1981). Although males are just as capable of being construed as fat it seems that females have more investment in being the right size and shape.

In the mental health field one encounters people who are in difficulty at various points on the spectrum from thin to fat. Although it is now recognised that obesity is not explicable solely in terms of some simple psychological mechanism, psychological factors are clearly at play: overeating and consequent weight gain are often associated with perceptions like 'no-one loves me' or 'I'm a failure'. In addition, the consequences of weight gain and obesity can lead to feelings of disgust and alienation if the person sees negative connotations of the obese state. Thus, although we don't have to regard obesity as primarily psychologically determined, for some people it can become the focal point of a disturbance in self-image which leads to the quest for psychological help.

The person who is described by the medical label anorexia nervosa also shares the construction that to be fat is a bad thing. The obese person may symbolise everything she despises: in particular this is often focused on the weakness of 'giving in', of lack of control. Of the various themes that have been advanced to account for the anorexic plight none has been more consistent than that of the need for *control* (e.g. Bruch, 1974). I shall elaborate on this theme later but suffice it to say that for the anorexic nothing seems to be more important than to have some control of her eating, her body and hence her weight. In contrast to the overweight unhappy person, the anorexic rarely seeks change herself. Whilst the concerned onlooker may view her as ill, if not at death's door, she will defend her position to the last with claims such as 'Can't you see the fat on me?'

In spite of the popular appeal of being just right in weight, some seem to attain it but still remain dissatisfied and disturbed. The term 'dietary chaos syndrome' (Palmer, 1979) is one of a number of terms which have been applied to those, mainly young women, who display all the anxieties and preoccupations about fatness as in anorexia nervosa, but whose weight is within normal limits. It seems that they also cherish the construct 'thin-fat' as a predictor of success, but curiously fail to consistently settle for one pole or other of the construct. Their weight frequently oscillates as they go through violent swings from food abstinence to enormous eating binges, interspersed with self-induced vomiting or some other drastic means of weight control. In fact it is tempting to conclude that they may not just be experiencing *dietary* chaos but may be close to *psychological* chaos. Unlike the anorexic and the unhappy obese person who in their contrasting ways have achieved a degree of certainty, their interpersonal experience may be confusing and unpredictable with food as a temporary haven with its familar pleasant associations.

A Personal Construct Theory Approach to Eating Disorders

My starting point for considering what construct theory has to offer to such problems is to emphasise that there is no *one* construct theory view. Like all of the problems discussed in Part Two we are starting with a medical construction and trying to look at people who have been so construed from a different and hopefully more constructive viewpoint. The chances are that if a person comes the way of a mental health professional then an illness formulation will have already been advanced. My aim as a psychologist is to seek a more fruitful line of enquiry: one which focuses on the person rather than pre-emptively opting for the conclusion that my client is anorexic, obese or whatever and therefore there is nothing more to say. When, in 1973, I began to research eating disorders I set out with a hypothesis, not of my own making I might add, but one advanced by my then supervisor Fay Fransella. Partly derived from her study of stutterers and also from some case studies of obese and anorexic patients using repertory grid technique, the following hypothesis had been advanced.

THE OBESE PERSON AND THE ANOREXIC MAY RESIST CHANGE BECAUSE LIFE IS MORE MEANING-FUL THAN IF THEY WERE TO CHANGE TO BEING NORMAL IN WEIGHT

I must confess that my attraction for working in this area was not born out of a fascination for eating disorders but out of excitement of being able to carry out research within a construct theory framework. In short, these disorders had little meaning for me and I found myself initially struggling to fit someone else's behaviour into someone else's construct system. In retrospect I feel that this was because the above hypothesis was not created from my own experience: in my clinical training I had seen just one 'anorexic' and that was at a case conference and I was thoroughly baffled by it: neither did I know anyone very well personally who had a major problem with obesity so I had a lot of learning to do. I now realise that I can only write about such problems now because I have spent a lot of time getting to know a lot of people who present with such difficulties. If I had attempted to stay with the above formulation in its blandest sense I would have been of no use to my clients nor have got very far with my research. Rather than being at pains to fit my clients into my hypotheses, I have increasingly tried to go beyond the stereotype and tried to understand them above all as people. By doing so I have indeed detected themes and these have formed the basis for some elaboration of the above general hypothesis. But without the ability to enter into a genuine relationship with the person, in which she can be taken seriously and recognised as a unique human being, such theorising is likely to be of no avail except perhaps as a means of offering some predictability to the otherwise perplexed clinician. Rather than advancing a highly articulate and elaborate technical theory I am more concerned with offering some relatively simple ideas which can be translated into creative possibilities for those who aspire to help those bogged down by weight.

I shall state three basic points which I feel have direct implications for the understanding and treatment of eating disorders.

1. It may be useful to approach the person who presents with an 'eating disorder' as someone who is aiming for some degree of predictability in her life.
2. The second question becomes one of what she is trying to predict. It is argued that both the concern with eating and the desire to control eating may become the main area in life where a person's predictions may be validated. The likelihood, however, is that where this arises there is a corresponding relative failure to predict people: this includes both self and others.
3. Therapeutic endeavours should primarily recognise the

person's need to maintain some predictability through eating or eating control strategies. The extent to which the client will choose to explore the personal (and by implication *inter*personal) side of her life will depend on the extent to which the client feels safe with the therapist.

The implications of these basic assumptions will be examined both in relation to research and practice.

Research

There is very little published research applying personal construct theory to eating disorders. The main impetus for research in this area has come from two contexts. First, in a series of case studies (Crisp and Fransella, 1972; Fransella and Crisp, 1970) there were indications that in both anorexic and obese subjects, relapse in the form of weight loss or weight gain respectively may be predicted by repertory grid measures of meaningfulness of 'normal weight'. Secondly, Fransella (1972) had also published her research on stutterers in which a series of stutterers had undergone a form of psychotherapy designed to increase the meaningfulness of being a verbally fluent person as opposed to being a stutterer. In the main part of her study 20 stutterers completed a series of Implications grids from which a number of measures were derived. Of the various significant findings, perhaps the most interesting was that increasing fluency was accompanied by a decrease in the meaningfulness of stuttering and an increase in the meaningfulness of fluency. On the basis of this finding, an analogous longitudinal study was planned with obese and anorexic patients undergoing treatment aimed partly at facilitating weight change.

An Implications Grid Study

This study was initiated by Fay Fransella with myself employed in the dual role of therapist and research assistant. Two groups of patients were studied: a group of 20 female in-patients diagnosed as suffering from anorexia nervosa and 20 obese females who were offered psychological treatment at out-patient level. Treatment was based at the Department of Psychiatry of the Royal Free Hospital, London. Half the subjects in each group were assigned to a behavioural approach and the other half to a personal construct approach to treatment. The study was complicated by the fact that all the anorexic patients were also undergoing nutritional treatment aimed at inducing weight gain. This treatment was successful in creating quite substantial weight gain, so that the psychological treatment could not be credited for this but was more concerned with the maintenance of weight gain after discharge. The obese patients, however, (with only one exception who was admitted to hospital) were more in control of their eating behaviour, so that it is not surprising that their weight loss was correspondingly more modest (mean loss 6.7 kg). Thus in both groups there were varying degrees of weight loss or weight gain, with some patients relapsing and others maintaining their weight change. It was therefore possible to relate individual differences in outcome to individual differences in construing. The latter was derived from two sets of implication grids.

Normal Weight Grids. Constructs were elicited from triads of people elements in which 'me as I imagine I would be at a "normal weight" ' was always one of the elements. From the resulting elicited constructs bi-polar 'normal weight' Imp grids were formed.

Present Weight Grids. In an analogous way constructs were elicited with the inclusion of a self element, 'Me overweight' or 'Me at my thinnest', depending on whether the subject was overweight or anorexic respectively.

Each subject completed both kinds of grid. An example of such grids can be seen in Figure 2.1 in Chapter 2. Two main measures were derived.

Meaningfulness. For both grids the number of implications (ticks in Figure 2.1) was counted and treated as a measure of 'meaningfulness' of either 'normal weight' or thinness or fatness.

Saturation. For both grids the ratio of the number of implications divided by the total possible in the grid. High scores on this measure (perhaps akin to the concept of tightness of construing) had previously been found by Fransella (1972) to be predictive of a greater likelihood of relapse.

Contrary to prediction, there was no evidence that normal weight was less meaningful than present weight for either the anorexics or the obese. It was of interest, however, that the number of implications on both grids were closely correlated, suggesting that the measures were tapping some more general features of interpersonal construing. In this respect it was significant that on both grids those anorexics who had had more than one hospital admission had less implications than first admissions. There was, however, some support for the importance of differential meaningfulness of thinness or normal weight. A higher initial number of implications on normal weight grids was associated with better weight maintenance amongst the anorexics. Furthermore, although the numbers of repeat-grids were too small to achieve statistical significance, there was a trend for an increase in meaningfulness of normal weight to be associated with a better outcome. In contrast to the stutterers, however, there was no evidence that the 'saturation' score was related to outcome.

Thus although there was some support for the meaningfulness hypothesis as far as anorexics are concerned, it seems to be not quite as simple as at first thought and is requiring of further research. In the case of the obese subjects, there was no support for the hypothesis, suggesting that this argument does not apply to all people with eating disorders. The obese were, however, more socially integrated and less appropriately viewed as ill than the anorexics. It is possible, therefore, that they do have an idea of what life is like for those who are normal in weight, but that it is an unrealistically rosy one and that by staying fat they avoid invalidating this view.

Following on from the above research project I chose to carry out a second study exploring further the construing of anorexics, this time using the more conventional format of rated grids rather than Impgrids.

A Rated Grid Study of Anorexia Nervosa

A further series of 20 female anorexic in-patients in the same treatment setting as above completed rated grids consisting of 21 elements and constructs. In contrast to the first study, there was no attempt to have separate grids for normal weight and thin construing but within the one grid a number of 'self' elements) e.g. 'me at the treatment team weight', 'me at my thinnest' etc.) were supplied allowing examination of the comparative meanings within the one grid. Furthermore the study differed in that the research did not involve a treatment component so that my role was confined to more of a kind of neutral observer. Perhaps for this reason compliance was somewhat higher and more subjects completed repeat grids. Grids were obtained on a maximum of four occasions: (a) on admission (n = 18); (b) at discharge (n = 12); (c) first follow-up (mean 2.2 months after discharge, n = 12); and (d) second follow-up (mean 7.9 months after discharge, n = 14).

The most striking initial finding was that the construing of the group as a whole mainly involved a contrast between 'me at thinnest' (evaluatively bad) and 'ideal self' (evaluatively good). This perhaps surprising finding is consistent with an earlier grid study of anorexics carried out by Fransella and Crisp (1979). Although the predominant evaluation of thinness in terms of the first component was negative, when grids were re-analysed restricted to the subject's own personal (as opposed to supplied) constructs using Slater's PREFAN programme (Slater, 1977) the third component revealed what may be described as 'implicative dilemma'. Here 'ideal self' was contrasted with several elements of which 'self at treatment weight' loaded highest. Thus although presenting many disadvantages to being anorexic, in terms of some constructs there are distinct disadvantages. For example, for one subject, becoming normal in weight meant becoming more 'conspicuous', which was something she definitely wanted to avoid.

From the point of view of the meaningfulness hypothesis there was definite support. Whereas 'me at thinnest' was very extremely defined, 'me at normal weight', although relatively positively construed, was far less extremely defined. Thus the anorexic's construction of a possible future as someone at a more normal weight is a far less certain matter than if she were to continue as an anorexic. In fact this was also borne out by the fact that grids completed after treatment revealed the only major change as a whole to be on their construing of 'me now'. Thus when they had become more normal in weight their construing of themselves was far more neutral or uncertain. It is not surprising then that many of the patients subsequently relapsed, perhaps retreating to the more predictable world of anorexia nervosa.

My main interest in conducting this study was to investigate the relationship between construing variables and outcome. A number of variables were significantly related to outcome so that I shall restrict my attention to those of particular relevance from a construct theory point of view: there was clear evidence that structural measures of construing at the outset of treatment were predictive of outcome as measured by weight maintenance after discharge from hospital. Both the degree of relationship between constructs and the way in which self was construed were implicated.

Using the percentage of variance accounted for by the first principal component as a measure of overall construct interrelatedness in grids, it was found that higher scores on this measure were associated with poor outcome. Using the language of construct theory I chose to call this particular indicator of poor prognosis 'tight' construing. What was of even more interest, however, was that patients with poor outcome remained consistently 'tight' in their construing on repeat grids whereas those with better outcome successively 'tightened' and 'loosened' their construing (Figure 7.1). This of course gives direct support for the importance of cycles of construing akin to Kelly's Creativity Cycle. Moreover, there was evidence that this cyclical pattern was not restricted to gross features of construing. First, measures of how extremely the various self elements were construed were obtained and it was shown that good outcome patients both started out with less extreme self-construing but also went through a successive increase and decrease in extremity of self-construing. Secondly, it was also shown that the meaningfulness of certain supplied constructs showed a similar trend. Of particular interest was the fact that between first and second follow-up a decrease in meaningfulness of the construct 'thin-fat' was highly associated with a good outcome.

Further details of the above two studies can be found in Button (1980; 1983b) and Fransella and Button (1983).

Other Grid Studies

Studies of clinical samples, of course, do have their disadvantages and we must await evidence about the construing of people with subclinical eating problems, as well as healthy people, before we can be clearer about the processes which are at work in leading to these distressing disorders. Fortunately, there are two unpublished grid studies of which I have knowledge. The first of these is an American study of 68 female undergraduates (G.J. Neimeyer, 1984), who completed a grid in which the elements were eating situations and the supplied constructs were described as 'affective' (e.g. 'feels guilty'). In addition, all subjects completed a 'Restraint Questionnaire' (Spencer and Fremouw, 1979), a measure of attitudinal and behavioural concern about dieting. Although 'high restrainers' did not construe themselves more extremely they did view themselves more negatively. Of particular interest, however, was the finding that high restrainers were less 'cognitively complex':

Figure 7.1: Change in Percentage of Variance Accounted for by First Principal Component over Four Occasions Among Two Subgroups of Anorexics

■–■ Poor Outcome (n=9), ●–● Good Outcome (n=9)

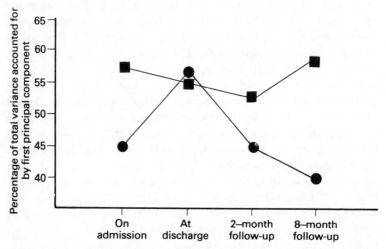

Source: Button, E. J. (1983a) 'Personal Construct Theory and Psychological Well-Being', *British Journal of Medical Psychology*, 56(4), pp. 313-21.

in other words they construe in a less multi-dimensional way. This is an important finding because it would suggest that the significance of this factor in my study is not just an artifact of dealing with an 'ill' population. It also begs the question as to the relationship between the negative self construing and the structural aspects of a person's construing.

A student I recently supervised (Munden, 1982) also carried out a grid study on a student population. She advertised in the university for women who had a problem with eating concern (n = 17) and compared them with a control group (n = 16) of female volunteers, mainly medical students. Subjects completed a grid in which the elements were all females and the constructs were elicited from each subject. She replicated the findings that those with an eating problem have a more negative view of themselves, in this case as measured by the distance between "self" and 'the sort of woman I would ideally like to be'. They also indicated that being slim would make them more like their ideal self, whereas the control group did not envisage any significant change if they were slimmer. There were not, however, any group differences in structural measures of construing so that we must be cautious before concluding that less multi-dimensional construing is *per se* the key factor predisposing females to an eating disorder. Clearly, however, there is no doubt that young women with an eating problem do construe themselves more negatively and further studies are required before we can tease out the processes involved. In that respect we might take heed from my own findings regarding cyclical changes in construing. Rather than looking at these young women's construing as fixed, we may get further by exploring their openness to movement, perhaps particularly as they deal with a 'negative' experience.

There are clearly many questions still left unanswered, but these few studies seem to give ample evidence that personal construct oriented enquiry has something to offer in helping us to unravel what have proved very resistant and distressing problems for all involved.

Practical Implications

I have earlier outlined some basic propositions as to the implications of a personal construct approach to helping people with eating disorders. I particularly emphasised the need to recognise the person's need for control (as represented by her eating concerns) and also of her likely difficulty in the area of person construing. I would now like to spell out some of the possible implications for how we approach helping them. My first principles are quite simple:

1. Respect her. This means not treating her as irrational but as a person with hopes, needs and fears like the rest of us.
2. Don't try and control her. Whatever your motives the chances are she knows all about 'controlling' relationships.
3. Be honest with her about the choices that may be available and how you think you can be of help to her.

The essence of my approach, therefore, is to concentrate initially on establishing the conditions for the formation of a relationship which may form a platform for the elaboration of her interpersonal life. This does not rule out the possibility that at some stage a more medically-oriented intervention may take place. In-patient re-feeding programmes may have the virtue of, at least in the short term, keeping the anorexic alive and giving her a chance to start again. I think it is crucial, however, that the timing is right and that her choice is maintained. At the end of the day if she chooses to hold on to her anorexic way of life then I have an uncompromising attitude that her choice be respected. This doesn't mean, however, that we assume her position is static. She may need time to weigh you up (pardon the pun!) before taking the chance of entering into a helpee-helper relationship.

With these general considerations in mind I have worked with a number of clients individually in order to try and help them become freed from the traps they have created for themselves. I have recently, however, become interested in the possibility of applying a group approach to such problems. It seemed to me that the obese, the anorexic and the bulimic all share problems in person-construing so that there may be a case for bringing them together in a group with a common focus on person construing. With this aim in mind, in conjunction with a colleague of mine, Margaret Campbell, I decided to set up an experimental group open to all people in the spectrum of eating disorders. Eight people eventually accepted the offer to participate in a 20 week group. They were all young women whose ages ranged from 19 to 30. They also varied considerably in weight from 38kg to 110kg: three were clearly underweight, three overweight and two were of more average weight. Most of them had had problems in the area of eating control for quite some time (range 2 to 18 years) and all of them had already had some previous psychological or psychiatric help. After assessment interviews in which several people were excluded either for practical reasons such as the timing of the group or for psychological reasons such as poor motivation or the need for marital help, the eight who accepted were all assessed in terms of eating behaviour and also completed a grid focused on person construing. Grids were personalised, but the following elements ('me', 'me as I would ideally be', 'me if I didn't have an eating problem' and 'me as others see me') were supplied as were the constructs 'slim-fat', 'sexually attractive-sexually unattractive' and 'in control-out of control'. It was also planned to repeat these assessments at the mid-way point of the group, at the end of the group and one year after the group began. The aim of the group was to help them elaborate *person construing* and was put to them as follows:

> Although all members of the group have had difficulty associated with weight and eating, we will not be emphasising weight change and we will be aiming more at helping you to learn ways of being yourself and attaining your goals other than through eating and weight control.

The group was partly modelled on Landfield and Rivers (1975) Interpersonal Transaction Group (see also Chapter 8, 10 and 15) which had a similar focus to our group and also introduced the notion of 'rotating dyads'. Essentially this involved paired brief interactions in which each pair was asked to talk to each other on some theme. The aim of these dyads was to help them to understand each other and hopefully this might generalise as a model for interaction outside the group. It was particularly envisaged that this procedure would help reduce threat. The themes of the dyads were varied but included 'what I like and dislike in people', 'situations where I feel at ease and ill at ease' and 'people who have been important and people who might become important'. In each dyad, subjects took it in turns to be the focus and had five or ten minutes each. The dyads formed just part of the session and all the sessions were at least partly with the whole group. At the midway point it was decided, however, to discontinue the dyads as there was a general feeling that we needed more time as a whole group. Whether in dyads or the whole group, however, the emphasis was on trying to *understand* rather than *judging* people.

It would be difficult to do justice to the multitude of complex and changing interactions and feelings over the life of the group. One thing is for sure. Like all therapeutic groups we were confronted with a variety of well-known issues. These included the obvious ones of trust, the role of group leaders, difficulty in containing feelings, hostility and other strong feelings between group members and insecurity surrounding termination. Like most groups we also had drop-outs and by the end we were left with five people. One of the drop-outs only missed the last few sessions but the other two deserve particular mention. Diane, an anorexic, had shown considerable anxiety about the group throughout. She told us that this extended to most situations where she had to face other people and that she got into a state of panic about it. The group tried very hard to help her deal with this, but after the twelfth session she didn't return. It seemed that her coping strategy was of avoiding situations other than those where she felt safe with people. In Kellyian terms this might be regarded as 'constriction' and fits into the overall framework I have applied to conceptualising anorexia nervosa.

Sally stopped attending after the fifteenth session, after having been arguably the most prominent figure in the group. Her construct system was very clearly in action, as evidenced by her considerable verbal contribution and searching for answers, feedback and direction. Quite early on in the group she asserted that she now realised that her weight was not so important and felt that expressing her feelings was the main problem. There was an impatience for change which was very reminiscent of Kelly's concept of 'aggression'. There was quite clear evidence also both from the group sessions and the grids that Sally was the most 'salient' element in the group, bringing out feelings of hostility, envy and hope in others. It became increasingly clear that Sally was beginning to define some kind of direction for herself and was becoming increasingly impatient with the resistance of some of the group members. It seemed as if, eventually, continuing with the group was inconsistent with her construction 'it's up to me to work at things — you can't expect other people to solve your problems'. Whether this was the right or wrong decision for Sally is not a matter for judgment from a construct theory point of view: freedom to choose amongst alternatives is for me very much a guiding construct and that extends very much to the entering and leaving of therapeutic situations.

Although there was quite clear evidence that the awareness of the limitations of a weight-oriented approach had permeated the group, there was also a fair amount of evidence of resistance to change or in Kelly's terms 'hostility'. This was most clearly expressed by Helen who had a very long-standing difficulty surrounding eating. During the later sessions of the group she came to place a lot of focus on me, on wanting practical answers for changing her eating. She had made it very clear that she saw her eating problem as being unchanged, if not unchangeable. In particular her stance was that because she was very thin, people thought badly of her and that until something could be done to help her put on weight she would not be accepted by others. Thus a lot of her focus when exploring interpersonal experience inside and outside the group was on evidence as to her difference and unacceptability to others.

At one point in the seventeenth session I 'lost my cool' and told her that I was fed up of trying to give her answers as to her eating, which was followed by a clear feeling of rejection on her part and her exit. She did return, however, following letters from various group members including myself, although her maintenance of her eating focus has remained undiminished and she has proved very resistant to a variety of subsequent developments which may have helped to broaden her horizons.

So what was learned or gained from this group? First and foremost I have had brought home to me the extent of limitations and handicap that such people experience and, as such, of the need to be realistic as to the difficulties of change particularly with such a short-term group. It has to be said of course that these young women had particularly long-standing difficulties and on the basis of my previous research it might be argued that earlier intervention may make change a less threatening prospect.

Although it would be wrong to conclude that the group was a startling success for all, I think we did demonstrate that change is possible with this group. Without wanting to generalise, the indications are from our group that the overweight and normal weight subjects were more open to the possibility of movement. All three 'anorexic' members showed considerable limitation in the interpersonal sphere and seemed more comfortable within the realm of their highly constricted world. It may well be, therefore, that they might benefit more initially from a more individual approach.

I think the second main message is that whilst the group may have invalidated their weight-oriented constructs this in itself is not sufficient to guarantee movement. Although we were in the group trying to help them develop alternative constructions the time span of the group meant that the period of elaboration of person-construing could be expected to mainly be a post-group process. The implication of this is that the giving up of a major part of one's construct system is inevitably associated with emotional disturbance as the person enters a state of transition. All those who changed expressed feelings of confusion and uncertainty and in at least three people depressive feelings were expressed, with one person taking an overdose. This was vividly expressed by Jennifer, one of the people who quite clearly changed. She recently wrote to me and told me of how she felt she had learnt a lot from the group, particularly in terms of realising that people can be just as likely to have problems irrespective of their weight. She emphasised, however, that she had consequently experienced a considerable feeling of depression, in her words . . . 'I feel as if my right arm had been cut off'. Terry had also redefined her problem, no longer seeing weight as the issue. She chose to see me further on an individual basis after the group had finished and the focus has mainly been on the forming of relationships with others. She no longer talks of the trouble with being fat but focuses on her ambivalence surrounding her simultaneous need for people and the threat and risks posed by close relationships.

Conclusion

I would therefore see interventions such as the above group as one way of freeing the person from the 'cage' (Bruch, 1978) that they have created with weight. But interventions should be viewed modestly and cautiously, in recognising that therapeutic movement is often likely to be longer-term and in some cases requiring considerable support as they enter into the potentially frightening world of people and relationships. Above all I believe that the abandonment or obsolescence of the weight theory will need to be mediated by a relationship with a person. This does not have to be a formal therapist but where we as professionals are involved we will need to take seriously our role and offer all the acceptance, understanding and above all care that we can muster. If we just treat her as an anorexic etc, with a problem that ought to be changed, we fall into the same trap as she does. Perhaps a question from Helen is a good thought to be left with! 'If I didn't have my eating problem would people really like me?'

8 PERSONAL CONSTRUCT THEORY AND ALCOHOL DEPENDENCE

Clayton Rivers and Alvin Landfield

Personal Construct Theory and Alcoholism: A Theoretical Perspective

Most of the theoretical thinking about alcoholism from the personal construct theory (PCT) point-of-view has been developed by later writers such as Landfield and Rivers (1975), Dawes (1981) and Glantz, Burr and Bosse (1981). However, Kelly (1955) did mention alcohol abuse and alcoholism in his writings. He pointed out that the person would experience *guilt* as he or she departed from the alcoholic role and that holding to the role would tend to prevent guilt. Kelly also cited Alcoholics Anonymous as one vehicle that might control the guilt of being dislodged from one's alcoholic role.

We begin our analysis of alcoholism with the utility of alcohol in social situations, where low intake might be seen as socially appropriate. It is this socially appropriate context that often provides the initial framework for later alcoholism and the elaboration of alcohol-related personal constructions. For example, consider the typical cocktail party. Not infrequently, this kind of social gathering involves unacquainted or minimally acquainted persons. In this setting, casually acquainted people may find it difficult to predict their own or others' social responses. One cannot so easily validate expectations and self roles. Alcohol, with its 'loosening' and 'dilating' effects more easily allows one to engage in superficial chit-chat and to feel his or her role being supported by the responses of others. Anxiety is lowered. One's constructs seem to be fitting the occasion. Thus, we see how alcohol can serve as a useful social lubricant and loosener of the personal construct system in a socially acceptable way. Unfortunately, the socially acceptable way can shift to a perpetual and abusive use of alcohol which the authors link to similar but more severe difficulties in social relating and the validation of one's personal construct system.

Elaborating on the theme of the foregoing paragraph, the disinhibiting effect of the drug allows a sense of social freedom and

169

comfort for the person utilising it. This particular effect of alcoholism, in PCT terms, could be seen as involving two processes, a *dilating* and *loosening* of the construct system. These processes of perceptual enlargement and a lessened need for predictive exactness can be associated with greater flexibility, spontaneity, creativeness, and, sometimes, grandiosity, impulsiveness, and confusion. The role of dilation and loosening in creativeness and confusion will be clarified in our later discussion of Kelly's CPC learning cycle.

Now the opposite of dilation is *constriction*, a process of narrowing the perceptual field in order to minimise apparent incompatibilities. This process can be illustrated by the socially inhibited person, one who takes few social risks. The person shares little of himself, observes only in a most limited way, and asks few questions. He or she cannot cope with any complexity of social information or situation. This person certainly does not encourage comfort in others.

Tightening, the opposite of loosening, means that the person becomes more exact, clear, and consistent about the events that support his anticipations. Taking an extreme case, a person may compulsively monitor another's gestures and conversation, trying to make definitive decisions about the other fellow's nature and one's relationship to him. An extremely tightened person does not rest easily with the ambiguity of incoming information. One of our recovering alcoholic subjects made others feel uncomfortable as he probed and questioned incessantly about 'exactly' what others valued. He was compulsively processing social information, but in ways that did not take into account the individualised expressiveness and somewhat unique personal viewpoints of others. His tight logic was most egocentric and was accompanied with much anxiety as he strained to locate the points of validation for his cynical expectations of life.

In this extreme illustration of tightening, we have noted constriction in our alcoholic's observations of others. He was not open to the alternative thoughts and feelings of others and he certainly was constricted in the valence of his anticipations, rigidly cast in their negative expectations. Although unhappy, and sometimes suicidal, he apparently found some satisfaction in evidence that supported his cynicism. However, alcohol provided a temporary vehicle for greater satisfaction. A drink or two encouraged him to choose Navy 'buddies' without discrimination. He could not feel part of any crowd. He became important and accepted in circumstances definable as superficial. His constrictively compulsive negativeness and exact questioning gave way to 'good' feelings, comradeship, and even grandiosity. His grandiosity sometimes took the form of leading others in pranks. Of course, drunkenness among Navy men is expected, even covertly approved by some officers. Heavy drinking can release tensions and even be construed as 'macho'. But, our subject drank too much for someone who wanted to become an officer. His work efficiency was decreasing and his home life was being adversely affected.

Pulling together some of the themes of our discussion, it would seem that alcohol acts as an agent for a temporary feeling of conceptual expansion. It also may act as an agent for a temporary loosening of the relationships between one's ideas and conclusions about self or others and the data one uses to validate them. One validates his expectancies loosely and somewhat inconsistently. In this phase of alcoholic loosening, almost any response can be construed as supportive of one's anticipations. If a person is looking for positive regard from others, he may find it. Of course, he or she might be intent on finding evidence for the opposite of positive regard. That can be found too. Thus, in this context of greater validation, anxiety is lessened. One's construct system seems to work better. Unfortunately, the person is not really able to play a *social role*. Kelly (1955) defined an effective social role as involving an awareness and understanding of the viewpoints of the other person. In our example of the Navy man, we did not observe much social role. His egocentric preoccupation with his own constructions precluded understanding and empathy for alternative constructions of others, drunk or sober.

Dawes (1981) makes the additional point that drug abuse allows the person to avoid the anxiety of confronting the situations which he or she cannot anticipate, a problem created by *insufficient elaboration* of the construct system. For the alcohol abuser who feels distant from people or who feels anxiety in the typical social situation, alcohol can act like an instant passport to the human race. Alcohol intake can reduce social distance instantly. It can change constructions from 'socially apart from people' to 'socially together with people'. As a result of imbibing high doses of alcohol, the person can achieve temporary reorganisation of his construct system since alcohol intake more readily allows fantasy to create new roles and new construct organisation.

Assuming for the moment that the alcohol abuser employs an insufficiently elaborated construct system for understanding people, including oneself, how is this person learning differently from others? Returning to our initial discussion of the concepts, dilation – constriction *and* tightening-loosening, it would seem that the person perseverates either at the level of tightness and constriction or, alternatively, at the level of looseness and dilation. In Kelly's CPC learning cycle, one shifts between a more open 'circumspection' that can involve dilation and loosening *and* a more closed 'pre-emption and control', identified with greater constriction and logical consistency in prediction. It is the free and continuous movement between the levels of circumspection and pre-emption-control that is needed for any creatively effective elaboration of the construct system. The alcoholic tends to get stuck at the one level or the other, movement between them facilitated only by a shift between the roles of drunk and sober.

Although we have stated that the alcohol abuser may find it difficult to elaborate his construct system effectively for social events, we must differentiate between sober relationships and drunk relationships. Even though the person may not be elaborating his system for ordinary, sober relationships, he or she may elaborate the alcohol-related role. For example, one can associate having sex only with alcohol involvement; getting through the work day only with alcohol; and, feeling that one can not accept social invitations unless alcohol is served. In other words, the person elaborates his alcohol role at the expense of his sober role. The loosely construing role practised with supportive alcoholic friends does not help much in understanding persons and situations outside the drug-related context. And, the more roles in one's life that become associated with alcohol abuse, the more difficult the recovery for the alcoholic individual.

That elaborative feelings within the drug-induced state do not carry over to the sober state is illustrated by the acute upset experienced by a recovered alcoholic who re-joined his old drinking crowd for an evening to test his sobriety. He recalled with a shudder, the frantic way that his host tried to force him to drink, as though the host were saying, 'If I can get you to drink, then I'm not an alcoholic.' He also recalled his utter boredom as he stated, 'They weren't really talking to each other. What the hell did I ever see in them?' In conclusion, the alcoholic's solution for dealing with life tends to bring only temporary satisfaction. It provides an uncertain validation for roles and relationships outside the alcoholic context.

An Overview of Relevant Research

The research on the alcohol-dependent person from the personal construct theory perspective is very sparse. Most of the existing research has been conducted during the past decade as the alcoholic and alcohol problems received more attention from both care-givers and researchers. In 1971, Landfield reported an exploratory study with five alcoholics. He found that three of these subjects had simplistic construct systems which were not very useful in making discriminations between people or for understanding and predicting behaviour. One of the other two subjects displayed a highly elaborate construct system, so complex that few similarities were seen between people or between descriptive constructs. Such extreme separations of people and constructs suggested fragmentation, confusion, and problems in anticipation. When the thematic content of his subjects was examined, Landfield (1971) found that the five alcoholics in this study relied heavily on constructs characterised by over-concern about responsibility and morality. In a study by Smith and Evans (1980) of 60 hospitalised alcoholic patients, such thematic concerns were not obvious. However, they did note the simplistic nature of their subjects' constructs.

Glantz, *et al.* (1981) also looked at the construct systems of alcoholics, comparing them to non-psychotic outpatients and normals. These researchers found significant group differences in both the structural and content measures of the subjects' construct systems. They found that alcoholics were more likely than the other groups to use 'approximate ratings', i.e. ratings which fall neither at the centre nor at the polar extremes. From these results they concluded that alcoholics may fail to declare a construct inapplicable and thus have an increased tendency to continue to apply constructs of presumed limited appropriateness. In the same study, alcoholics defined situations in terms of emotions to a lesser degree than non-psychotic, non-alcoholic patients. There were also some additional problems. For example, these researchers suggested that alcoholics may have increased problems resulting from their lower use of interpersonally oriented constructs. As a result, other people would be less likely to be sources of gratification and more difficult to understand and cope with.

Although these researchers found alcoholics to be oriented to direct impact of events, they seemed to have available only a moderate usage of constructs they felt would facilitate predicting and controlling events. They also had fewer value designations to indicate the desirability of events and changes. These construct characteristics, coupled with a tendency to persist in the use of constructs which have marginal applicability to the situations they are construing, only exacerbate their inability to predict and control events. Glantz *et al.* concluded that alcoholics use alcohol to (1) attempt to change their world by altering their own perceptions, (2) attempt to increase the efficiency of their behaviour (under the assumption that alcohol will increase the efficiency of their behaviour), or (3) reduce the negative feelings resulting from a lower level of coping ability.

Several studies have used a personal construct methodology to investigate self-perception in the alcoholic. Hoy (1973) used provided constructs (and a standard set of photographs) to investigate how alcoholics construed themselves in terms of several contrasts. These included 'weak character vs. strong character', 'alcoholic vs. moderate social drinker,' and 'not like I am vs. like me in character and personality.' The pattern of relationships among the construct pairs was such that the subjects did not *as a group* construe themselves as alcoholics, either denotatively or connotatively, although there were significant relationships for individuals. While not describing themselves as alcoholics, they construed alcoholics as being weak in character, sexually frustrated, lonely and unhappy (but not necessarily solitary), not especially interested in food, and as feeling suicidal. The relationship of self construal to treatment outcome was not explored in this study.

Heather, Edwards and Hore (1975), in a more sophisticated study of self construal, utilised specific outcome criteria, i.e. abstinent after six months, improved after six months or relapsed after six months. Using a standard set of provided constructs (which included elements representing aspects of self constructions and role constructions of drinking) they derived a factor designed to differentiate subjects on the basis of the way they identified themselves in relation to alcoholism and styles of drinking. They found that the successfully treated patients were the ones who made a clearer distinction between alcoholics and others. It is also important to note that Heather *et al.* found that the *relapsed* group had either (1) made the highest gains in self respect (which may reflect overconfidence), or (2) made the least gains in self respect (which could mean they view themselves as hopeless failures). These investigators also suggested that those patients excluded from both the conventional world and from the deviant subculture of alcoholism may feel lost and relapse in order to regain their deviant status and a sense of belonging somewhere. Another important finding in this study was that the patients who showed the most change in construing themselves relative to their drinking (towards either more or less identification of themselves as alcoholic) were more likely to relapse.

Book (1976) studied the changes in how alcoholics rated personal constructs while in treatment. Using Landfield's (1971) modification of Kelly's rep test, he measured the changes in the elicited personal constructs of 40 alcoholics between the first and last week of a 30-day treatment programme. Confirming the prediction, as a group, the patients used their counsellors' personal constructs significantly more meaningfully at the end of treatment than they did at the beginning of treatment. However, contrary to prediction, these changes were not found to be positively related to ratings of improvement made by the patients' individual counsellors at the end of treatment. In fact, there was a non-significant trend in the opposite direction. Another hypothesis that failed to be confirmed is that there would be a relationship between counsellors' final ratings of patient improvement and the mutual meaningfulness of initial ratings that the counsellor and patient made of each other on their own personal constructs. Further data analysis indicated that patients, as a group, changed significantly in the direction of more meaningful use of their own personal constructs as well as those of the counsellor from the beginning to end of treatment. However, the most changes in degree of meaningfulness occurred in the patients' ratings of the personal constructs of the programme's founder. Book interpreted this to mean that the programme milieu, insofar as it reflected the personal construct system of the person who founded the programme, is more powerful than the influence of the individual counsellor who sees the patient two or three times a week.

Additional data analysis by Book revealed that 30 patients changed in the direction of more-positive ratings of themselves during treatment. However, there was no significant relationship between these changes and counsellors' ratings of patients' improvement. Since the issue of whether counsellors' ratings were valid predictors of improvement could not be answered, this question was left unresolved in Book's study. However, he did speculate that the lack of relationship between meaningfulness changes and improvement could be due to the impulsive shift of patients in a short-term intensive treatment programme. More specifically, he suggested that this phenomenon might represent what Kelly (1955) described as the foreshortening of the circum-spection phase of the 'Circumspection-Preemption-Control (CPC) Cycle'.

In a later study, Blum (1980) used a self-construing inventory (developed by Professor Monte Page, University of Nebraska-Lincoln) to study changes in self-esteem and the relationship of those self-esteem changes to the positiveness of various sober and drinking roles in 50 male alcoholic in-patients in a 30-day treatment programme. This was the same treatment programme utilised earlier by Book (1976). Blum examined both changes in self-esteem and the relationship of the alcoholic's self-esteem to his ideal self and his perception of the positiveness of various drinking roles. While previous research had demonstrated that the self-esteem of the alcoholic improves as a result of treatment, Blum wished to establish whether the degree of agreement between the alcoholic's newly developed self-esteem and his ideal self was related to the alcoholic's anticipation (expectancy) for the role of sobriety. He used scores on the MMPI and counsellor's prognostic ratings of subjects as outcome measures.

Blum's prediction that positiveness of self, ideal self and the role of the recovered alcoholic would correspond closely in the good prognostic group was confirmed only when the counsellors' prognostic ratings were utilised as the outcome criteria. Blum also hypothesised that the good prognosis patients would develop a negative relationship between their self positiveness and their perception of their past drinking roles. This prediction was also confirmed. Both of these changes in perceptions of self and drinking roles showed dramatic changes across the 30-day treatment span. The poor prognostic group showed none of these changes. Blum concluded his summary of the research by noting:

> These results suggest an important issue to address in treatment is the alcoholic's expectations for sobriety and how they conflict with his ideal values. While raising the alcoholic's self-esteem may be a necessary factor in recovery, without the development

of positive, meaningful role expectations for sobriety and a correspondence between ideal self and the newly entered role of recovering alcoholic, prognosis for long-term sobriety might be poor. (1980, *ii-iii*)

This observation by Blum of the alcoholic's need to reconstruct events, paralleled the observations by Fransella in her study of stuttering and stutterers. As she notes, 'So the stutterer has to find out what life will all be about when he becomes fluent. The central theme of this theory is that *the road from stuttering to fluency* is paved by reconstructions' (italics hers, 1972, p. 70). If we substituted the words *alcoholic, sober, drinking* and *sobriety* for *stutterer, fluent, stuttering* and *fluency* in the above statement it would fit the alcoholic as well, suggesting that the goals of change for these two disorders may be much the same even if the contents of constructions are different.

Finally, basing their research on Kelly's sociality corollary, Landfield and Rivers (1975) assumed that the alcoholic feels alienated from others and that alcohol may be a method of bridging social barriers (or of avoiding more profound social interactions). More specifically, it was hypothesised that their group procedure, designed to facilitate interaction between unacquainted people, would lead to the following consequences for group members: (A) an increase in their ability to predict other group members' responses, (B) an increase in their positive feelings toward group members and (C) an increase in their expectations of positive feelings from group members. A secondary prediction (D) was that positive feelings toward the 'group in general' would be related to an increased positive feeling toward 'people in general.' Hypotheses (A) and (C) were confirmed for all alcoholic subjects; hypothesis (B) was confirmed for 13 out of the 15 alcoholic group members. The secondary hypothesis (D) was confirmed for all but two of the alcoholic group members, i.e. of the eight members in one group and five in the second who showed a positive change in group expectations, there was also an increase in their positive expectations for people in general. We will elaborate on the potential clinical significance of this group procedure in the next section.

Treatment Issues and Personal Construct Theory

In this section we will outline several issues which seem implied in
the PCT approach to alcoholism. Where appropriate, we will use
the Interpersonal Transaction group (IT) (Landfield and Rivers,
1975) to illustrate how these issues were or could be dealt with using
this treatment strategy. Due to space limitation, we will not attempt
a detailed description of the group procedure, except as it bears on
the specific issues under consideration. For a more detailed description of the IT group procedure, the reader is referred to the original
article and to Landfield (1979).

One final note: this chapter represents the continued development of our thinking about alcohol abuse and PCT since 1975. The
reader will not be surprised, then, to find that many of the conceptualisations described here were not present in the original article
(Landfield and Rivers, 1975).

The Alcoholic has Major Difficulties in Social Interaction

He or she seems to apply inappropriate constructs in the attempt to
understand and predict people. Because of this difficulty, the
person experiences a continual invalidation or lack of validation
and, hence, feels anxious in his interactions with other individuals
when he is sober.

Now a major thrust of the IT group is to reduce the threat of
invalidation for our alcoholic subjects. First, we attempt to reduce
the ambiguity of the typical group treatment situation by having
each person talk with each other person in the group, in pairs, for a
structured length of time. We further reduce the ambiguity of group
treatment by providing, in most sessions, specific topics for discussion in the conversational pairs. Finally, we reduce potential
invalidation by stressing with group members that they should listen
carefully to one another and to try understanding each other's
viewpoints *without* confrontation, criticism, or by questioning the
logic of the other person. Although members share their thoughts
and feelings with others, they need not share to the point of great
discomfort. Further, it is expected that, on the same discussion
topic, group members will share different things with different
people. In other words, we allow for discrimination in one's
sharing.

This focus on sharing with discrimination and listening and responding without confrontation and criticism seems to lower the

anxiety of group members. Moreover, these instructions seem to maximise social interactions early in the group. In this context of sharing and careful listening, the person begins more effectively to use others as sources of gratification.

The Recovering Alcoholic Needs to Accept as Positive the Role of Sobriety and to Relegate Alcohol Use to a Less Important and Even Negative Position in His Life

This means that the alcoholic who has elaborated his alcohol using role, in positive ways, must begin to experience a greater elaboration and positiveness from his sober role. He or she needs to experience validation through the sober role. This shift in focus of elaboration requires an increased capacity to endure the 'threat of change'. In regard to this point, Kelly hypothesised that a construction of change and a more hopeful view of it might facilitate change.

To create a more constructive view of change, the IT group procedure includes sessions that focus on change. For example, 'Talk about wise and unwise decisions that have been made and could be made in the future. Share your thoughts and feelings about why I should drink the way I do and not drink the way I do. Discuss myself in the next six months — things I plan to do and the way I want to be and feel.'

As we noted elsewhere (Landfield and Rivers, 1975; Landfield, 1979), many changes occurred in how the people viewed relationships and themselves over the 20 sessions of the IT group. However, our experience with the IT group suggests that we may need more sessions for alcoholic members that focus on the commitment to change issues; e.g. 'In what ways do I need to change and in what ways do I need to remain the same? What will I find most difficult about the sober life and what will I find most difficult about the drinking life?'

The Alcohol Abuser Seems to Get Stuck at One Level or Another of the CPC Learning Cycle

This cycle between circumspection and pre-emption-control, encompasses the alternative processes of dilating-constricting and loosening-tightening. Circumspection seems linked with dilated and loosened construction. The pre-emption control phase seems linked to more constricted and tightened construction. We have theorised that the alcoholic tends to get stuck at one or the other of these levels. Alcohol provides the primary vehicle for shifting to the level of dilated and loosened construction, a level at which the person is less likely to experience invalidation.

The IT group tends to facilitate a more appropriate use of the CPC cycle, with greater movement between levels of construction, *in the role of sobriety*. Within a session, the first dyadic discussions seem more circumspective. Later dyads seem to show more pre-emption and control. In other words, the IT group members begin to function at both levels of the cycle. Over the span of the IT group sessions, they tend to get 'unstuck' from one level of function and without the use of alcohol.

The 'value' session is of particular interest in this respect. In this session, subjects are asked to discuss, 'what is it I value and what is it I don't value.' The struggle and lack of clarity that mark the first dyads give way to more assured and clearer statements in the later dyads. The freedom to think through and to share within a supportive context seems to facilitate greater movement along the learning dimensions of dilated-constricted and tightened-loosened construction.

Now one might question the absence of *direct* criticism and invalidation in the IT group. However, we contend that listening to the differing views of others can serve as sources of validation-invalidation of one's construct systems, sources of validation that tend to minimise defensiveness. After all, one is not being forced to change. Moreover, it is the constructs of sharing, listening, and changing that tend to take on a shared superordinacy for group members. Process constructions become centrally valued, providing a security of stable meaning in the midst of concrete change.

The More a Person's Life is Involved with Alcohol, the More Difficult it is to Establish Sobriety and an Effective Non-drinking Life

As we have noted, the person must learn to appreciate the positive values of a sober role.

As Kelly has noted, sobriety means losing a 'core role'. While many professionals hesitate to use Alcoholics Anonymous (AA), one could reconstruct the admonitions of AA as 'new constructs' for the recovering alcoholic. These provided statements often seen as trite by the professionals, include sayings like, 'Easy does it; One day at a time,' etc . . . One way of seeing the utility of these statements is that they provide *temporary* constructions to help the alcoholic deal with the immediate sense of chaos and fragmentation that can occur during the early stages of recovery. However, it is critical that the person develop new constructions for the sober role if he is to achieve the level of adjustment necessary for a full and productive psychological life.

All of these issues we've discussed in terms of alcohol abuse, could be resolved in other ways and be reflected in other forms of human and psychological problems. What makes the use of alcohol virtually unique as a solution to these human difficulties is that it constitutes a ready and almost instant temporary solution to the person's problems. Once it is selected as the method of choice, it is difficult to overcome because it effectively and efficiently (albeit temporarily) deals with the person's problems.

In summary, we have attempted to outline our perception of how alcohol problems develop in terms of personal construct theory. We have also attempted to review the research that has been produced using this theoretical stance. Finally, we have attempted to show how PCT can be translated into treatment strategies. Nothing has impressed us more in writing this chapter than the fact that PCT has great potential for contributing to the future theory and treatment of alcohol abuse. While the realistic space limitations of this chapter have made our effort only a modest overview of PCT and this problem area, the struggle we had in selecting what we have presented suggests that much more can and will be written from the PCT point-of-view in the future.

9 CONSTRUING DRUG DEPENDENCE

Andrew Dawes

Theoretical and Research Aspects

The Field of Drug Dependence and the Position of Construct Theory

As is true of most areas of psychopathology there are numerous approaches to the aetiology and treatment of drug dependence. The models presented cover a variety of disciplines and within each discipline evidence of our uncertainty in this area is visible in the multiple frameworks on offer. As Gambino and Shaffer (1979) have commented, there is very little unity of understanding which has led of course to the lack of integrated approaches to treatment and research (Nathan and Lansky 1978).

Gambino and Shaffer suggest that any comprehensive account of drug dependence needs to incorporate four factors which are summarised as follows:

1. Individual differences in choice of drugs, patterns of usage, personality of the user and experience of drug effects
2. Motivational factors
3. The context of drug use and other social aspects
4. The mediation of drug effects by physical, psychological and situational factors.

Clearly such an account would be multidisciplinary, and the contribution of a psychological framework such as personal construct theory (PCT) would address itself primarily to point (1) above. It would stem from an analysis of how PCT could make sense of the individual's construction of the drug experience, how being drug dependent can become an elaborative choice which resists change, and finally how knowledge of this sort when individualised can guide treatment. PCT should not simply present another account which adds little of substance to our already overstocked market. To me its particular use lies in its ability to address the structure of an individual's understandings of his or her position, because it is only by taking this into account that a rational approach to manage-

182

ment can proceed.

The research literature relating PCT to drug dependence is not well developed as yet. More work has been carried out in the field of alcoholism, for example Rollnick and Heather (1980), which focuses on the alcoholic's construal of self and the implications of this for treatment. In the area of drug dependence my own work (Dawes, 1979; 1981) has focused on developing a PCT account of drug dependence which will be outlined here, while the work of Viney, Westbrook and Preston (1984) has discussed the drug addict's experience of self and its implications for treatment. Penrod and Epting (1981) noted that differences in cognitive differentiation are evident in groups of stimulant and depressant abusers such that the former are more differentiated than the latter suggesting that this may relate to their reasons for choosing a particular drug of abuse. Finally certain clinical studies of drug-abusing subjects using repertory grid studies are mentioned by Slater (1977) and by Ryle (1975).

While the PCT literature is underdeveloped in this area, research on altered states of consciousness (Ludwig, 1969; Ornstein, 1972; Tart, 1971) and on the determinants of drug response (Barr, Langs, Holt, Goldberger and Klein, 1972; Carlin, Post, Bakker and Halpern, 1974) provides useful support to the position to be advanced in this chapter. Their contributions will be noted as we proceed.

Having outlined the potential contribution of PCT it is necessary to place it within the context of current accounts. This will not be an extensive or critical presentation which is beyond the scope of this work and accounts of that nature may be found in Glatt (1974) and Madden (1979). Greaves (1974) provides a useful classification of current frameworks within the psychiatric tradition. These approaches are:

1. The *Acquired Drive position* followed by Berjerot (1972) based on the drive reduction position, which posits that the need for drug state takes on the characteristics of an acquired drive which the individual seeks to repeat.

2. The *Avoidance position* followed by authors such as Collier (1972) which is the corollary of the first position stating that dependence is due to the avoidance of withdrawal effects.

3. The *Metabolic Disease position* of Dole and Nyswander (1967) which argues that certain persons have an inherent tendency to

enjoy certain drugs and that the presence of the drug substitutes for an underlying deficiency.

4. The *Conditioning position* which is based on classical and operant learning models of reinforcement. This position is supported by Wikler (1965).

5. The *Automedication position* focuses on the notion that drug dependence is an active choice of a way of coping with stress, and which is seen as adaptive to the individual (in the personal sense of the term). A particular drug or drug experience is discovered through experimentation which is found to help the individual cope with life in a less distressed manner. Adherents of this position generally suggest that the individual was psychologically disturbed prior to the onset of dependence. Major supporters are Greaves (1974) and Wurmser (1972).

No doubt each of the above positions has something to say in terms of its particular range of convenience. The approach that seems more attractive from a PCT point of view is the Automedication position, due to its acceptance that the individual is given credence for active involvement in his condition, and also due to its openness to developing understandings based on the person's own frame of reference.

There are however two possible lines of attack which flow from this position. On the one hand, the person's *drug* of choice may be viewed as a clue to the reasons for dependence, while on the other hand one might focus on the individual's *experience* of choice. The first option has given rise to category system (e.g. ICD 9 or DSM III) based searches for personality clusters linked to particular classes of drug and is reflected in the work of Schoolar, White and Cohen (1972), Hartman (1969), Wieder and Kaplan (1969) and the PCT work of Penrod and Epting (1981). While this approach may seem logical according to normal psychiatric practice, and while it may be relevant for certain classes of drug, it tends to assume that all users of a particular drug will construe the experience in a similar way and that this will therefore suggest aetiological and treatment possibilities based on commonality of personality structure. While there is some support for this contention in the work of those noted above, the picture is complicated by evidence concerning the individuality of responses to drugs at the physical level (Weil, 1975) and at the psychological level (Barr *et al.*, 1972; Tart, 1971). In addition Rounsaville, Weissman, Wilber and Kleber's (1982) observation that opiate addicts comprise at least three classes of person and Feldman's (1968) earlier observation that heroin addicts who did not relapse after treatment often became skid-row alcoholics, lends further support to the contention that there may not be a clear relationship between drug type and personality type.

It is for reasons such as these that I favour a position that focuses on the *experience* which is sought after rather than the *drug* type. The importance of understanding the addict's experience is also stressed by Viney *et al.* (1984), and from a PCT point of view it makes sense to start at the level of the individual's personal theories concerning what he or she is up to.

Up until now the terms drug dependent and addict have been used rather loosely. It is important to note that the literature is strewn with different interpretations of these constructs and related notions such as physiological as against psychological dependence and tolerance. In construct theory terms these notions all represent ways of apprehending reality which are open to revision and in addition have ranges of predictive utility. It is beyond the scope of this chapter to debate the relative merits of the various positions on these matters.

For present purposes drug dependence is seen as a category of excessive behaviour which is characterised by the compulsive and repeated seeking of a particular variety of drug-induced altered state of consciousness (ASC). This would include alcohol but as this volume follows conventional nosological practice, it is dealt with in the preceding chapter. We are not concerned as to whether dependence is physical or psychological. No doubt both understandings have their place (e.g. Collier, 1972). What we are concerned with is the individual's construal of the role which particular drug-induced ASC play in the maintenance of a particular state of affect or cognition, and his or her rationale (in terms of construct structures) for remaining dependent. The term addict will be reserved as a social category for those whose drug dependence is construed as having the socially dysfunctional consequences attendant on a pattern of 'total personal involvement' (Chein, Gerard, Lee and Rosenfeld, 1964). Those who can avoid such involvement which includes close contact with the drug subculture, potential police contact and the threat of declining social position, would not carry the 'addict' label.

Drug Dependence as an Elaborative Choice

In this section, I intend to outline a model which attempts to make more of the notion that drug dependence is a coin with two very different sides. On the one hand it may be viewed as a self-destructive and mal-adaptive approach to life which on occasion can result in death. On the other hand, from the drug-dependent person's point of view, this path can be seen as adaptive in the sense that it helps elaborate aspects of the individual's construct system, which would not be possible in the drug-free state. The model presented here acknowledges both sides of this coin, and will be informed by work which has focused on the study of altered states of consciousness (Ludwig, 1969; Ornstein, 1972) and on the determinants of drug experiences (Barr *et al.*, 1972; Carlin *et al.*, 1974; Tart, 1971) within PCT particular reliance will be placed on the work of Hinkle (1965), Kelly (1955) and Tschudi (1977).

The drug-dependent person's first exposure to drug use is likely to be at a social gathering in which the initiate is taught to appreciate the drug experience (Becker, 1953). When a drug is taken for the first time as Becker (1953) and Tart (1971) have shown, the individual's fantasies concerning what will occur, will affect his experience. This is what is referred to as the individual's 'set'. This set may be seen as a group of loosely held constructs which will guide the appreciation of the drug experience. As Becker points out it takes time for the individual to anticipate the effects of the drug correctly, and the individual's fantasy may pre-empt the kind of sense he makes of the initial experience. Thus the degree to which emerging sensations are interpreted as drug effects is affected by the individual's prior constructions which may be invalidated if the predictions fail. This can result in such a degree of 'loosening' (with a drug such as LSD) that chaos may ensue as in the development of a psychotic episode. The important point here is that drug effects are interpreted.

The initial contacts with the drug experience (both social and psychological aspects) are thus likely to be important determinants of the likelihood of continuing to use drugs. If continuing has limited implications for the elaboration of the individual's construct system (Hinkle, 1965) then it is unlikely that this will occur. For those who find that the early contact enables them to anticipate some aspects of life in a more satisfactory manner, the path to dependence is open. This may include an ability to attain a 'cool' image associated with drug usage in certain communities (Feldman, 1968).

As the user begins to appreciate the effects of drug use, Kelly's framework would suggest that a separate construct sub-system begins to emerge (according to the Fragmentation Corollary) which we can regard as a new construction of the self as intoxicated or 'high'. Mair (1977b) has suggested that we all possess a sort of 'community of selves' which is a set of subsystems about ourselves. We can see the 'drugged self' as being a new member of this community. This new subsystem enables us to anticipate certain events which have limited implications for us when 'sober', but which may be important for the individual to negotiate. These include actual situations such as social gatherings or they may involve states of mind such as depression. It is important to note that while the Organisation Corollary in Kelly's system posits that the subsystems (or fragments) are linked at superordinate levels, the different subsystems need bear no logical relationship to one another and may function independently (Landfield, 1971). Thus there is not likely to be transfer of coping abilities which are developed when the drugged self system operates to times when the individual is utilising the sober-self to negotiate the same issue. As Partington (1970) has noted, alcoholics construe themselves as completely different people when drunk and sober.

It is argued then that the drug state, through the production of an altered level of awareness due to physiological actions (e.g. the depression of central nervous system activity or the control of somatic correlates of anxiety) leads to possibilities for reconstruction. The drug state in effect alters the 'elements' of the individual's internal and external environment, thus altering the construction processes involved in their apprehensions.

For example, the businessman who can only maintain a successful performance on the job by utilising prescribed anxiolytics, is no less dependent on his drug than the person who is dependent on cannabis in social gatherings. The businessman uses his drug to construe events which do not have clearly developed linkages within a particular system when he is drug-free. He therefore avoids the anxieties which would accompany the realisation that the events concerned are beyond the range of convenience of his system. When he tries to give up his drug, he finds that his 'regnant' construct 'effective businessman' is at variance with what he perceives himself able to do when drug free — i.e. perform poorly.

In general what I am arguing is that as the new subsystem is elaborated, the individual's ability to act in the problematic situation when drug free is likely to decrease, as the implications for doing so also decrease according to Kelly's choice corollary. Why try and tackle an area which has limited implications when drug free, when you have discovered a new and easily managed method? The drug-facilitated reconstrual of a particular set of events or aspect of self, extends the previous repertoire for dealing with problematic situations to such a degree that he sees no meaning in acting in such situations without the drug experience. In the extreme case of heroin dependence, one's whole construal of drug-free life is so miserable by comparison with the drugged state that there are clearly few implications for this option. As Viney *et al.* (1984) have noted in their study of addicts, these people displayed a high degree of anxiety and threat towards the drug-free life. In Kelly's terms this indicates that they could not construe it adequately and that many constructs which they did hold were likely to be invalidated. This observation has clear consequences for therapy which will be taken up briefly at a later point.

The gains which are obtained from the drug may be costly (Tschudi, 1977), but such costly gains are outweighed by the elaborative potential of drug usage. Thus the paradoxical nature of drug dependence as being both destructive and adaptive becomes intelligible. As Tschudi remarks: 'Having elicited the pay off (of drug dependence in our case), it is not facetious to ask "do you really want to change"?' (p.325).

In order to become drug free, drug-dependent persons would have to learn to reconstrue the situations or aspects of self which initially promoted drug use as an adaption. Since these factors have in the past had limited or negative implications (Hinkle, 1965) for the extension of the individual's system and because people resist change in the direction of reduced implications, due to the anxiety which this generates, they will tend to resist change and therefore be difficult to contain therapeutically. This of course is a common observation with respect to the prognosis of drug-dependent people with a long history of having found in drug-dependence, a 'solution' to their difficulties Sells and Simpson, 1976; Wurmser, 1972).

Practical Aspects

What are the implications of this framework for the practical setting? We can perhaps address this question with some remarks regarding therapeutic intervention with help from a case illustration.

The first implication is that it is essential that the automedicative aspect of the drug dependent person's habit be considered seriously. From this it is clear that there will be commonalities as well as idiosyncrasies in reasons for automedication, suggesting that these people require focused individualised treatment programmes aimed at assisting them to reconstrue those aspects of the environment and the self which they have learnt to construe more effectively when drugged. Arguing that drug dependent persons need therapy X or Y treats them in a 'constellatory' manner which belies their individual experience of themselves and their treatment (Viney *et al.*, 1984).

Due to the threat and anxiety which accompanies reconstruction, it is necessary for a climate of support to be present. This is perhaps optimum in therapeutic communities of the sort described by Sugarman (1974) in which the members have commonality of experience. The rider to this is that opportunities for the design of individually-based treatment options must exist. In addition it is necessary that the individual has construed himself as having need of treatment and is not there under duress. Evidence of this motivational aspect may be obtained from reports of the person himself and outsiders as to behaviour indicating intent to remain drug-free. In addition programmes such as Day Top (Sugarman, 1974) may require the individual to perform certain tasks to demonstrate motivation while remaining drug-free outside the community. Although Kelly does not have a specific account of motivation as such, the process outlined thus far is a means of estimating the degree of elaboration of the individual's need to change. Another way of assessing this factor might be through the use of a repertory grid in which one might employ the distance between elements such as 'self' and 'people in need of treatment' as a way of estimating likelihood of positive engagement in treatment. Something of this sort has been proved useful by Rollnick and Heather (1980) with alcoholics.

Finally this approach suggests that treatment and research endeavours should flow from a knowledge of the user's drug experience of choice rather from the drug type *per se*. This does not discount the validity of physiologically based treatments (Dole and Nyswander, 1967) for those whose likelihood of responding to psychological therapies is low. Indeed an important contribution of PCT could be in just that area through the provision of assessment techniques which measure resistance to change (Dawes, 1979; Hinkle, 1965) and also the individual's 'psychological mindedness' (McPherson and Gray, 1976). The latter authors' study gives support to the contention that those whose construal of their condition is more 'psychological' than 'physical' and whose system is relatively 'permeable', are likely to accept psychological therapies whereas the 'physical' construers are not. We can waste a great deal of time in treatment by attempting to force people to give up their constructs concerning their condition and accept our own professional notions, when the nature of their construct systems is such that change is impeded by rigidity of structure and a closely linked implicative network. Unless we can train them in the use of psychological constructs (which may be an option) we should perhaps treat them with methods which are closer to their understanding of life.

I want to end this chapter with a brief illustration of how, using Tschudi's (in 1977) method of mapping implicative dilemmas, we can show how a person may utilise his drug automedicatively in order to overcome his dilemma, but at the same time becomes trapped by this solution when he attempts to change to a drug-free life. This approach is useful when exploring the constructs of the patient before attempting therapy and follows on an earlier process of elicitation of constructs relative to the patient's problem using conventional grid methods. Tschudi's 'ABC' method requires the person to express firstly his reasons for wanting to change from state A1 — A2 the more desirable position. These reasons are expressed in terms of the advantages of being at state A2 and are denoted B2. The disadvantages of remaining at A1 are denoted B1. Finally, he is asked the seemingly absurd question 'what are the *advantages* of remaining as you are, and then the disadvantages of changing'. The answer to this question provides C2 and C1. In conducting this inquiry, the person may be required to give all the reasons he can think of (known as Laddering — Hinkle, 1965) at each level.

James was a 31-year-old man who had a long history of drug dependence and a very disrupted childhood. He used various drugs depending on their availability and their ability to stimulate the automedicative state which he needed. James would prefer to use cannabis to induce a 'calm confident state' in which he was not 'bothered by what people thought of him' in order to cope with social conversational situations which normally made him feel 'tense and inadequate'. He stated that he wanted to leave drugs, and expressed surprise that I could ask him for the advantages of *not* doing so. This is how the ABC inquiry proceeded:

Situation; social conversational setting

A1	A2
When high self construct	*When drug free self construct*
Calm and confident	Tense, self-conscious
can handle anything	feel a fool

Disadvantages of taking drugs	*Advantages of being drug free*

B1	B2
I will never learn to cope with difficult situations when sober.	I would not make a fool of myself
I will get sick from drugging	Could get to know others in a more genuine way.
	People would respect me more.

Advantages of taking drugs(A1)	*Disadvantages of being drug free (A2)*

C1	C2
I can be more assertive.	I can't keep a conversation going and feel a fool.
Nothing can touch me.	
I appear intelligent and confident.	Don't know what to do with myself.
I seem to know what to say.	Feel very tense.
I can gain respect from others.	Want to get out of there.

This of course is not the whole story, but it illustrates part of James' dilemma. He wants to engage with others, he wants respect and so on. He has discovered an easy route to these desires through drug use. Changing to a non-drugged state while having potentially positive implications, is not possible because he does not know how to conduct himself.

It would obviously be a gross oversimplification to say that one could plan psychological intervention on the basis of the material presented above. A full assessment embodying nomothetic and ideographic considerations would be necessary. The nomothetic aspects of the assessment would take account of how our patient compares in general terms with others with a similar history and make up so that the appropriateness of a particular course of management could be determined with reference to outcome

research. Thus for example the patient's history of personal relationships would guide the decision as to whether to embark on
long-term individual psychotherapy. Malan's (1979) work suggests
that people with a history of an inability to form lasting personal
relationships do not do well in therapy of this kind. The 'tightness'
or 'looseness' of the patient construct system is another variable
which could help us predict the likelihood of his being vulnerable to
stress to the degree to which invalidation of his previous approach
to life could lead to his 'loosening' his construct network to the point
of becoming psychotic. Finally nomothetic information would
indicate whether he is a candidate for psychologically oriented
therapy at all, and if he is, it would suggest the setting within which
this could take place, i.e. an out-patient clinic, a general psychiatric
ward or a therapeutic community.

Earlier in this section I have argued against the practice of
treating drug-dependent persons in a 'constellatory' manner, and
would regard the nomothetic aspects of treatment planning outlined here as being 'propositional' in nature and as being based on
an assessment which embodies a wide ranging description of social
and personality functioning. Having described the individual in
terms of a set of nomothetic professional constructs, the idiosyncratic aspects of his drug dependence and its automedicative
function come to the fore in designing an individualised programme
of intervention to be carried out within the treatment context
defined by nomothetic considerations.

James, the patient in our example, indicated that he had a major
difficulty in the area of social interactions. His difficulty was such
that it validated notions which he had about himself as being
someone who is not worthy of respect. Thus certain 'core' aspects of
his construct system were affirmed by his poor social performance,
which involved the use of more 'peripheral' constructs. These 'peripheral' constructs embodied the various acts and rituals involved in
behaving appropriately in informal social situations. James' poor
knowledge of the rules and acts involved in playing this social game
did not allow him to anticipate events of this sort too well, which led
to anxiety which was combatted with his drug.

There were two major therapeutic foci evident in the brief vig-
nette derived from Tschudi's (1977) method. The first concerned
his poor self image and the second was indicated by his social
inadequacy. In planning intervention with James we had to take
account of the fact he had shown evidence of a marked character

disorder since he was a young teenager. His 'core' negative identity had had ample validation during his life. A repertory grid focusing on personal relationships indicated that his world was peopled by folk who did not understand him and whom he felt had let him down. The only ones who seemed to understand him were his drug-taking friends who of course validated his perspective on life.

These facts indicated that he would not easily build up a trusting relationship with an individual therapist, although one could clearly see his need for fairly major personality change. In addition the 'tightness' of his negative self-image together with its long incubation, would counter-indicate change in this form of therapy (Malan, 1979). It seemed as though a greater likelihood of change in core role construing would occur in a context in which his negative approach could be invalidated in a setting which provided support for his active attempts to reconstrue his position in relation to others. He was referred to a therapeutic community in which the above process formed an integral part of the daily routine.

While sharing many aspects of community life with his fellow residents, it was also necessary to address his particular social skills deficit as this 'peripheral' problem served to validate his negative self image. The social skills training model reported by Trower, Bryant and Argyle (1978) and Spence and Shephard (1983) was therefore seen as an appropriate way of helping him elaborate this aspect of life and hence reduce anxiety and the need to self-medicate. Finally success in this more 'peripheral' area of functioning was likely to assist in the validation of an emergent and more positive identity.

James remained in the community for a period of six months, and was able to improve his social behaviour to the point where it no longer generated anxiety. This ability did have the effect of enabling him to put himself across in a more positive manner to others which led to greater validation of his emerging more positive self-system. However the system came under threat when he re-entered the outside world and he required continuing support through visits to the community. This highlights a major problem with intensive therapeutic community programmes. The residents may learn to reconstrue various aspects of self while embraced by the community, but these constructs may not be sufficiently elaborated for use outside, i.e. they are too context-dependent. This is why the planning of the individual's return to the community is such a crucial component of treatment (Sugarman 1974).

A personal construct approach to drug dependence stresses therefore the importance of a careful assessment of the individual before and during treatment. This should occur at both nomothetic and ideographic levels, and repertory grid technique is most valuable for the latter purpose in particular. This approach suggests in addition that models of understanding the drug-dependent person's predicament must take account of his or her particular drug experience. Psychological accounts of the development of this form of behaviour are perhaps better developed outside the nosological system of psychiatry, and should start rather with an examination of common patterns of automedicative experience which may or may not be based on the use of particular drug types.

10 DISTURBED RELATIONSHIPS: A PERSONAL CONSTRUCT VIEW

Robert Neimeyer and Greg Neimeyer

Despite its strongly idiographic orientation, it can be argued that Kelly's clinical psychology is also inherently a social psychology, since it builds the importance of interpersonal construing, 'commonality' between persons, and especially 'sociality' or role construction into its assumptive structure and therapeutic techniques. Given this fundamental social emphasis, it is crucial that any personal construct discussion of 'mental health' and its contrast — whether denoted as 'disturbance,' 'disorder' or 'psychopathology' — reflect the interpersonal milieu in which the individual 'personal scientist' formulates, tests, and elaborates his or her construction of reality. Seen in this light, disturbed relationships do not represent a distinct classification of disorder, but instead reflect processes that underlie and sustain numerous specific conditions (e.g. depression, schizophrenia, marital disharmony). This chapter is written to direct attention to these general processes, to consider their therapeutic implications, and to review and stimulate research relevant to them.

For heuristic purposes, we have discriminated the broad field of relationship disturbances into four categories — disrupted relationships, negative relationships, absence of role relationships, and disorganised relationships. Each is defined by a characteristic *mode of relating* to (at least some) other persons. In doing this, we have emphasised the *construing processes* that are associated with each, rather than attempting to treat different categories as necessarily different in 'type.' One implication of this conceptual strategy is that the reader may see some familiar diagnostic groups (e.g. depressives and sociopaths) discussed under the same heading (absence of role relationships), while others will be distributed across a number of categories. For example, organising the discussion along process lines may help to dispel the 'uniformity myth' that typifies many discussions of marital disturbance. From the present perspective, the conflicted marital relationship may be disrupted, negative, disorganised or even absent. Thus, we will be

195

distinguishing among relationship disorders on psychological rather than nosological grounds. Although our emphasis on distinctive features of construing associated with each class of disorder may strike some readers as highly cognitive, we will emphasise equally the salient *negative emotions* that characterise each class, and illustrate them through the use of clinical examples. Finally, we will sketch some assessment and intervention strategies for these conditions, tethering our recommendations to research findings whenever possible.

A Taxonomy of Disordered Relationships

The contribution of interpersonal relationships to psychological health is difficult to overestimate. As Stringer and Bannister (1979b, p. xiv) have noted, 'for Kelly, the person . . . was only constituted in relations with others; constructs were chiefly available through interaction with others and obtained their meaning in the context of that interaction . . . ' In a very real sense the individual *depends* on others, not only to support and extend a construction of reality (Duck, 1979a, b; 1983; Neimeyer and Neimeyer, 1982), but also to create and maintain a sense of self (Mead, 1934; Stringer and Bannister,1979b). When close relationships are severed by divorce or death, for example, individuals experience a partial disintegration of the self (Weiss, 1975). This disintegration blurs the classical distinction between the personal and the interpersonal and underlines the position that it seems 'impossible to disentangle psychological disorder from social relationships' (Button, 1983a, p. 317).

The importance of interpersonal relationships in Kelly's (1955) theory is implicit in the sociality corollary, which indicates that the extent of an individual's understanding of another limits his or her ability to develop a *role relationship* with that other person. For Kelly (1955, p. 98) 'the role refers to a process — an ongoing activity. It is that activity carried out in relation to, and with some understanding of, other people that constitutes the role one plays . . . ' Elsewhere it has been argued that the particular *type* of role relationship is defined by the predominant construct subsystem which is engaged in the interaction (Neimeyer and Hudson, 1985; Neimeyer and Neimeyer, 1982). The sports pal, work colleague and close friend therefore evolve from shared activities in recreational, professional, and personal areas, respectively. Each of these relationships has a unique 'trajectory' (Delia, 1980) insofar as they do not aim at the same relational target (e.g. personal intimacy). Nonetheless, as is implicit in Kelly's (1969d) discussion of dependency, every relationship has a vital function to serve in helping individuals to expand particular aspects of their construct systems.

As Kelly's (1955) metaphor of the 'personal scientist' implies, individuals strive to predict and anticipate the events with which they are confronted. They do this by elaborating a construct system that provides them with increasingly useful interpretations of experience. These interpretations are forged within a social context (Adams-Webber, 1979a; Crockett and Meisel, 1974). Only by testing and retesting their constructions against the behaviour and attitudes of other people do individuals extend and define their understanding of interpersonal experience. From this it follows that people develop relationships in part out of a need to elaborate their construct systems (Duck, 1973a, b; 1977, 1979a; Neimeyer and Neimeyer, 1982). Especially through close role relationships, individuals strive to make the world more meaningful, predictable and understandable.

On Healthy Relationships

Because personal relationships 'have the characteristic of attempting to move forward another's construction processes' (Stringer, 1979, p. 107), they can be viewed as enduring partnerships. Close relationships operate as forms of intimate colleagueship in which two or more personal scientists collaborate in supporting and extending one another's critical life investments. This support derives in part from developing intimate relationships with others who share common constructs for interpreting experience (Duck, 1973a, b. 1979a), who apply those constructs similarly to mutually known acquaintances (Neimeyer and Neimeyer, 1981a), and who organise or structure their systems similarly (G. Neimeyer, 1985a; Neimeyer and Neimeyer, 1983). For example, two interactants could support one another's view of social reality by sharing the construct 'trustworthy vs. untrustworthy' as an important way of seeing people, and by agreeing with each other as to which of their acquaintances was worthy of trust. Together with a shared understanding concerning the nature of their relationship (c.f. Duck, 1982; Ryle and Lipshitz, 1981), this similarity confirms the viability of the individuals' perceptions and contributes to more satisfying friendships

(Duck, 1973a, b; Duck and Allison, 1978; Neimeyer and Neimeyer, 1982) and marriages (Neimeyer and Hudson, 1985).

But as Duck (1979b, p. 6) has noted, 'individuals will, over and above the search for similarity, be searching for ways in which their partner can help develop or elaborate their system for them.' One means of extending the construct system, while at the same time assuring high levels of mutual understanding, is by subsuming or incorporating the differing viewpoints of intimate others (Neimeyer and Hudson, 1985; Neimeyer and Neimeyer, 1982; Thomas, 1979). For example, the husband who has in the past discounted the importance of his wife's same-sex friends may come to appreciate the centrality of those relationships in defining her identity as a woman. In this case, he simultaneously extends his understanding of same-sex relationships and comes to understand his wife more deeply.

In developing successful role relations, there are certain aspects of the construct system that are most vital to understand. In a careful discussion of sociality, Duck (1983, p. 47) notes that 'there is a crucial and indispensable element to the construction of the other person's psychological processes and . . . this indispensable element involves . . . construing the person . . . in a way in which the person does him or herself.' Extending this argument, Williams and Neimeyer (1984) found that individuals developed more satisfying relationships with others who they felt accurately understood the way they viewed themselves and their desired direction(s) of change. This may suggest that successful relationship development is also characterised by the ability of partners to understand and support personal changes in what each other perceives to be elaborative directions.

Positive Emotions. McCoy (1977, 1981) distinguishes between positive and negative emotions on the basis of the person's awareness of the outcome of his or her social predictions. Since the individual strives to make the 'world more predictable, and for this purpose develops a construct system, *positive emotions are those which follow validation of construing. Negative emotions follow unsuccessful construing*' (McCoy, 1981, p. 97). Partners remain *contented* so long as they can meaningfully construe the course of their relational process. As this process provides continued validation for progressively more central aspects of their systems, partners may experience *satisfaction*, *happiness* and *love* respectively. The occasional experience of *anxiety* and *doubt*, following from incidental changes in the course of the relationship, are effectively handled by revising constructions to accommodate this reality. Against the backdrop of continued support and development, partners maintain a shared perspective on the meaning of their relationship (cf. Duck, 1982) and therefore jointly negotiate a successful relational course.

Disrupted Relationships

Because 'an essential aspect of relationships is that they are . . .continually unfolding, developing, moving, dynamic and variable' (Duck, 1979a, p. 281) partners must be willing to revise their constructions of one another. A failure to do so denies the dynamic reality of the relational process and of each partner as a living being (cf. Duck and Sants, 1983; Leitner, 1985). Because both partners keep changing, even if their views of one another do not, maintaining static views of their relationship can lead partners to grow apart 'such that original levels of similarity and communication support are not adequately sustained' (Duck, 1979b, p.6). This can set the stage for the *disruption* of a once satisfactory relationship that previously offered validation and extension to both partners.

Relationship disruption is frequently observed in long-standing marriages in which one spouse begins to develop in a direction unanticipated by the other. By pursuing a college degree after spending years as a homemaker, for example, a wife may develop new interests and commitments that do not easily fit her husband's once accurate image of her. Unless both parties can modify their constructions of the relationship to accommodate these changes, both may feel undercut or invalidated in the roles they are attempting to enact toward one another. Numerous developmental challenges over the course of relationships (marriage, birth of a child, career changes, retirement) pose the potential for disruptions of this kind.

In marital therapy such changes in the course of the relationship are usually made clear in the intake session. When a relationship history redirects the confused and angry partners to earlier times, they often re-experience a glimmer of the support and optimism which characterised their budding relationship. Comments such as 'We just don't seem to have anything in common anymore' betray the more recent invalidation they have suffered.

The consequence of this lack of common ground for the maintenance of friendship has been illustrated by Duck and Allison (1978) in a study of lapsed relationships. They found that after a year of communal living, individuals who chose not to continue living together in more personal quarters the following year shared fewer constructs than those who did choose to live together. Of these continuing relationships, those that lapsed before an additional eight month period showed still less similarity along psychological constructs than did continuing relationships. Extending these results, Neimeyer and Neimeyer (1982) found that 60 per cent of all 'deteriorating friendships' (in which partners became less attracted to each other over 20 weeks of interaction) also showed low levels of similarity in applying their constructs early in the relationship, whereas only 4 per cent showed high similarity. Likewise, in marital relationships the inability to see 'eye to eye' disrupts healthy relationship development. Dissimilarity in the way spouses describe others, especially along their important constructs, is related to marital dissatisfaction (Neimeyer and Hudson, 1985). When, for example, a husband views his closest opposite-sex friend as 'trustworthy' and 'caring' and his wife views her as 'manipulative' and 'flirtatious', their constructions are mutually invalidating and disrupt a supportive relationship. The level of the disruption depends, among other things, on the centrality of those constructions for the spouses and on the implications they carry for their images of themselves. In marriage, as in friendship, the lack of support at deeper levels of the system disrupts the relational course, leaving partners feeling confused, hurt or angry.

Negative Emotions. The negative emotions which accompany relationship turmoil can be understood as a direct consequence of the type of relational disruption. Particular events, such as the return to school for one spouse or the birth of a child, challenge both partners to revise their relational constructions. They may gradually experience *anxiety* to the extent that the relational course flows outside the range of convenience of their current constructions. Or the more sudden realisation that events cannot be adequately understood from within the current system may *startle* (McCoy, 1977) or *threaten* partners, signalling the need to reconstrue the relationship.

But these reactions are not inherently destructive. Anxiety, for example, is a precondition for making revisions in the construct system. It portends inevitable change which, if incorporated into the relationship, gives rise to an expanded understanding of both oneself and one's partner. A disrupted relationship becomes disordered at the point that one or both partners cannot engage in this essential revision.

The individual who does not revise constructions to fit new experience is left with three choices: to discount the invalidations and recast the same social 'experiment' (try again), selectively attend to only those events which are consistent with the original belief ('constriction'), or force the other person to act in a manner consistent with these beliefs ('hostility'). Recasting the experiment is likely to become frustrating for everyone involved, as when the adolescent repeatedly implores her parents to recognise that she is no longer a helpless child. Her subsequent behaviour is either consistent or inconsistent with this claim (probably both). In response, her parents can design more suitable social hypotheses (e.g. by gradually allowing her to regulate her own dating behaviour) to test the validity of the construction of her as 'more adult.' Or they can constrict their awareness of her behaviour to those aspects which support their existing constructions of her (e.g. her failure to make curfew). This constriction may relieve the parents' *fear* and *threat* occasioned by the need to revise their own core role structures (as parents of an 'adult' who no longer needs them in the same way). But it will also frustrate, bewilder and anger the daughter whose emerging constructions of herself do not meet with the relational validation vital to their development.

The third alternative to constructive revision is still more disruptive to relationship development. In the case of *hostility*, instead of revising the outmoded construction, the person 'takes further steps to alter the data to fit his hypothesis' (Kelly, 1955, p. 512). In this case the concerned parents may attempt to preserve their constructions of their daughter by applying to her a set of unrealistic expectations which she is sure to fail (e.g. 'If you're so grown up, why don't you pay the bills around here!'), thereby fabricating validational support for their current construction of her as immature. This hostility 'freezes' (Leitner, 1985) the relationship, disrupting further growth or maturation.

Negative Relationships

Compared to disrupted relationships, in which a relatively healthy developmental process has run aground, negative relationships are typically more destructive. In this more stable relational style, partners are engaged in a *sustained* and often *intimate* relationships marked by a preponderence of negative emotions. For example, in the negative marital relationship, the lack of perceived similarity between spouses at any significant level robs both partners of the direct *consensual validation* that undergirds healthy relationships. In the optimum marriage, commonality between partners at the level of their superordinate constructs (i.e. their central values and ways of viewing life) provides extensive validation for each partner's 'core structure,' giving rise to the experience of love and happiness (see McCoy, 1977). In contrast, the negative relationship is sustained by powerful *validation by contrast*. Partners profoundly support the basic validity of one another's systems by embodying the non-preferred poles of each other's constructs. Thus, the wife who places great stock in cultured behaviour can support her system not only by admiring the wit and social grace of some acquaintances, but also by deploring the unsophisticated and ill-mannered behaviour of her husband (cf. Duck, 1977, 1979a). In extreme cases, contrasting oneself with an intimately known but actively disdained other can provide the major source of self-definition. Complaints that one's partner is stupid, unpredictable, and sloppy may be coupled with the self-affirming implication that one is intelligent, reliable, and neat.

Little systematic research on the nature of negative relationships has been conducted, either within construct theory or within the larger field of social psychology. One exception to this statement is the work of Neimeyer, Banikiotes and Ianni (1979), which examined the relation between self-disclosure and interpersonal construing. In general, they discovered that subjects construed most meaningfully those people with whom they had intimate disclosing relationships. There was only one exception to this rule: disliked figures were construed very meaningfully, despite their being low targets for self-disclosure. The finding that these disliked relationships were construed in extremely clear (albeit negative) terms is compatible with the argument that they help provide definition for the perceiver's construct system.

More direct evidence for this view derives from the recent work of Leitner and Klion (1984). In their study, subjects were asked to rate 15 individuals (five liked, five neutral and five disliked) along a series of personal constructs and to designate any of the figures as 'loved' or 'hated.' Results revealed that hated individuals were rated as meaningfully (as reflected in extremity of the ratings) as loved ones, and as significantly more meaningful than those who were merely disliked. Thus, to an even greater degree than disliked others, hated others seemed to anchor the perceiver's constructs by embodying their negative contrast poles.

A study by Ryle and Lipshitz (1976a) of a dissolving marriage illustrates the fixed, reciprocal roles that tend to characterise negative relationships. This was particularly true from the perspective of the husband in their case study. When the marriage was 'going well,' he rated himself as caring and supportive on the grid, and his wife as isolated, oppressed and rejected. When things were 'going badly' this situation precisely reversed; he saw his wife becoming supportive, whereas he became hopeless, rejected, and isolated. This tendency to 'slot-rattle' from one pole to the other of an unchanging relational axis behaviourally validates the idiosyncratic network of complementary roles that Procter (1981) has termed the 'family construct system' (see Chapter 16). A similar dynamic is apparent in Ryle's (1967) case study of a 19-year-old woman, Susan, who attempted suicide when her boyfriend, Brian, challenged her rigid construction of him as weak and herself as strong by threatening to leave her (see Chapter 6).

As both of the above examples illustrate, negative intimate relationships can be remarkably resistant to change, even though in a superficial sense, they may be 'unrewarding' to one or both interactants. While this state of affairs may seem paradoxical when viewed in straightforward reinforcement terms, it is quite comprehensible from a construct theory perspective. Such relationships tend to persist (even in the face of treatment) because they often serve to validate both (a) the self-image of one or both partners, and (b) the basic framework by which the entangled parties construe close relationships. Frequently, *guilt* (in Kelly's sense) further militates against the dissolution of the bond, to the extent that one or other of the parties defines his or her 'core role' in terms of maintenance of the relationship ('If I left her she'd never survive on her own, and I'm not that kind of person').

Negative Emotions. As in disrupted relationships, negative relationships provide the arena for a number of painful and unpleasant emotions. The dominant affect, however, is *contempt*, which entails the perception that the other's core role is comprehensively different from one's own (McCoy, 1977). As McCoy (1981) observes, contempt can be seen as 'positive' from the standpoint of the perceiver insofar as it reaffirms the validity of the individual's current system — albeit at the expense of one's partner. Other salient negative emotions include *guilt* (discussed above) and *threat*, when one's core structure is massively challenged by the partner's threatened exit from the relationship, as in the case of Susan and Brian studied by Ryle. *Anxiety* is not particularly prominent, since the relationship typically is clearly — if negatively — construed within one's existing system.

Absence of Role Relationships

In contrast to disrupted or negative relationships, the *absence* of role relations signifies an enduring difficulty in effectively construing other people *as people*. This deficiency restricts interpersonal development to those less intimate relationships which can be played out in light of a superficial or circumscribed construing of the other. Deeper role relations (e.g. close friendship, marriage) are frustrated by the limited nature of interpersonal understandings; limitations imposed by certain restrictive features in the content and structure of the person's psychological processes (cf. Duck, 1983, p. 50). Among the best-studied of these features is 'cognitive complexity', which can be understood as 'the number of different dimensions of judgment used by a person' (Tripodi and Bieri, 1964, p. 122). Several lines of research converge to suggest that the development of productive role relationships is jeopardised by reliance on simplistic forms of interpersonal construing.

For example, Applegate (1983a) has argued that social cognition undergoes a characteristic development from concrete and global to more abstract and complex conceptions over the course of experience. He further reasoned that poorly developed interpersonal construct systems should adversely affect the quality of communication in the context of interpersonal persuasion. In keeping with this rationale, he found that more 'complex' perceivers, when placed in a situation involving a conflict of interest, utilised a larger number of different persuasive strategies, were better able to adapt their communication to the listener's perspective, and made greater effort to create and maintain a positive interpersonal relationship. In contrast, the interactions of less complex persons showed higher levels of relational inflexibility, insensitivity and negativity. Less complex individuals apparently pursued their persuasive goals more doggedly, without modifying their approach to better fit the listener's viewpoint. In all, the results of this work offered 'consistent evidence supporting the argument that individuals with more developed construct systems evidence a more complex strategic orientation in their persuasive communication with others' (Applegate, 1983a, p. 200).

These findings prompt interesting questions concerning the relationship between cognitive complexity and social competence, where the latter is understood as the ability to adjust one's constructions of social experience 'as the demands of the situations change and different needs become salient' (Reid, 1979, p. 236). Because more complex persons are better able to adopt the perspective of others (Olsen and Partington, 1977), they may be better able to discern information regarding social expectations and to modify behaviour accordingly. In contrast, less complex persons may be hampered by a limited ability to adopt others' viewpoints and hence display more limited behavioural repertoires in social interactions (Applegate, 1983b).

Some of the clinical implications of this reasoning for the development of role relationships are suggested by work on Machiavellianism, psychopathy, and delinquency, where similar deficiencies in complexity of social construing have been linked to the inablity to form genuine role relationships. For example, Delia and O'Keefe (1976) reasoned that the interpersonally manipulative and emotionally distant characteristics of Machiavellians might be due to their inability to understand others as *people*, viewing them instead only as a means toward an end (cf. Leitner, 1985). Results of their two-part study supported this reasoning in that significant negative correlations were noted between Machiavellianism and cognitive complexity along psychological constructs. More recent work by Sypher, Nightingale, Vielbhaber and Sypher (1981) has qualified these findings by failing to note a significant relationship between Machiavellianism and *overall* interpersonal complexity. Insofar as they neglected to distinguish psychological from non-psychological constructs, however, the authors allowed that 'it may still be that low Machs, while no more interpersonally complex, utilise more "psychological" and fewer "non-psychological" constructs that their high Mach peers' (p. 219).

Further evidence bearing on the relationship between features of the construct system and the ability to develop effective, positive role relationships derives from Widom's (1976) study of psychopathy. Groups of psychopaths and controls were asked to construe different social situations and to predict how they thought 'other people in general' might view these same situations. Results indicated that the construct systems of the psychopaths were consistently idiosyncratic. They also showed significant misperception about people in general, failing to distinguish between their own and others' perceptions. In other words, psychopaths 'do not think people think differently, and hence, they make little effort to modify their own construct systems' (Widom, 1976, p. 622). Results were interpreted as indicating a deficiency in the psychopath's ability to take the role of others, which in turn blocked the establishment of more meaningful role relationships.

A similar argument has been advanced regarding other disorders. Hayden, Nasby and Davids (1977), for instance, found that emotionally disturbed boys had simplistic interpersonal construct systems that hampered their ability to respond appropriately to social interactions. They found that the better a boy was able to view a situation from another child's perspective, the more appropriate was the child's behaviour, again implicating the ability to subsume another's constructions with more productive role relationships. In a similar vein, delinquency has been linked to the juvenile's inability to enter into role relations. From their analysis of several cases of delinquency, Miller and Treacher (1981) concluded that delinquent boys have difficulty in understanding and identifying with positive adult role models because they possess poorly developed interpersonal construct systems.

Negative Emotions. A range of emotional experience may follow from this set of conditions depending on whether role relationships are entirely absent or merely curtailed. In the latter case, the individual may experience a chronic sense of emptiness, since his or her germinal core role is deprived of the consensual validation that follows from meaningful involvement with others. Such persons may also experience *anxiety* when confronted with interpersonal events that lie beyond the range of convenience of their underdeveloped systems for social construing. For instance, the college freshman whose system is inadequate for anticipating the complexity of heterosexual situations may become acutely anxious when faced with the social demands of the collegiate environment. One response to this situation might be *constriction*, or 'drawing in the outer boundaries of his perceptual field' (Kelly, 1955, p. 477), perhaps by withdrawing from social interactions and absorbing himself in his studies. In this case he retains the ability to anticipate experience only by restricting the events to be interpreted (cf.

Button, 1983a). This can lead to a continued cycle of constriction and isolation: the more he constricts, the more isolated he becomes, and the fewer persons with whom he interacts, the less often he will encounter events which force a revision of his constricted system. A process of this kind may be operative in depression, where constriction at the level of the construct system may be associated with sensed distance from other people (R. Neimeyer, 1984, and Chapter 4).

In cases of greater dysfunction, such as psychopathy, anxiety may be minimal because the individual lacks a more abstract psychological approach to relationships (viewing them in terms of loyalty or sensitivity to others). Instead, others are viewed in more concrete, egocentric terms (e.g. bearing on their wealth or availability) which permit fairly accurate, if shallow, predictions of their behaviour. The pickpocket who enacts his 'role' with shoppers in a crowded market does so on the basis of his understanding of them as 'easy marks,' not on the basis of an appreciation of their humanity.

Similarly, the absence of *guilt* in psychopathy also follows from an underdeveloped, concrete core role structure. Not having organised his identity along psychological lines, the confidence artist does not feel dislodged from a self-image in which trust and respect for others figure highly. Instead, he experiences *satisfaction* (McCoy, 1977) as the result of having validated his construction of himself as 'clever' or 'successful.' In such cases the experience of anxiety or guilt might be viewed as a positive indicator that germinal personal or social constructions are being ordered along more humanistic lines.

Disorganised Relationships

Like the absence of role relationships, the experience of disorganised relationships is usually pervasive, in that they stem from an individual's *general* deficit in social construing, rather than a *focal* difficulty in construing one or a few other persons. Duck (1984) points out that in cases of such 'pre-existing liabilities . . .the relationship is not itself the problem: rather it is one of the constituent partners who requires detailed attention.' Both the failure to construct role relationships and the tendency to schematise them in only a disorganised way represent liabilities of this kind.

As is true of the disorders discussed above, the experience of a disorganised social world is a matter of degree, ranging from the interpersonal confusion of the obsessive to the chaotic relationships of the thought-disordered schizophrenic (cf. Button, 1983a). Despite their manifest dissimilarities, the common denominator in these disorders is the failure of the person's construct system to provide a coordinated framework for social perception, one that permits an integrated, coherent interpretation of complex social phenomena.

Specifically, Landfield (1980a; 1982) has argued that a vulnerability to 'chaotic fragmentalism' of interpersonal experience is a function of construction systems that are *highly differentiated* but only *poorly integrated*. Construct systems are considered differentiated if they comprise a great many 'functionally independent' discriminations, as when construing an acquaintance as 'sharp' rather than 'dull' carries no implications for whether she might also be 'studious' rather than 'lazy,' or 'well-read' rather than 'illiterate.' In the limiting case, operating on the basis of such a system might permit one to make a number of *specific* attributions to other people, but without being able to fit them together to form a meaningful overall schema within which one's discrete impressions make sense. What is lacking is the ability to integrate constructions of another's behaviour through the use of what Kelly (1955) terms permeable superordinate constructs (e.g. intellectual vs. non-intellectual'), higher-order dimensions that link together a number of subordinate implications.

Rigdon and Epting (1983) have provided a clinical illustration of social perceptual disorganisation in their case study of an obsessive client, Jay, who presented for therapy with a paralysing inability to act decisively regarding his personal relationships or career choice. A grid study of Jay's interpersonal construct system was performed, and his ratings of several important figures in his life were analysed by three different scoring methods. The conclusions drawn from the grid study were consistent across methods: Jay appeared to have a highly differentiated system for making minute distinctions among people, but lacked the flexible overarching constructs needed to integrate his numerous specific ways of viewing others and himself. As Jay himself formulated his problem in therapy, 'I have thousands of ways to focus on details, but no way of standing back to get the overall picture.' Reflecting on Jay's apparent fragmentalism, Rigdon and Epting (1983, p. 255) noted that it was 'small wonder he had such difficulty deciding what to do in a world he perceived as chaotic'.

Controlled investigations have been conducted of the interpersonal perceptions of individuals displaying various levels of conceptual disorganisation. Studying an essentially normal sample of college students, Neimeyer and Banikiotes (1980) found that individuals who engaged in inflexible levels of self-disclosure across contexts varying in intimacy tended to employ construct systems marked by high differentiation but low integration. Thus, more disorganised social perceivers seemed less attuned to subtle cues indicating the appropriate intimacy level of disclosure. A second study by Neimeyer, Neimeyer and Landfield (1983) also examined interpersonal deficits associated with varying levels of system fragmentation and integration. Subjects in their study participated in 20 weekly Interpersonal Transaction groups (Landfield, 1979), during which they engaged in carefully regulated dyadic self-disclosure exercises. Grid testing was administered after four and eighteen weeks of interaction, along with a task requiring each group member to make predictions regarding the way that each of the others construed him- or herself. As predicted, individuals who were high in differentiation but low in integration were the least accurately predicted by other interactants, followed by highly differentiated, highly integrated targets. Persons who were relatively undifferentiated social perceivers, but who were highly integrated were most easily predicted. This finding is consistent with Leitner's (1985) contention that 'the confusion and disorganisation associated with chaotic fragmentalism . . . will hinder others in their attempts to understand the fragmentalist.' Construct system structure of *predictors*, however, was unrelated to predictive accuracy, and the effect of target structure held only after four, and not eighteen weeks of interaction. In combination, these studies suggest that even the low levels of fragmentalism found in these non-psychiatric samples are associated with difficulties in understanding and being understood by other persons, at least in the initial stages of acquaintance. Not surprisingly, the greater levels of disorganisation found in clinical samples can have more serious consequences.

The suicidal individual is a case in point. According to personal construct theory (Kelly, 1961; R. Neimeyer, 1984), self-destructive behaviour becomes likely under two main circumstances: depressive fatalism and anxious indeterminacy. The former often represents a deliberate choice predicted on the conviction that the future offers no real prospect of change in a hoped-for direction; in all significant respects, it seems utterly predictable. In sharp contrast, the latter reflects a desperate bid for certainty in a world that has become totally unpredictable. This condition of total anxiety is closely linked to construct system disorganisation as discussed in this section, in that the ability to interpret and anticipate social experience depends on an intact system of interpersonal construing. Evidence in support of this position is reviewed in Chapter 6.

Finally, a large body of literature has demonstrated the existence of conceptual disorganisation or 'loosening' in schizophrenic thought disorder (see Adams-Webber, 1979b, and Chapter 3 for reviews). Not only is serious fragmentation characteristic of the construing of schizophrenics compared to other diagnostic groups (Bannister, 1960; 1962), but it also is specific to the area of *interpersonal* construing, with construing of physical objects left relatively intact (Bannister and Salmon, 1966). Bannister has advanced a *serial invalidation* hypothesis (see Chapter 3) which may help explain why loss of construct system structure is focal to the social realm. In keeping with theories emphasising 'double-binding' communications within the schizophrenic's family (Berger, 1978), Bannister argued that conceptual disorganisation could result from having one's interpersonal predictions repeatedly disconfirmed. By employing a highly differentiated system in which no construction carries any implication for any other, the schizophrenic may minimise the short-term costs of having his or her hypotheses about other people invalidated, but only at the long-term cost of living in a shifting and fragmentary social world.

Negative Emotions. Despite the obvious differences in severity of disorders included in this section, the dominant affect associated with all of them is *anxiety* (Kelly, 1955), the awareness that the social world with which one is confronted is too complex to be anticipated on the basis of one's current construct system. In the case of obsessives this anxiety may be masked somewhat by their heavy reliance on incidental, verbalisable constructs that appear remote from affective experience. But even in such cases, the general avoidance of intimacy suggests a protective withdrawal from close relationships so as not to undermine the fragmentary social constructions they do have available. As Fransella (1974) has suggested, the apparently tight and organised construing of the obsessive may be limited to the area of his or her symptoms, leaving the domain of interpersonal construing much less structured and more anxiety-provoking.

Threat is less salient in individuals with disorganised relationship schemata, since their core role structures may be less accessible to their acquaintances, and for that reason less assailable by invalidating circumstances. On the other hand, such persons may often experience vague *bewilderment* (McCoy, 1977), as the peripheral and disjoint constructions by which they interpret the motives and behaviours of others shift to accommodate repeated invalidation.

Assessment and Psychotherapy

The literature on which we based this review derives from diverse sources, ranging from social psychology to personality theory. While some of this literature derives from clinical case studies and research in psychopathology, few authors have discussed the implications of their work for the general assessment of relationship disorders, and still fewer (e.g. G. Neimeyer, 1985b; Procter, 1981) have made specific recommendations for treating relationship disturbances. For this reason, we will try to summarise some of the ramifications of current research for assessing and treating such cases, emphasising those techniques that seem particularly applicable to *relational* as well as *individual* disorders.

Assessment

The great majority of personal construct research into disordered relationships has utilised some variant of Kelly's (1955) Role Construct Repertory Grid or Repgrid. While a heavy reliance on this set of techniques is by no means limited to relationship research (R. Neimeyer, 1985c), the Repgrid seems uniquely suited to the study of role constructs, those dimensions bearing on social behaviour. The very form of the instrument (eliciting personal constructs used to construe important persons in the respondent's life) indicates that Kelly 'realised the necessity for a construct system to operate within a socially defined context' (Stringer, 1979, p. 100).

Since one of the primary advantages of grid technique is its considerable flexibility (Neimeyer and Neimeyer, 1981a), it is not surprising that the instrument has been adapted to study a broad range of processes associated with relationship disturbance. For convenience, we will organise our discussion under two main headings corresponding to individual and genuinely relational applications of the method. In addition, we will briefly mention the utility of a number of non-grid techniques in promoting understanding of disordered relationships before moving on to a discussion of therapeutic implications of the above literature.

Individual Grids. In contrast to relational grids, which are administered jointly to the members of a marital, family, or acquaintance network, individual grids can be completed by a single member of such systems as well as by the entire group. While such grids do not permit a comparison of the respondent's constructions with others in his or her network, they none the less can provide a great deal of clinically relevant information regarding the individual's problematic social construing. For this reason, they may be especially useful in assessing persons with absent or disorganised role relationships, where pre-existing individual liabilities militate against relationship success. Kelly (discussed in Neimeyer, 1980) has provided an example of the use of an individual grid to clarify relationship problems.

Kelly's client, Cal, had presented for therapy with a host of occupational and personal difficulties. The interpersonal dimensions of these problems did not become evident, however, until Kelly administered him a Repgrid in their sixth treatment session. Introducing the administration as 'kind of a formal exercise to give me some better understanding of how you see things,' Kelly first asked Cal to designate figures in his own life that fitted a standardised list of role titles. Even Cal's responses to this apparently simple task were clinically revealing. For example, unusually long pauses followed Kelly's request for the names of Cal's parents; he had to 'stop and think' of how he referred to them before giving an answer. Similarly, Cal baulked at providing the names of a girlfriend and ex-girlfriend, since 'no one came close to occupying that place.' Cal appeared equally remote from a number of other figures on the list, thereby reflecting in miniature the absence of significant role relationships in his life. The impoverishment of his interpersonal construing was just as clear in the concretistic constructs Cal used to construe the figures (focusing on their success, age, or social position rather than their personalities), and in his inability to construe many of the people under either pole of many of his constructs. These findings gave Kelly several leads which he then pursued in their subsequent therapy.

Structural scores derived from individual grids (see Chapter 2) can also illuminate some of the personal dimensions of inter-personal disorders. For example, Bannister and Fransella's (1966) Grid Test of Schizophrenic Thought Disorder yields measures of the differentiation of the respondent's system for construing other people (intensity) as well as the stability of that system across time (consistency). Together, the two scores permit an assessment of the extent to which the individual has available only a disorganised and shifting framework for interpreting social experience. Other structural measures also can elucidate relationship disturbances. Grid measures of 'identification' (similarity between the construing of self and others), for instance, have been used to study the inter-personal estrangement poignantly felt by depressives (R. Neimeyer, 1984 and Chapter 4).

Relational Grids. In addition to providing information concerning the psychological world of each individual in a relationship, relational grids permit the assessment of *dyadic* or *systemic* features of a marriage, family, or group that cannot be inferred from knowledge of its constituent members. The 'emergent properties' (Duck and Miell, 1984) measured by such techniques include the relative importance of each partner's constructions in determining the network's consensual view of the social world, similarity between or among the associated individuals, and the ability of members to take one another's perspective.

Bannister and Bott's (1973) *duo grid* allows assessment of the first of these factors. In a marital context, for example, constructs are first elicited from each spouse, and then combined into a grid that the couple completes jointly. By correlating spouse's individual ratings with those completed together, the clinician can determine whose view is dominant in the marriage (i.e. whose individual ratings correlate more highly with the joint ratings). In their own use of the instrument, Bannister and Bott found that the lopsided dominance between spouses helped explain a good deal of the couple's sexual dissatisfaction.

A related format has been described by Thomas (1979). In this *exchange grid* partners complete grids individually, rating a variety of people (including self and partner) along each of their elicited constructs. They then trade grids and perform similar ratings using their partner's dimensions. Comparison of the instruments yields a measure of 'social distance,' defined as the difference between ratings of self and other role elements analogous to the 'identification' scores on depressives mentioned above. G. Neimeyer (1985a; Neimeyer and Hudson, 1985) has employed similar methodology in his clinical research with dysfunctional couples. By asking spouses to rate themselves and both sets of their parents on their own and one another's constructs, he has derived measures of their degree of similarity in construct system content, application and structure. By detecting significant discrepancies between partner's views, the method helps provide an explanation for relationship disruption and points out areas requiring intervention. In addition, it assesses the degree of *accurate empathy* shown by each spouse for the other's perspective, since ratings predicting the partner's views of particular figures can be compared to the ratings actually performed by the partner.

The closely related *interpersonal perceptual grid* of Childs and Hedges (1980) allows an in-depth analysis of conjoint therapy through the use of Slater's (1972) principal components programme. It extends the above-mentioned methods by having partners perform ratings of themselves from three different points of view: the direct perspective (the way I see myself), the meta-perspective (as my spouse sees me), and the meta-meta-perspective (as my spouse thinks I see myself). Among other things, the results of this grid form can be used to identify spouses' ability to adopt one another's viewpoints and to pinpoint particular areas of misunderstanding. Methods of this kind can be useful in treating the negative relationship, where the disparity between an individual's self-evaluation and the way she believes her partner views her may be especially large.

A further extension of grid technique has the *relationship* itself as its focus. Ryle and Lunghi (1970) have replaced the traditional individual elements on the grid (e.g. your mother) with relational elements (your relationship with your mother), permitting a direct comparison of the extent to which partners concur in their perception of their interaction (cf. Duck and Miell, 1984). An additional advantage to this procedure is its specificity. In the traditional grid, information may be lost by disembedding figures from their relational context. For example, a wife may view her husband as typically 'generous' but may be painfully aware of his 'stinginess' in relation to her. She also may not reciprocate this stinginess, highlighting the purpose of distinguishing between 'self to spouse' and 'spouse to self' relationships. Other adaptations of this general technique allow the measurement of convergence between partners' views with the *double dyad grid* (Ryle and Breen, 1972, a, b; Ryle and Lipshitz, 1976a) and of changes in spouses' joint perceptions of their marriage over the course of conjoint therapy with the *reconstruction grid* (Ryle and Lipshitz, 1975; 1981).

Finally, relational grids can be applied to interpersonal networks that transcend the marital dyad. Thomas (1979), for example, has devised a *socio-grid* procedure that maps grids completed individually by group members in sociometric form, indicating visually who construe things more similarly. The extensive research into friendship formation (e.g. Duck, 1973a, b; Neimeyer and Neimeyer, 1981a, 1983) also has generated measures that help predict what pairs of interactants out of an initial pool of acquaintances will be likely to develop successfully and what pairs are candidates for eventual relationship disruption.

As Kelly (1955) suggested, the distinction between assessment and psychotherapy is often a hazy one. Thus, some grid techniques may serve clearly therapeutic as well as diagnostic ends. A case in point is Bonarius's (1977b) Reptest Interaction Technique or RIT. In this application of grid method, interactants take turns 'interviewing' each other using a Repgrid format, openly discussing and recording their perceptions of the various role figures throughout. Designed as a 'getting acquainted' exercise, the RIT has been used in studies of self-disclosure (Eland, Epting and Bonarius, 1979; Neimeyer and Banikiotes, 1981) in a way that combines experimental control with a more natural information exchange. As a relatively structured, non-threatening means of seeing the interpersonal world through another's eyes, the RIT and similar methods may be a valuable form of intervention with persons who have few, or only disorganised role relationships with other persons.

Non-grid Techniques. Despite the popularity of grid technique in personal construct theory, it would be a mistake to identify the theory only with this method (see Chapter 2, and Neimeyer and Neimeyer, 1981b). In assessing interpersonal difficulties, for example, a number of alternative methods have proven useful, ranging from elaborate rating tasks to very informal strategies of questioning in the course of psychotherapy. While space considerations preclude our covering these strategies in detail, we will mention a few of them and their potential clinical utility.

One of the more formal techniques of this kind is the 'disagreement analysis' developed by Slater (1983). The method requires two or more persons holding conflicting views on an issue first to record arguments for their own positions, and then to rate the similarity of each of their arguments to those of the others. Mathematical analysis of the resulting matrix of ratings discloses previously unrecognised areas of agreement, and helps pinpoint the essential points on which the individuals differ. Use of the method would seem especially promising in negative marital or family relationships, where the verbal profusion of disagreements may cloud the therapist's (and the clients') understanding of which conflicts are most crucial for intervention.

A somewhat less formal non-grid method has been used extensively in communications research. Crockett's (1965) Role Category Questionnaire simply requires the respondent to write an impression of liked and disliked others within a specified period of time. Analysis of these free-form descriptions provides an assessment of the respondent's 'cognitive complexity' (the number of distinct interpersonal constructs used) and 'abstractness' (the use of constructs at different levels of superordination). Low scores on both measures have been associated with inflexible and poorly adapted communication strategies (e.g. Applegate, 1983a, b), processes that militate against the development of significant role relationships, as discussed above.

Kremsdorf (1985) also has used written assignments as a means of clinical assessment, requesting that spouses write a description of their marriage from the standpoint of an intimate, but sympathetic outsider. As in Kelly's (1955) selfcharacterisation technique, the descriptions can be perused for the major construct dimensions each partner uses to organise his or her view of the relationship, and for indications of where each spouse's construing of the marriage becomes problematic. Kremsdorf points out that this exercise can provide the opportunity to develop a modified 'marriage contract' which can allow the relationship to develop along new lines.

Lastly, it should be remembered that the most important 'assessment' to take place during treatment may be spontaneous and informal, rather than deliberate and well structured. Often, this will take the form of questions or observations regarding the nature of the therapeutic interaction itself, since as Leitner (1985) observes, 'the difficulties the client has in roles will most likely be manifested in the relationship with the client.' Using this awareness, Kelly (described in Neimeyer, 1980) would often ask the client to describe their relationship, or to discuss himself from the therapist's perspective. Enactment techniques of this kind can be especially valuable for the client with few significant role relations, since they can both highlight his impoverished interpersonal construing, and provide encouragement for his trying to 'get inside' the perspectives of others.

Psychotherapy

Like assessment techniques, therapeutic interventions can be classed into those that focus on the individual and those that treat the relationship itself. This is not to say that a convenient 'package' of techniques can be prescribed that corresponds to individualised versus more relational disorders. For example, there may be times when the partners in a 'negative' marriage (clearly a relational disturbance) would better be seen separately in order to reduce the immediate conflict that would arise in conjoint sessions. Conversely, it may be beneficial to refer the individual with few significant role relationships to group therapy, where preliminary trials at construing the motives, feelings and behaviours of others can be attempted. Recognising that clinical decisions of this kind will influence the implementation of any change strategy, we will simply present a number of therapeutic techniques that seem broadly compatible with the research outlined above.

Individual Techniques. In general, construct theory's emphasis on commonality and sociality as the basis for productive role relations gives strong warrant to seeing the partners to a relationship disturbance jointly. Occasionally, however, close attention to personal rather than relational difficulties will be called for, and these are sometimes best handled in the context of individual therapy, at least initially. A case in point is the spouse who seeks therapy alone, with considerable ambivalence about whether the marriage should continue. Since therapy for such a spouse may represent little more than an effort to legitimise the demise of a relationship that has already lapsed — to provide it 'grave dressing' in Duck's (1984) apt phrase — the work of therapy may entail more individual attempts to 'sort out' the meaning of the old relationship than collaborative attempts to re-establish it. While conjoint sessions are often useful in such cases, they may be more effective once the therapist has clarified the initial agenda of the presenting client.

Turbulent, negative relationship problems may show almost the reverse trajectory. Such couples will often present together, their 'cry for help' precipitated by a recent verbal or physical conflict. If such couples prove unresponsive to attempts to establish them on healthier grounds (see below), it ultimately may be more beneficial to both partners to help them disengage from a relationship that indirectly validates the construing of both parties, but which offers little direct validation to either. Much of this work of disengagement is best conducted individually. Interventions useful at this point include exploring with each partner his or her own anticipations regarding close relationships, with the goal of making them more realistic prior to the initiation of new intimacies. Additionally, since the loss of even a negative relationship represents an important 'discontinuity' in one's construing of oneself (Rowe, 1984), the therapist will need to help each client reestablish a sense of identity independent of the marriage. Frequently, this will entail experimenting with new forms of social behaviour, 'distributing dependencies' across several relationships rather than concentrating them all upon a single individual (cf. Kelly, 1969d).

The use of therapeutic *enactment* that typifies personal construct therapy (Kelly, 1955; R. Neimeyer, 1980; 1985a) can be especially useful in dealing with relationship problems. By encouraging the client to address an interpersonal problem 'as if' she were someone else (e.g. her spouse, an imaginary person who is comfortable relating to people), such techniques can serve as vehicles for training in prosocial skills (e.g. appropriate self-disclosure, conflict negotiation, assertiveness), as well as opportunities to practise taking the role of another.

A related imaginal technique has been discussed by Crockett (1983) in the context of his research in impression formation. Crockett observed that if subjects were given a suitable induction procedure, they often were capable of enacting either pole of commonly used constructs. For example, some subjects were instructed to recall in detail a time that they were feeling very relaxed, confident, and interested in a social interaction, and then to act as if they felt that way now. Other randomly designated subjects would be asked to imagine and enact the contrast — feeling tense, unsure of themselves and uninvolved. What was striking was the ease with which both sets of subjects could do so, convincingly enough that detached observers accurately recognised the condition to which they were assigned. More impressively, their interaction partners were able to perceive the person's behaviour accurately (e.g. as involved and self-confident), even when they had been told to expect the opposite behaviour from them. Although a straight-forward change strategy of this kind is likely to be unworkable in some cases (e.g. when the subject has never had an experience of genuine self-confidence), it may have potential as a means of cog-nitively 'priming' clients for behavioural change in many circum-stances.

Strategies that aim directly at validating and extending the individual's interpersonal construing may also be indicated. Ban-nister *et al.* (1975, discussed in Chapter 3), for example, have experi-mented with a 'serial validation' therapy to reverse the disorgani-sation of schizophrenic thinking. By first identifying 'islands of structure' in which the client retained some degree of integration and stability in his or her concepts about people, and then behaving so as to prove these ideas correct, the therapists tried to help the client rebuild a more workable framework for understanding others. Rigdon and Epting (1983) also report the conceptual ela-boration of a less disturbed, but still socially confused obsessive client. As a consequence of therapy, the client developed a super-ordinate dimension, 'venturesome vs. non-committal', which helped him understand his own inconsistent interpersonal be-haviour in a more integrated way.

Finally, it bears emphasising that the careful examination of a client's emotional experience is among the most important strategies of intervention at the individual level — even if other parties in the relationship are being seen as well. Whenever the therapist becomes aware of a vivid emotional reaction on the part of the client to some turn in the relationship, it is vital to discover what the emotion *means*. Thus, *anxiety* experienced by a client is not seen simply as an irritant to be reduced, but as a signal that some aspect of the client's problematic relationship(s) is so minimally construed that it cannot be anticipated in sufficient detail (Kelly, 1955). The elaboration of the system into these underdimensioned domains can be accomplished through both therapeutic discussion and the assignment of relevant readings as homework. The client who is anxious about developing sexual relationships, for instance, might be asked to read any of a number of excellent self-help manuals on the topic. On the other hand, the individual who is feeling *threatened* by his spouse's development of new friends might be helped to examine what part of his core identity appears to be undermined by his partner's social reorientation. By understanding the implications of the client's affect in terms of the awareness of imminent change in his or her construct system (Kelly, 1955; McCoy, 1977), the therapist can implement interventions that address both the emotional and reconstructive processes at issue.

Relational Techniques. Whereas the individual techniques discussed above attempt to change interpersonal processes by altering a single person's perception of or behaviour in a relationship, relational techniques work directly with two or more members of a dysfunctional social system. One advantage of this approach is that it permits modification of behavioural exchanges that leave interactants feeling mutually invalidated and poorly understood. While some of the techniques useful here are widely current in the practice of couples and family therapy, others stem uniquely from a personal construct approach.

Among the former is the use of behavioural monitoring, an integral feature of behavioural marital therapy (Stuart, 1980). In its standard application, spouses in therapy are asked to observe and record positive behaviours that their partners display toward them between sessions. An adaptation of this technique can help personalise the assignment and focus the monitoring on those specific behaviours that are most problematic for the couple. This requires that the therapist first understand in some detail both the *positive constructions* each partner has available to place on the other and what each would consider to be the *evidence* for these interpretations. For example, a wife may complain bitterly that her husband is 'uncaring'. To help the couple focus on potentially positive aspects of their relationship, the therapist might elicit the contrast pole of this construct by asking, 'What is the opposite of that?' or 'How would you describe someone who was definitely *not* uncaring?' (see Landfield's, 1971, discussion of the 'pyramid procedure'). The wife's response (e.g. 'I guess the opposite would be being involved') suggests a more hopeful direction in which the wife may wish to see the relationship move. Next, the therapist needs to determine the 'concrete representations' that she takes to be 'prototypic' of this abstract attribution (Crockett, 1983). Simply stated, the therapist must elicit the wife's view of what behaviours imply 'being involved.' Often, this can be done simply by inquiring, 'How do you know that someone is involved?' or 'How does an involved person act?' Her reply ('an involved person would listen to me and talk with me') provides a clearer conception of what she would consider evidence for this sort of behavioural change on the part of her husband. Rather than being asked to observe and record general positive behaviours displayed by her spouse, then, she might be instructed to record instances in which he responded to her attempts to initiate conversation. Specific, tailor-made assignments of this kind can often be helpful in breaking the cycle of withdrawal that characterises disrupted and especially negative relationships.

A second elaborative strategy entails orienting the partners in a disrupted relationship to the superordinate values they continue to share. As Neimeyer and Hudson (1985) observe, spouses who seek treatment often present a host of complaints about relatively concrete or subordinate dissimilarities (e.g. 'I like to keep the house looking nice, but he makes it look like a pigsty'). In the 'laddering' technique, spouses are asked to trace the implications of such presenting problems to their 'core role structure' (G. Neimeyer, 1985b). In reply to the therapist's question, 'Why is it important that your husband keep the house clean?' couples usually ladder upwards towards shared superordinates such as 'It would show he respects and loves me.' Partners are often relieved to discover that they are looking for the same things in their relationship at more abstract levels, thereby setting the stage for therapeutic colla-boration.

Enactment strategies, discussed earlier under individual tech-niques, also can be adapted to foster change in couples or family therapy. Kremsdorf (1985), for example, has successfully used Kelly's fixed role therapy approach in treating a deteriorating marriage. After assessing the dominant constructs by which each partner construed their relationship, Kremsdorf drafted a role sketch for each spouse designed to facilitate more adaptive inter-actions and expand their constructions of their marriage. For the husband, who cast himself as the 'leader' in the marriage, this entailed writing a description of an imaginary character who was 'interested in learning about people.' For the wife, who saw herself as the 'passive' victim of her husband's domination, a sketch was written which emphasised the character's 'assertiveness.' The spouses were then instructed to enact their respective characters for three weeks, with frequent in-session role plays directed at helping them discuss, from the standpoint of the new roles, progressively more demanding topics (e.g. household chores, relating to their parents, sexual behaviour). Although the roles were consciously abandoned after the specified period, both partners appeared to gain new behavioural skills, and — more importantly — to recognise that old interaction styles could be changed through spontaneous experimentation.

Not all relational enhancement techniques require the existence of pre-established intimacies. Duck and Miell (cited in Duck, 1979b), for instance, tested the success of different acquaintance strategies derived from the social psychological literature. They gave pairs of unacquainted subjects the task of getting to know each other, instructing one group to look for, focus on, and discuss thoroughly the similarities they found between themselves. A second set was told to focus only on dissimilarities, and a third was asked to follow a filter sequence derived from Duck's earlier (1973a) work (establish similarities at superficial, then progressively deeper levels of construing). Of these prescribed strategies, subjects in the filter condition ended up liking each other much more than those in the other conditions. While the Duck and Miell study was not aimed at remediating relationship problems, coaching in explicit acquaintances strategies may prove useful for individuals who are relatively unskilled at establishing close role relationships.

Finally, Landfield's (1979) Interpersonal Transaction (IT) group procedure holds promise as a technique for treating absent or disorganised relationships (cf. Button, 1983a). The IT group typically consists of a specified number of weekly group meetings, during which members engage in progressively more self-disclosing contacts with each of the other members on a one-to-one basis (see Chapters 8 and 15). Preliminary research on the IT format indicates that group members typically increase in their ability to interpret meaningfully one another as persons (Landfield, 1979), their mutual attraction to one another (Neimeyer and Neimeyer, 1983), and their capacity to take the role of other group members accurately and empathically (Neimeyer et al., 1983).

Conclusion

In this chapter we have attempted to present the disparate personal construct research on dysfunctional relationships by organising it under four headings, focusing on disrupted, negative, absent and disorganised role relations. We are aware that this classificatory system, like any other, has its limitations, and that the complexity of human beings will ultimately render it inadequate. Certainly, in our own clinical experience, few relationships conveniently fit one and only one category. A single relationship may be constituted by individuals who have a background of absent or disorganised inter-personal bonds, may become disrupted as major dissimilarities between the partners come to the fore, and settle into resigned negativity as a poor alternative to still more threatening relationship dissolution. But we hope that the heuristic model we have formu-lated will provide a starting point for clinicians and researchers dealing with the complexities of disordered relationships.

In particular, we see an urgent need for clinical research that would clarify the constructive, emotional and interactional processes that sustain disordered relationships, and the way in which such styles of relating contribute to other psychological disorders. Regrettably few of the assessment and treatment recom-mendations presented above are firmly grounded in empirical studies, leaving the construction of integrated treatment approaches wholly to clinical intuition. With the increasing partici-pation of personal construct psychologists in the larger fields of social psychology and couples and family therapy, we look forward to a time when the outlines provided by current empirical research will begin to be filled in.

Acknowledgement

Work on this project was supported in part by funding to Memphis State's Center for Applied Psychological Research granted through the Centers of Excellence Program of the State of Tennessee.

11 CHILDHOOD DISORDERS OR THE VENTURE OF CHILDREN

Joyce Agnew

It is through the experience of being responded to lovingly, of being nurtured and stimulated, of being valued for who he is that the child's capacity to co-respond develops. His awareness of his self-hood, of his unique and separate identity, increasingly informs and is informed by his sense of others and of his relatedness to them. So he is enabled to reach out to form connections, to enlarge his capacity to contribute to and receive from the world. Becoming human, he encounters pain and distress in a variety of forms. He comes to know something of such experiences as grief, rage, jealousy, frustration, isolation, of being rejected or excluded, of being devalued. Hopefully he will be helped by those around him to make these a part of his living experience in ways that strengthen his understanding of himself and of his connection with others. For some children, however, this movement towards integration may be impeded or hindered. For others it may scarcely be possible. For them, the world they experience is corrosively ungiving, rejective, punitive, even violent so that their vision of themselves and others, their potential for relationship is dislocated, distorted or damaged. They may thrust themselves destructively into the world or with-draw from it, fragmented and fragile. The impact of their behaviour within the family, school or community is such that professional help may be sought. Unfortunately, the nature of that help may be determined not by the child's needs but by the particular point at which he collides with adult ordering of the world. He is accordingly a social, psychiatric, legal, educational problem or he reflects problems within the family. 'Disorder' is involved somewhere along the line. How it is construed carries important implications for the therapy, treatment, management of, disposal, control, remediation and care of problematic children.

224

Construing Disorder

The Medical Model

The diagnostic system and process of child psychiatry is an analogue of that of physical medicine. Disorder is a term within a language system that is purportedly specialist, a specialist language being characterised by a well-defined, stable and publicly agreed-upon terminology with discernible implications for work in a professional field.

Psychiatrists seem to agree that only a few rare conditions such as infantile autism and childhood schizophrenia can be termed as mental illnesses. The vocabulary of symptoms, syndromes, pathology, diagnosis, prognosis continues to be used meta-phorically as a language for understanding the psychological problems of children, problems acknowledged as being rooted in their interpersonal relationships within their family, school and other social environments.

The limitations of a unitary medical language to deal with the changing complexities of children's behaviour and its effect on the adult world is reflected in the extent to which medical diagnosis invokes other language systems, notably developmental psy-chology. Disparate factors such as 'biological' or 'psychosocial' are also nominated as associated with, or aetiological to, psychiatric disorder. This translates the technical and empirical considerations of medical diagnosis into interpretative and evaluative ones, open to contamination from personal, social, political, economic, moral and other non-technical factors. Within physical medicine, disorder is a relatively 'tight' construct. Within the less integrated framework of the multi-axial system of classification of child psychiatry, which assumes multi-causation, the term 'loosens' and its predictive linkage to treatment is less discernible. It may, however, be reified into a thing, a condition the child has. A diagnostic term may be used as if it offered an explanation by giving a name. So the child is encopretic because he soils becomes he soils because he suffers from ecopresis. Diagnosis may also be used pre-emptively so that no reconsideration, alternative construing of the child's problems becomes possible and behaviour that is counter to his 'disorder' may be ignored or misinterpreted.

Disorder and Development

The concern of developmental psychology is to describe the

changes and continuities of human experience and behaviour over time, to offer modes for understanding and explaining the processes of differentiation and integration that superordinate the orderly transformation. It is not a unitary discipline but subsumes a range of separate theories which isolate off as crucial different aspects of development — cognitive, behavioural, affective. Each theory characteristically has evolved its own terminology, favoured methods of research and theory building, and model of the child, since developmental psychology seems to have become almost synonymous with the study of child development. Since each theory constitutes a discrete multi-dimensional system, it would require a major synthetic leap of the imagination to integrate them.

There are, however, some common assumptions. Development progresses in an orderly sequence through definable stages and phases, each of which involves the combination of social and constitutional influences. At each phase previous development is not only added to but transformed into more complex, highly differentiated levels of functioning and in turn becomes a growth point for the next stage. Progress is not, however, smooth or even. Both Piaget and Erikson see each phase as requiring the resolution of a dialectic crisis. Set-backs, reversals of direction, deviations and difficulties are essential to development. The unproblematic child is a mythical being.

In this framework, disorder is some form of dis-order of development. The central point in question is not, as in the medical model, developmental disorder as a specific syndrome or secondary to a primary disorder or the guideline to discriminating normal and abnormal. It is what are the particular developmental issues intrinsic to the dis-order. From this stance, the knowledge of developmental process and of the psychological context necessary for growth serve not only as criteria for achievement or failure but reflexively suggest the means of re-directing dis-order, of restoring it to proper order.

Disorders as Social Threat

To survive, all social groups require to impose some degree of order on their members by prescribing certain values, standards and conventions. People, including children, who contravene or disrupt the social structure are seen as problems and may be liable to censure, moral condemnation, punishment and removal from the group to institutions of social control.

Children require to be trained into and adjust to the norms and authority structures of the group to which they belong, to learn the appropriate social behaviours and right manner of relationships. Where the process of socialisation fails, the child may be seen as disordered mainly because of his impact on the order of the world around him. This may range from the child's causing concern for parents because of episodes of stealing, lying, disobedience, aggressive outburst, to his leaving behind him a trail of defeated adults impotently raging at the intractability of his defiant and destructive behaviour. Such children are likely to be considered to be in need of care and appropriate control.

The designation of children's socially disruptive behaviour as a disorder may serve to allow us, as adults, to deny the possibility that their dis-ordering behaviour is a legitimate, courageous and even necessary response to the unacknowledged disorders of society, e.g. the refusal of a child to attend a school where he is consistently devalued and dehumanised, where what he is offered has no relevant meaning for his life, or the dis-ordered reaction of children to conditions of cumulative deprivation. Moreover, the adult culture gives little credence to what children have to say about things. Their notions are childish (except perhaps when they dare to comment on the Emperor's new clothes). In spite of the folklore of 'out of the mouths' or 'becoming as a little child', there is little genuine space given to the depth and point of their questioning or wisdom of their comment and answering. If additionally a child is stigmatised as disordered, he may well again be denied since protest on his part may be seen by adults as further evidence of his state of disorder.

Disorder as Personal Threat

There may be ways in which children are relevant to some vision we hold of ourselves. The child is a kind of proof, an exemplar, of hopes and beliefs we hold dear at a superordinate level, deep in ourselves, as part of our 'core role structure'. The beliefs may not even be made explicit. The child may equally invalidate our beliefs, call them into question and so disorder our personal and familial ordering of ourselves and the world, e.g. the child who insists on being sexually explicit in an inhibited family. For some teachers the child's disobedience may be seen as a personal threat because of the nature of their own issues over being obedient. If you choose to live your life out in terms of the expectation 'you must do what you are told', by your boss, the State, your next door neighbour, your relatives, the demands of being in a state of graceful obedience may only be tolerable because they are seen as a necessary part of the order of things. The child's disobedience demonstrates that obedience is not of its nature (following a well-known precedent over the consumption of an apple). The child, therefore, is seen as deviating from his proper nature, not as manifesting another aspect of our nature, confronting us with possibilities that run counter or obliquely to those in which we have invested. He is out of order.

The Elaborative Choice

How people concerned with children choose to construe disorder, to define, understand and explain the psychological problems presented by them is governed by the kind of theoretical framework they endorse and how they use this to provide the rationale and techniques for promoting psychological change. One dimension of this choice is between an approach based on eclecticism and one grounded in a single theory. The former may be chosen as offering the possibility of comprehensiveness of understanding, flexibility within discipline, freedom of experiment within an open system. Commitment to a theory may be rejected as a commitment to dogmatism, orthodoxy and prescribed movement within narrow boundaries. Alternatively, eclecticism involves choice and the basis of this choice itself constitutes a superordinating secret theory. This inarticulated theory may have its own consistencies or it may be made up of a number of theories arbitrarily jammed together in disjointed and uneasy alliance along with a few personal prejudices and flashes of wisdom dignified as theory. Similar issues inform the construction of the multi-axial systems of classification or assessment in which eclecticism is formalised. The central dilemma is how to relate, rationalise, integrate diverse conceptual and language systems, and operationalise the multi-dimensional model in terms of action and the help provided for children.

To be useful in the venture of therapy with children, a theory should offer an integrated conceptual system from which propositions regarding the nature and explanation of psychological problems can be derived and modes of inquiry generated. It should also offer general propositions about psychological change to provide guidelines and directions for creative encounter with children. It should, in other words, provide for the professional the basis from which he can anticipate the greatest possibility for moving in directions that elaborate his work.

Personal Construct Theory is one such theory, offering the supports of a rational and consistent system of thought and the excitements of therapeutic eclecticism. Framed at a high level of abstraction, within a unitary language, it is a theory of the nature of man. From its tenets it should be possible in any area to derive implications. Some of its implications for working with problematic children are offered in the next two sections of this essay.

A Personal Construct Theory Model of Childhood Disorder

Personal Construct Theory is pre-emptively a developmental psychology. Within it children as persons are dignified with the same 'scientific' capacity as adults to live their lives expressively or restrictively, collaboratively or conflictfully, in relation to or isolation from others, within or beyond the unique patterning of meaning that is their personal construct system. There are no stages or phases of development, no end to it, nor are children ascribed a special concessionary place. All that can be said of the constructional processes of persons can be said of the child. We require no special language, arguments, considerations in seeking to understand his way of being in the world, his child-hood. This is not to imply that there are no issues of special interest within construct theory with regard to children. Salmon (1970, pp. 197-221), starting with a critique of theories of personality development, has offered the beginnings of an alternative psychology of personal growth based on construct theory and has developed this theme in terms of the social life of children (Salmon, 1979, pp. 221-32). The issue of the increasing differentiation of children's construing systems with age and the movement to psychological forms of interpersonal construing has been a focus of investigation (Barratt, 1977; Honess, 1979), while a comprehensive survey of the use of grids with children has been produced by Salmon (1976, pp. 15-46). The interplay between mothers and their children was explored from a theoretical point of view by O'Reilly (1977, pp. 195–219) and the application of construct theory in the context of parent training programmes described by Mancuso and Handin (1980, pp. 271–88). Ravenette (1977, pp. 251-80; 1980, pp. 36-51) in devising imaginative procedures for interviewing children and in his advocacy of counselling work with teachers has firmly grounded construct theory in the day-to-day practice of a Child Guidance Service.

Being a Child

Personal construct theory's model of the child is that he is concerned with creating meaning in order to anticipate the world and its ways. To do this he poses questions, carries out experiments and evaluates their outcome. This view accords particular significance to both behaviour *and* emotion and disclaims the usual contrast. Emotion is defined within the theory as the construct system in a state of actual or impending change. So the child when anxious is facing a situation which he can only construe in part and the implications of which are unclear. 'What will happen to me if my mummy and daddy separate?' Through his behaviour the child represents a proposition to be tested, he poses a question. By acting in accordance with his hypothesis he tests its validity. His behaviour allows him to know. There is no guarantee that all his experimental ventures will be successful or easeful. Behaviour is not a question of observable movement but of a stance, an en-actment in order to find out. Indeed, some of the child's experiments may be notable for their lack of desired observable movement. He refuses to eat, sleep, speak. Unless we know something of the nature of the child's experiment, we may find ourselves in a position with him analogous to that which might result from a group psychotherapist rushing into a Trappist monastery with offers to help the inhabitants with their communication problem.

Not only is behaviour experimental. It represents an 'elaborative choice'. A primary area of elaboration for the child is his construing of self. Bannister and Agnew (1977, pp. 99-125) comment on the act of construing of self in the following terms:

> The ways in which we elaborate our construing of self must be essentially those ways in which we elaborate our construing of others, for we have not a concept of self but a bi-polar construct of *self – not self* or *self – others*. The ways in which we respond to validation or invalidation of core role constructs and the strategies by which we test out the implications of self are part of our repertoire for construing our world as a whole. If "a person's processes are psychologically channelised by the ways in which he anticipates events," then events can be anticipated by being seen as *relating to – not relating to, destroying – creating, flowing to – flowing from, constituting – being no part of*, Self.

Disorder and the Construing of Self

A starting point for constructing a model of disorder from within construct theory would be, therefore, that however disordered or distorted a child's behaviour may appear from the outside, it carries its own unique sense for him and centrally for his construing of his self. There are a number of ways in which disorder might be related to a child's theory of self.

If a child is to elaborate actively, to undertake great explorations, he can only do this from a basic sense of continuity, from having a sense of himself as being historical in contrast to his sense of being here and now, or in the future. A child's sense of continuity develops out of a sense of his own history; it is constructed from specific replications and repeated themes. History is continually rewritten from the point at which he is, so that what is salient, pivotal or obscure can alter. It is not a chronological account of events but a way of viewing himself. For the small child his continuity may be held in terms that make little sense to the adult — 'I had a green jersey.' 'There was a butterfly and a flower.' 'I had cider with Rosie.' It may be lodged in the continuous qualities of a particular house or things you could do. 'There was a cupboard with pans. I was a cupboard opener and rattler of pans.'

Loss and deprivation are forms of disorder of continuity. It is not to minimise the trauma and devastation of these for children to suggest that at times we are too concretistic in our definition of what is lost such as 'mother'. This is to make the loss too bound into an element. The question is not how to replace mother but how to restore the particular continuities held by her motherliness. Children in care frequently suffer from such disruptions by replacement in another home or family which it is assumed will be continuous with the last one but which may in fact deprive the child of what was uniquely continuous for him.

Piagetian psychology would seem to suggest that in the hierarchy of constructs 'self' is superordinate. The child dwells in the land of egotism. This can present problems for a child if, for example, his over-arching sense of self is located in the dimension of good – bad, with self at the bad end, which he continues to elaborate extensively and apply in a pre-emptive way. 'I am bad and nothing but.' This leads to correspondingly pre-emptive construing of others in relation to him so the world is hostile, persecutory, censuring and nothing but. The child may be so threatened by experiences that seem to carry implications for his being 'good' that he locks himself intransigently and hostilely into proving to himself and others that it could not be so.

Dorothy Rowe (1978) in re-construing the experience of depression has pointed to the metaphors and myths which are the pivots that inform our lives, the axioms that become a life script. These are given and received in childhood and formed into propositions which are implicitly enacted by the child. 'I have no right to be born.' 'I mustn't show my feelings.' 'As long as I do my best — all the time.'

There are ways in which adults deal with a child that may lead to problems for him as to where he places self in the hierarchy of his construct system. Extreme institutionalisation within a regime that frowns on any display or assertion of individuality, extreme inconsistency in the validation — invalidation given by parents to the child, 'double-binds', mystifies and fragments the sense of self. His behaviour and his self-hood are truly dis-ordered. The child who lives out a symbiotic existence with a mother fearful for his safety, isolated from the outside world by his school refusal, becomes a non-self, merged indissolubly with the other. The extremely 'enmeshed' family provides a similar context for uncertainty about the boundaries of self – non-self. There are parents who chillingly and with smiling altruism undercut their child's experience. 'You don't really mean that.' 'Your only hope of coping with the world is to refer to us. We will tell you what is true for you.' The attack on the child's self is primary. He may choose to loosen his constructs to such an extent that he liberates himself by setting up a cloud, thus proving his parents were right all along — he does not know. He can accept the parents' construction but at a devastating cost to his self or he may try to creep between the cracks of the family ethos by behaviour antagonistic to it.

Disorder of Relationship

The child's self-theory is elaborated through the extension and definition of the construct 'self – others', which includes the relationship of self and others. Within personal construct theory, the commonality and sociality corollaries deal specifically with this area. The former focuses on the question of shared meaning while the latter establishes the terms of interpersonal interaction as each person's understanding of the other, although only one person needs to be engaged in such an effort to play a social role.

Our attempts to bring up children seem on the whole to be biased towards inducing commonality rather than encouraging sociality.

The emphasis seems to be that to be part of the world, to grow into it, the child should share, copy, acquire communal constructions rather than learn ways in which people can communicate, relate, negotiate, while still entertaining different constructional systems. Commonality about the nature of the physical world can relatively easily be established. The common construing of interpersonal relationships tends to be more hazardous and as grids have indicated it may be open to question whether we share as much commonality as we pretend.

In terms of disorder, the question can be asked of how might a child fail to develop communal constructs and what might happen as a result. One situation that could cause or contribute to such a failure would be marked inconsistency in what is presented to the child as common constructs – either within the family or when the culture of the family and of the school or community are markedly different. For the child to acquire commonality, constructs must be available, articulated and open to exploration. The child in a family that does not talk much or does not talk much about feelings has to play guessing games. Commonality may be expressed in action by the family but unless the basis of the commonality is pointed out, the child may find it difficult to pick up. Disorder of commonality is likely to manifest itself as a child marching to the beat of a different drum, such as the 'old fashioned' child. The child working from a system of low commonality is likely to experience increasing isolation, so that he has no understanding of what others are engaged in nor they of him. He is truly isolated and open to victimisation. Since it is easier for people to come together through commonality, he may be under enormous pressure to conform.

In order to move to the exploration involved in sociality, some degree of commonality is necessary. If the constructs of those around the child are confused or unusual, it is more difficult for the child to make sense of them. Similarly if the constructs are not articulated or enquiry is illegal, e.g. by being seen as impertinence, a primary mode of developing constructions about others' constructions is ruled out.

If the child has consistent difficulty in construing others' constructions, the complaints are likely to be around his not being able to make relationships. Autism can be construed as an extreme form of failure to construe the constructions of others and indeed of engaging in commonality. We may see the child as arbitrary, selfish, whimsical. He is likely to experience us in much the same way. The problem here is a two-way affair. Jackson and Bannister (1984), however, were able to differentiate within a group of children regarded by others as problematic or hard to understand, those who experienced themselves as confused or unsure from those who were self-confident, their actions being guided by a clear but possibly 'original' view of themselves. We cannot assume, therefore, that because a child is experienced by others as confusing that he shares this experience. When there is extreme failure in the development of sociality as may be the case with some very violent children, adults may end up dealing with the child physically as an object to be maintained. There can be no relationships, no basis for contracts, negotiation or communication between.

Disorder and Elaboration

The superordinate construction within personal construct theory for all forms of problem or psychological disorder is that they are essentially failures in elaboration. Within elaboration, Kelly distinguishes two processes, 'extension' and 'definition'. The choice between them is between security and venture, between clarifying or confirming what we already know and moving into lands where for us mystery, if not dragons, be. The choice is not, however, between one or the other since the processes operate cyclically. Extension starts from an area of definition and in turn may inform the definition. Extension also requires the punctuation of definition if it is not to become chaos.

Disorder may arise out of a child's pre-emptive commitment to either end of the construct. The child engaged in non-stop extension without the benefit of definition will be experienced by adults and other children as wild, overactive, distractible, unable to concentrate. In Kellyian terms he may be described as 'aggressive'. For others involved in his active and massive experimentation the effect is likely to be devastating and infuriating as he rushes through a shifting world or flits randomly.

Children who take up an ensconced position in impermeable definition live in a highly structured, rigid and brittle world, vulnerable to the threat of novelty and change and impervious to their excitements. They include the timid, fearful, withdrawn children, the overconforming 'good' children who are so open to fragmentation with adolescence. They include also the children who seek to maintain the predictability of their world by recourse to magic ritual and compulsive action. Faced with the inevitability of change, such children may lock themselves into a hostile stance against the arguments, persuasions and reassurance of parents and others.

Elaboration is primarily based on choice within a dichotomy. For a construct to work well for us in anticipating, both ends require to be elaborated since the richness of meaning of a construct lies in the contrast. Children on the whole are lively explorers of contrast. Part of what may become problematic between the child and adults is that the latter tend to be in a hurry to have the child make his choice in favour of one pole, leaving the other as a dark patch. The way the construction is put to the child assumes the placement of elements. It comes as a package deal with the superordinate implications laid out. So the child should be obedient and good. To be disobedient, rebellious, independent is naughty and forbidden. The contrast remains inarticulated and unexplored so that if the child does decide to venture experimentally, his experiment with the 'submerged' pole is likely to be badly formulated, sweeping, without direction and troublesome to others. There may be ways of allowing children to illuminate the forbidden alternative by rephrasing the experiment in ways acceptable to the adults, e.g. the seaside may be considered as one such rephrasing of how to experiment with dirt and water and shouting.

Our culture is made by adults for adults with little space for what is of the child. Certain modes of construction are favoured by adults so that the child's strategies, the balance of his modes of construing, ways of anticipating are not represented in our society and may even be seen as anomalous.

Adults' lives tend not to be lived fully in the here and now but to gain direction from long-term anticipation which is shaped by their capacity for superordinate construing. The child's commitment is more likely to be to short-term anticipation. He has to learn how to move to the longer term and to do this he has to develop both a language and methods. If he is not helped to do this within the family or in other social contexts, he may well be trapped in repetitive cycles, the nature of which he cannot see and which for him do not validate what they do for other people. For the adult the situation proves something, which the child does not seem to grasp. For the child the adult's reactions are inexplicable. 'Look, can't you see? Of course every time you push him, he hits you. You started it.' If a child is particularly given over to the joyful immediacy of short-term anticipation, he may present problems for others who end up complaining about his impulsiveness, his sudden changes of mood, his inability to tolerate frustration.

At early stages children are happily engaged in elaborating all kinds of non-verbal modes of construction. They smell, taste, touch the world. They become their own songs and the measure of their own dance, and grow truly visionary with images. There comes a point, however, when the adult world begins to push them towards verbal construing, communication and to knowing through words. Some children may be loth to surrender their initial modes of construction and move to adults' expectations. They may be regarded as suffering developmental delay in speech and language, or be described at school as underachieving, lazy, forgetful, a dreamer or a truant. In such cases it may be enlightening to look to see what modes of construction the child is still committedly elaborating, and rather than see him as disordered, explore the implications of seeing him as moving a vote for an alternative culture. Perhaps if we adults were more prepared to enter and follow children's modes of construction, negotiating with them through a kind of simultaneous translation, then we might all benefit from having a wider vocabulary and as adults we would not suffer the handicaps and disorders of our over-commitment to words.

Implications for Therapy

Like all systems of construing, the model of childhood disorder is not a device for labelling but the guidelines to action. Its implications for work with children require to be worked out as personal construct theory offers no set procedures for therapy. What it does offer is a stance from which to be creative, from which to generate and incorporate modes and methods of work. It is directional rather than directive.

If all psychological disorders are construable as failures of elaboration, with the child caught in static repetitive experimentation, the purpose of the therapeutic encounter is to enable him to move from restrictive and damaging forms of being in himself and with others to resume creative elaboration, to reach beyond what he knows into new areas of self discovery and growing relationship to others.

All therapy based on construct theory is an educative venture based on re-elaboration carried out through experimentation and reflection. The modes and methods of work are based on alternative construing, movement in modes of construction, the use of the propositional voice. Working with children in this language is in some ways easier than working with adults since children are natural construct theorists.

The Natural Construct Theorist

Part of the task of working with adults in therapy is to support experimentation based on 'as if' thinking but adults tend to want to nail down the furniture, to test out the immediate anticipatory value of their constructs. In this sense adults are more impulsive than children. Children are more willing to stay with the ongoing experiment, not tie it to their history or to the immediate situation. There is no problem in being a deep sea diver without water. Children are prepared to live through a series of inventions and to explore them, not needing to prove, to have instant validation, but to live with loosened constructs, to follow emerging pathways wherever they go. It is as if they are ready to hitch-hike their way through the galaxy without a guide. Compare the ease with which children can move into elaborating alternative roles in what we call play with the cumbersome conventions of fixed role therapy with adults. Fixed role therapy requires much negotiation, written scripts and frequent support for its enactment.

It is not only that children move pioneeringly across the terrain. They have a disconcerting capacity to become airborne. One moment you are engaged in rollicking with the elements of life, the toy truck stuck in the sand, the sound of rain on the window, water gurgling down a sink, and suddenly the realm of discourse is moved to a show-stopping level of abstraction that leaves you wondering who is the simple and who the complex construer. You find yourself striding the firmament of superordinacy, questioning the axioms of your life. So Peter cleaning out paint jars in a sink and watching the rainbow of colour — 'Why should so much beauty be wasted?' or Fiona after months of killing off her mother and burying her unrepentingly in the sand, sitting back in calmness and saying, 'Now I know how to love my mother even though she doesn't like me.' Perhaps we adults tend to engage with life in an intermediate agreed level of explanation, causes, consequence, a sort of middle earth which serves to cushion us against too frequent and painful meeting with our superordinate commitments. Perhaps because of the nature of their experience, 'disordered' children require more urgently to deal with the superordinate issues of the human condition.

Concrete thinking may in fact be characterised by rapidity of movement up the hierarchies rather than a lack of abstraction. And yet is
not this an essential ingredient of the world of fairy tales, where one
moves effortlessly from wolves that eat our grandmothers, christen-
ing parties that go wrong, old crones with a strong interest in
cooking, to notions of the nature of power, death and violence,
love, wealth and themes of leaving home, proving oneself, being
part of a reconstituted family? Only, living happily ever after is not
elaborated. Perhaps if it was, the world would be a different place.

The Child-Therapist Relationship

The therapist as a caring adult carries particular responsibilities for
the child's well-being. The relationship is not one of parity. Adults
and children are not equal in our society. The therapist carries the
experience of having been a child herself and of seeing the child as
being in progression. She requires at times to sketch in pathways
and perspectives, to articulate experience missing for the child.
While she creates space for the child and space between them, she
also provides bounds, safety nets, so that the child does not undertake more than he can bear. At the same time she does not avoid
what the child implicitly feels because he might not be able to cope
with it. He already is. The issue is whether he does so alone or is
enabled to make of it an experience in sharing.

Therapy is dialogue though not a dialogue confined to words, an
interplay. This is in contrast to much of adult conversation with
children which is basically a monologue concerned with rule-
following. Even if the child disputes or is distressed by the adult's
pronouncements, his outcry may not be heard but be met by a
repetition of the monologue in elaborated form. Dialogue is a
two-way process within which questions can be posed and answers
found and both be changed in the sharing. It assumes that the
contribution of each is valid and worthy of response. In this,
therapist and child are in a relationship of parity. For both there are
risks and neither knows where dialogue may lead them. The experimentation is dual.

The definition of the locus of disorder being between the child
and others implies that therapy must involve both child and
therapist attempting to understand each other i.e. therapy is based
on both assuming a social role towards the other. To do this each
may have to learn how to be more articulate for the other. It is in the
nature of 'role relationships' that if I wish you to change your

constructions, I must show you how in your terms you can work to the elaboration I am offering. To influence each other we must connect our constructions no matter how old or young we are. The language of the therapeutic dialogue is accordingly the language of negotiation. Negotiation is about alternative construing and requires some construing of the other's constructions. It assumes that neither party has a monopoly on infallibility or rightness. Negotiation both settles the issue and teaches the child about negotiation. The method becomes the results.

Personal construct theory does not accept the fragmented complaint. What is at issue is not the problem but the whole person. This reading is often not accepted by adults who remain bounded in their defined problems. The child is already on the therapist's side in this. He sees his encounter with the therapist as being about him. What he brings along is himself and the engagement is accordingly personal and total. The closeness of the relationship is likely to be made explicit because of the child's demand and assumption that the therapist will deal with all of him, that it all comes down to what he feels himself centrally to be. 'Do you like me or love me?' 'Can I be your baby and marry you?'

Play Therapy

The traditional format for long-term work with children is play therapy. The convention of the session within a specially equipped room serves to define for both child and therapist that this is a time and space for the child, in which he may disclose his inner life of feeling and thoughts with an adult fully present for him. The structure offers the child the choice of how he will express himself and through what kind of relationship with the therapist, through conflict, struggle or closeness. It allows him to run through constructs 'propositionally' with a fair amount of articulation and symbols marking out the process.

The therapist too works from a propositional stance, drawing on a variety of strategies for promoting elaboration, such as 'slot-rattling'. Margaret, aged ten, with two alcoholic parents, had for two years risen at six a.m. to wash, dress and feed two younger children. The extent of her experience and commitment to what she saw as 'having to take care of the kids, be responsible for them', unfolded over several sessions of anxious and unwavering re-enactment with dolls in the playroom. Part of the therapist's task was to help her view herself in terms of her own contrast pole of 'needing to be taken care of, a bigger person is responsible'. In creating this kind of change for herself, Margaret assigned to the therapist the caring adult role in innumerable permutations of 'playing house' while she experimented with various forms of being a child being cared for, from babyhood to ten.

Elaboration may also be promoted in play therapy by extending 'the range of convenience' of an existing construct. For Billy, all life was construable as solo warfare. His only possible allies were the members of his large family who were dispersed through a variety of caring institutions. He had, however, derived some notions of fair play in competition and cooperative effort through his keen participation in games. These notions, however, were restricted to this area of activity. We began to consider what might happen if life was construed in the same terms as games. The starting point was the twists and turns and moments of meeting between us as we struggled to design and construct two miniature theatres, one for each of us. The nature of 'fairness between' was constantly in question as we moved between disagreement and conflict on one hand and sharing and reciprocal help on the other. We experimented with ways of separating the idea of competition from that of annihilation and of experiencing co-operation, not only as a strategy for survival but as carrying its own kind of joy. Through this process, Billy was able to begin to risk a reconstruction of his disablingly isolated life style.

Children can be helped too by shifting from the level of non-verbal to verbal construing, e.g. Jamie, who consistently soiled at home, used puppets to contact his rage at his parents' apparent favouring of a younger child. He began by smacking two adult puppets with increasing fury. He then amplified this action with a roared commentary on their sins of omission. In the final stage he transformed this monologue into a dialogue among the puppets which indicated the possibilities of his forgiving them if only they would be good from then on. At this point, outwith the play sessions, the implications of 'not soiling' were worked out with the aid of a star chart. This helped Jamie to differentiate between the two poles, to clarify and build up the construction of 'soiling – not soiling', by specifying what could be anticipated. Most crucially both parents quickly established a family ritual round the giving of stars which made clear for Jamie their love and appreciation of him. Within three months he had stopped soiling.

Kelly (1969f, p. 231) proposes further techniques of psychotherapy. These have been further elaborated and illustrated with clinical examples by Karst (1980, pp. 169-76).

Children in Groups

It is curious that while much is made of the importance for children of their membership of a peer group, relatively little advantage has been taken of this in therapeutic practice with children as distinct from adolescents. Similarly, there seems little acknowledgement of this aspect of children's learning in the organisation of institutions to which children may be sent for care. For the child in residential care the structure of the community becomes the locus of his experimentation with self and others. It is supportive of his growth to the degree that it allows him to reformulate and try out alternative constructions, to negotiate and explore avenues usually ignored. When the possibility of the child's having an active influence on his setting is ruled out of court, all change must be prescribed as change within him and in the direction of 'adjustment' to the structure of the institution. The issue of peers and groups becomes incidental. There may be an assumption that at the end of the day only adults are likely to be of sustained good to children. Left to themselves children will only fight or play. A second line of argument may be that children are not sophisticated enough to interact with one another at the level necessary for therapy. This seems nonsensical since children will interact with each other at a level that is elaborative for them. Moreover, the social images of children together are scarcely encouraging — the Lord of the Flies vision of children as powerful and certain to revert to savagery, the image of children as a gang with a social structure excluding of adults and potentially anti-social. There may also be a fear that disordered children may become more disordered through close contact with children similarly diagnosed.

The Magic Garden. The Magic Garden (Agnew and Peacey, 1982) was a venture in finding ways of working with children as a therapeutic group. The children happily proved to be untrammelled by the problems of an adult therapy group, which filters itself through a network to do with being a therapy group. There were six, aged five to ten. Four were girls. All came from 'deprived' backgrounds. They were selected arbitrarily as the children within an in-patient unit not due for discharge within the six weeks during which the group was to run. It turned out that all six had lost a parent by death or separation in the previous four months. The themes of endings and loss were accordingly there in our beginnings . The group was held weekly for about an hour and a half in a softly lit room, completely empty except for a green rug.

The process of the group was designed to encourage fluency of construction without too much insistence on the niceties and to enable the children to take advantage of their own modes of construction. It was hoped that the experience would allow each child to discover the richness of his ideas and the power of his action and that we would all learn something about touching each other's worlds. The two therapists provided the context of the Magic Garden to which the children in their active elaboration committed themselves. Superordinate problems and issues were built into the framework of each session and articulated for the children. This served to raise their level of awareness of what they were engaged in. They could then match this against the outcomes they created, e.g. the theme of friendship was a dominant one, how to be one, what it's like to have one, how to make friends. The ending was known to be an ending. It could, therefore, be visualised and seen to be related to what went before.

The garden was introduced in detail as a changing place where the familiar and unfamiliar lived together. The roses and pansies grew beside flowers of fire that danced on the end of their stem. The dogs and cats lay down with white unicorns and green dragons, and so on. The children were first invited to move about the room to explore the garden. The younger ones did so with more ease and confidence than the older and it was they who made the first find — a green hedgehog. The finding of animals gave way to the discovery of trees and plants. This led on to movement, the children unfurling great branches and delicate petals and sending down stubbly roots. Flowers sprouted everywhere.

This first session was characterised by a follow-my-leader type of exchange. An idea passed in orderly exchange from one child to another with surprising variation. The two less-confident children tended initially to keep close to the adults but this need lessened as the session went on. The children took over a bit more and we ended sitting on the green rug, which thereafter became the symbol of the garden. It felt as if we had been out on our separate searches and were coming back to recognise our links with one another. The children sang and acted familiar nursery rhymes. Words came back — Mary, Mary quite contrary — and beautifully new expressive ones — Miss Muffet on her 'puffet'.

The second session centred round helping the children to listen to their own inner dialogue. The 'Spirit of the Garden,' a new introduction responsible for supplies and quickly accorded wheels by the children, had distributed beautifully painted eggs around the garden to be looked for and chosen. As one of the adults began to speak of how the inside of the egg could be listened to, the children spontaneously lay down on the floor and curled into a foetal position. They listened and then began to whisper of the secret inside. One was filled with singing birds, another had wall to wall carpeting and for the youngest it was simple — 'There's the whole world inside my egg.' As the children came back to the rug, we were aware of one's isolation and the clingingness of two. We were more on our own than together. The children themselves brought us back to the familiarity and sharing of the nursery rhyme sequence. They began with Humpty Dumpty!

The central idea of the third session which was about reconstituting a rainbow from bubble solution foundered on being too complex for the children. An alternative theme was supplied by a child after excited trials at bubble blowing through a wand. 'We can talk to each other with bubbles.' And so they did, catching each other's fragile globes to make one into a pair. They became bubbles themselves, were blown along by others or caught very gently.

The next two sessions were more tightly structured to encourage the children to engage in joint ventures. The theme of the first was that frightening things can become good things, that how a person is outside does not always match how he is inside, while in the second we explored the nature of celebration. Adults and children were provided with puppets, the therapists taking the roles of King and dragon. There was in the garden a bag of gold coins which belonged to a grumpy King who scoldingly insisted that his pet, Snapdragon, guard it fiercely. The treasure could only be gained by six true friends who had through their friendship the joint ability to make a friend of Snapdragon. Snapdragon actually did not want to be fierce. He wanted to have friends. The first task for the children was to demonstrate their affection for each other. This was quickly established. Squeaky voices spoke nicely of each other through the animal puppets and hands were clasped. A few shy kisses were hazarded. They then faced the business of making friends with Snapdragon. They rather lost their group identity at this point and looked round uncertainly, but the youngest led them forward. He said the dragon had a nice smile. That broke the ice. Snapdragon looked shy and coy as one by one the children complimented him. Soon he and the children were happily moving to the treasure, leaving behind a complaining King.

The children had been very affectionate and open throughout the session. We seemed to have moved closer with the noise level in the room lower than in previous sessions, as each child gained a hearing without a struggle and was responded to.

For the fourth session, Snapdragon's Party for His Friends, each child received a colourful invitation card for himself and a friend that could be seen only by him. When they came to the party, the child had to speak about his invisible companion. Each of them did so confidently and sensitively. The party was an orderly affair, each child seated with his unseen friend. The King repenting of his bad temper was allowed to join. There were a variety of specialities for the children, Dragon Juice, fruit and sweets shaped like stones which were shared without fuss. The talk was mainly about the feast, the children easily providing ideas and suggestions as we ate and drank toasts. The predominant feeling was of contentment, sharing and friendship.

The children were aware that the next session was the final one. The Spirit of the Garden had provided a long roll of paper, which was secured to the floor. The children readily accepted our suggestion to remember back over our adventures and to draw them on the 'Map of Things That Happened'. Very soon the paper was covered with their memories. Each child brought a new twist, something forgotten by the rest or a shared recollection. The time grew vivid for us as we worked. People did not appear for quite some time but then each was given space. The group seemed confident. No-one lagged from giving of themselves. As each of us drew out our ideas, the map became a tapestry, a visual representation with spoken commentary of the time so richly spent together.

The children orchestrated the finale. We joined hands and proceeded singing round the room as if visiting old haunts and delights and in joyous celebration of ourselves and us. The children left quietly in their own time, each carrying a paper flower. As we adults sat silently in the empty room, feeling sad, the youngest child came back in. Without acknowledging our presence, he kissed the rug and said, 'Good-bye, Magic Garden.'

There was another magic garden to which we adults have said

good-bye. For George Kelly, its story, as an attempt to come 'to grips with that perplexing something that makes man human', was worth retelling more than once in relation to the venture of psychotherapy (Kelly, 1969e, pp. 165-88; 1969g, pp. 207-15). Eden in construct theory terms was a place and time of successive choices for man. The first choice was between loneliness and companionship, the second between innocence and knowledge, the third between good and evil. Kelly, I am sure, would have found pleasure in the corroboration of his views, so elegantly given by a young client of mine. He was heard in the clinic waiting room explaining to another child who was there to see a paediatrician, 'Oh no. She's not a doctor. She's a special kind of friend who helps me decide whether I'll be good or bad.'

12 MENTAL HANDICAP: PEOPLE IN CONTEXT

Hilton Davis and Cliff Cunningham

By historical accident, mental handicap (or alternative terms) is included as a psychiatric category of which there are a range of definitions and subcategories. The American Association on Mental Deficiency, for example, defines mental retardation as 'subaverage general intellectual functioning which originates during the developmental period and is associated with impairment in one or more of the following: 1. maturation, 2. learning and 3. social adjustment.' (Heber, 1959).

Whatever systems are considered, in principle the diagnosis is generally made on the basis of; 1. the age of onset, 2. intellectual performance and 3. deficits in adaptive behaviour. In practice, however, it can still be argued convincingly that it is intellectual performance alone that is the effective criterion (Seltzer, 1983).

Considering this situation functionally, such systems do have administrative and scientific purposes in that they identify people to be provided with appropriate resources or included in research. However, little else is achieved and there is the ever present danger of labelling and pigeon-holing, which can both stereotype the individual and elicit stereotyped action from treatment resources. In Kelly's (1955) terms the attempt is made 'to cram a whole live struggling client into a nosological category' without specifying the 'lines of movement open to a person'. In other words such efforts do little to delineate the needs of people so diagnosed or to indicate effective intervention. Whatever remediation is to be suggested, it is interesting to note that it is likely to be neither psychiatric nor medical, but educational.

As currently used, albeit unintentionally, mental handicap is a superordinate 'constellatory' construct in that by defining a disorder, the person as a whole is defined in all aspects. The person so labelled is, therefore, generally unintelligent, socially inept and even, as was the view at one time, ineducable. At worst, the construct may be used 'pre-emptively' so that the individual is nothing but mentally handicapped. In either case, the person is seen as pathological in all aspects; he/she is a collection of disabilities and

246

not, first and foremost, a *person* who also has a handicap. Weakness is emphasised and strengths ignored. Because of intellectual impairment, all other characteristics of being a person, having individuality and being valuable are dismissed. Such classifications also focus upon the individual and by implication deny the social context generally, but particularly the family. Yet the family must be seen as an integral part of the situation and crucial to the solution.

This chapter will first consider current frameworks used in mental handicap and state the case for personal construct theory as a viable alternative that is easily communicated and understood by parents and diverse professionals alike. Research results will then be described before finally exploring the implications of the theory for working in this area.

Theoretical Frameworks

The more obvious theoretical frameworks in the area of mental handicap fall into two broad categories: medical/physiological and intellectual. Within the medical/physiological framework, important contributions have been made in terms of classification of a number of distinct syndromes and in identification of underlying physical pathology and aetiological factors. The prime example is Down's Syndrome and the discovery of the chromosomal abnormality associated with it. Such findings have had some therapeutic impact as in the case of the early dietary treatment of children with phenylketonuria. However, the major advance has been preventive, as in the ability to screen for disorders such as Down's Syndrome and spina bifida during pregnancy and the efforts to increase immunity to rubella infection.

Since an estimated 80 per cent of people with mental handicap have no obvious physical pathology, and since medical intervention is of little value even when pathology has been diagnosed, more psychologically oriented understanding is necessary, if remedial intervention is to be undertaken. In general, the common theoretical approaches are almost entirely concerned with intellectual functioning, reflecting the classification schemes discussed earlier. Within this general orientation, however, one can identify a number of different frameworks.

Intelligence

To begin, there is the global, psychometric framework in which the concept of intelligence, as a generalised ability, is central. This has had enormous influence within society in terms of both assessment and classification, but it is difficult to see any explanatory signifi- cance. Since the most that has occurred is a number of contradictory factor-analytic classifications of the types of ability, all that has been achieved is a dubious structural descriptive scheme which neither enables the prediction of intellectual dysfunction nor its remedia- tion and which perpetuates the notion of generalised impairment.

Information Processing

The second major orientation has derived from general experi- mental psychology. It has been concerned with the detailed investi- gation of specific information processing systems available to the person with mental handicap with an emphasis upon discovering deficits. Although a vast body of research is now available, the level of understanding is once again descriptive. Little is known about the development of the information processing systems and therefore little help can be offered in terms of specific efforts to facilitate improvements.

Developmental Theory

There are several frameworks that emphasise developmental delay as opposed to specific deficits. Many of these tend to be purely descriptive and are associated with developmental testing. However, some theories do seem to offer more than a structural view. The theory of Piaget is a main example. This traces the development of intellectual functioning from the first movements of the child to the complex logicomathematical operations of scientific thinking. Like other approaches, it has suggested ways of assessing different levels of intellectual function. However, given that Piaget attempts to specify how change occurs in terms of concepts like 'equilibration,' 'assimilation' and 'accommodation', it is most sur- prising that the studies reviewed by Klein and Safford (1977) are almost exclusively concerned with structure and not with ways of encouraging change. Other reviewers such as Fincham (1982) and Smedlund (1977) conclude that the theory is of little practical use because of, for example, the lack of conceptual clarity, the arti- ficiality of tasks and its focus upon abstract structures as opposed to the child's behaviour in context. Brown and Desforges (1977) dispute its usefulness in terms of its failure to consider alternative hypotheses, the evidence against Piaget's description of stages and the lack of empirical support for the postulated processes of change. Thus, there is still no clear understanding of how change may be brought about.

Learning Theory

The only approach to have been of predictive value is that based upon the principle of operant conditioning. Although it has not provided guidance in terms of curriculum, it has given a highly beneficial and relatively simple method of analysing the relationship between behavioural and environmental events in ways that generate methods of facilitating behaviour change (e.g. Yule and Carr, 1980). Mental handicap is not seen as a gross, necessarily innate, non-remediable characteristic, and socio-environmental factors are manipulated to produce change. However, major disadvantages of this approach are that it is unable to consider the *experience* of people with handicaps or the *communications* between them and people such as parents and professionals who work with them (Davis, 1984).

Common to all these theories is the neglect of non-intellectual characteristics. Concepts such as personality, temperament, motivation and emotion are not even indexed in many major texts (e.g. Craft, 1979; Matson and Mulick, 1983). Nevertheless, some studies are available in which a variety of variables have been assessed using such methods as questionnaires, projective techniques, and the semantic differential (Clark, 1974). There is a small body of work on the self-concept (Schurr, Joiner and Towne, 1970), but little progress has been made in recent years (Gowans and Hulbert, 1983).

That there is this paucity of work is most surprising since personality and motivation are acknowledged to play a role in many cognitive tasks (Clarke and Clarke, 1974a). Zigler (1966), for example, has provided evidence to support the view that performance differences between people with mental handicap and controls arise because of differences in motivation associated with impoverished experience and social deprivation. Cromwell (1963) has emphasised the role of failure experiences and the generalised expectancy to fail. Excitability has been related to performance in discrimination tasks and social interaction (e.g. Beveridge and

Evans, 1978). With Down's Syndrome infants strong concurrent relationships have been found between affective variables (e.g. expression of positive and negative emotion), self-recognition scores, and developmental quotient (DQ). These also predicted at a significant level DQ scores at 3 to 5 years (Motti, Cicchetti and Sroufe, 1983). Relationships have been found between a positive self-concept and, for example, academic achievement and paired associate learning (e.g. Wink, 1963). Nooe (1977) has even shown self-acceptance to correlate more highly than IQ with the degree of independent living achieved. Such findings not only endorse the importance of considering all aspects of people, but these latter studies in particular emphasise the significance of the person's own views of themselves starting in the earliest months of life.

It is this that is emphasised by personal construct theory. Unlike the other frameworks, it particularly respects the person sufficiently to pay attention to his/her own frame of reference. It does not imply a negative view of the person with mental handicap or emphasise pathology. On the contrary his/her strengths are emphasised. The person with mental handicap is construed as someone attempting to make sense of events in order to anticipate and therefore adjust to them. He/she is seen as fundamentally motivated and operating like all other people and not qualitatively different. Those with mental handicap make discriminations, build a set of constructs which are organised in some way and have the function of enabling anticipation and regulating behaviour.

The theory also has the advantage of being described systematically in clear ways which directly imply the appropriate assessment procedures that may be used. However, unlike many alternative theories, personal construct theory is predictive in terms of suggesting ways in which changes may be brought about. In this respect it is similar to the learning theory approach, but is more useful in that it can accommodate behaviour modification within its own framework whilst not ignoring the individual's experience. Where alternatives consider a limited aspect of the mentally handicapped person *per se*, personal construct theory can cope with the person as a whole, and in relation to other people such as parents and professionals. The Sociality Corollary enables one to make sense of the interaction between people with mental handicap and, for example, their parents without recourse to additional theory. Indeed, this aspect is stressed. Since parents or their substitutes are crucial to any possible remedial endeavours, the fact that they can be considered in the same terms as their child is a major strength of this theory and an advantage over alternatives. That the professional is also construed in the same way (i.e. as someone construing the people she/he is working with) enables one further to consider the vital therapeutic importance of the relationship between the professional and both the person with mental handicap and his/her family. This gives the theory both pertinence and parsimony.

Construct Theory Research

Having made such strong claims, it has to be pointed out that there has been very little empirical investigation. Reference could be made to autobiographical (e.g. Boston, 1981) and biographical (e.g. Hannam, 1980) information about people with mental handicap and their families. The work on parental attitudes and reactions (e.g. Waisbren, 1980) and studies on their self-concept may also be seen as relevant. Nevertheless, to date very little research has been conceived and conducted within a construct theory framework.

Only three completed studies of how people with mental handicap construe others were found. Wooster (1970) supplied both elements (photographs of strangers) and constructs to adolescents in an ESN residential school. Oliver (1980) used photographs of familiar people to elicit constructs from adolescents with Down's Syndrome. Barton, Walton and Rowe (1976) elicited both elements and constructs from 26 patients who were mainly in-patients in a hospital for the mentally handicapped and had been referred for assessment because of behaviour problems.

All the studies showed not only that grids could be completed by people of very limited intellectual ability, but that the process was both useful and meaningful. The results made sense of what was known about the person and frequently suggested specific and realistic therapeutic goals for individual patients. Barton *et al.* suggest that this technique may be limited in value for people with an IQ lower than 50, though further exploration is needed.

Oliver (1980) found that individuals had a very small number of highly interrelated clusters of constructs and this was confirmed by Wooster (1970) who found significanlty fewer clusters than for matched controls. The simplicity of the construct system is further indicated by the very high proportion of variance accounted for by the first component in the analyses conducted by both Oliver (1980) and Barton *et al.* (1976). They also both found a tendency for elicited constructs to be 'concrete'. Wooster (1970) showed that the people with mental handicap had less stable constructions of themselves and fewer significant relationships with other constructs when the self construct was stable. Barton *et al.* (1976) found no relationship between IQ and either the number of elements and constructs elicited or the variance of the first component. There were, however, interesting relationships between the content of constructs elicited and the type of ward environment in which the person lived.

The usefulness of personal construct theory in working with families of children with mental handicap has been discussed (Cunningham and Davis, 1984a; Davis, 1983, 1984; McConachie, 1982), but again there has been little empirical research. McConachie (1981) found that parents of children with a handicap had a significantly 'tighter' set of constructs about their children than parents with normal children. Constructs about teaching, controlling the child, and his/her independence did not differ in importance. A parent teaching course made no overall statistically significant changes in the grids, though there was some evidence of specific change, for example in terms of the perceived importance of teaching.

In the preliminary analysis of a recently completed study, Davis, Stroud and Green (1984) found that the language behaviour of mothers in interaction with a handicapped child was similar whether asked to play freely or teach the child. Mothers of normal children, however, behaved differently in the two situations, suggesting that parents with a handicapped child construe themselves in a teaching role more generally. Nevertheless, in comparing the same mothers using repertory grid techniques and a child characterisation sketch (where the parent is asked to describe the personality of their child as fully as possible), the most remarkable feature was the lack of difference in the ways they construed their children whether or not the child had mental handicap. In general parents used the same kinds of constructs with the same kinds of frequency. This is important because it runs counter to the assumptions implied in the literature that by being a parent of a child with mental handicap you are immediately different from other parents in a whole range of ways. For example, Waisbren (1980) and Worchel and Worchel (1961) found more negative parental feelings for handicapped children, but this is disputed by Davis, *et al.* (1984). At its extreme, this tendency assumes pathological functioning in these parents almost by definition (e.g. Cummings, 1976). As Seligman (1979) has said about parental reactions, 'The focus of the published literature is on pathology (what is wrong) to the virtual exclusion of ego (coping) mechanisms' (p. 63).

The only other study using construct theory methodology found in the literature is that of Myatt (1983). This provided only illustrative data concerning the way professionals construed their clients involved in a Portage scheme, which is a home visiting programme to instruct parents in the use of behavioural methods. Although the elements of the grid were children, it seemed that they were construed not in terms of their own characteristics, but in terms of their diagnostic category, the programme success and the mother's attributes such as her understanding, motivation and ability related to the treatment programme. Thus, despite the limited empirical work, that which is available supports the applicability of the model to child, parent and professional.

Implications for Practice

Since it will be impossible to cover all aspects, we will focus mainly upon the area of early intervention to exemplify and explore the implications. We have chosen to do this, because it fits in with current trends of a community orientation, as opposed to large institutions, and with relevant services beginning as early as possible and oriented towards facilitating parental efforts and resources. There has been a gradual movement away from the pre-eminence of the professional towards a situation of partnership between professional and parents. Such a change necessitates the development of new skills in professionals who are from a wide range of disciplines and working in conditions of totally inadequate manpower. As a consequence, it is particularly important that there should be a general framework that is relatively easily communicated to make sense of the complexities of interacting effectively with families and people with handicaps.

The Professional

In the area of handicap generally, criticisms of the services not only concern the lack of resources, but also professional inadequacies in communication skills and lack of sensitivity, compassion and understanding (Cunningham and Davis, 1984a). It has been argued, therefore, that many of these criticisms can be remedied by fostering professional relationships with parents that are based upon a collaborative partnership model, as opposed to the model of the professional as the expert (Cunningham, 1983). Not only does personal construct theory endorse this position in a fundamental way, it also provides a very general framework for facilitating consideration not only of the person with a handicap but also their parents, the professionals and the complex interactions between them. As such, it may provide a useful guide both for the professionals' actions and the parents'.

Kelly construed the client-therapist relationship in psychotherapy as analogous to that of a research student and supervisor, who work together, contributing different but complementary expertise to their research endeavours. In the same way, if we see the parents as having expertise about their own child and the professional as having a more general expertise, then the parents are more likely to be respected and treated in a way that fosters their self-esteem. This will, therefore, facilitate their ability to adapt to their situation and to behave as effectively as possible both in general, and also in terms of the development of the child.

As Davidson (1982) notes 'An increased sense of self-efficacy partly determines the persistence with which coping behaviour will be sustained' (p.425). The role of the professional is to facilitate the actions of the parents; it is of no value to demonstrate his/her own competence, if by so doing the parents are made to feel incompetent. Bronfenbrenner (1975) cautioned against practices that indicate to the parents that 'someone else can do it better'. Just as it is the research student who does the research, so it is the family who help the child. If the supervisor took over, the student would fail, as will the family, if the professional dominates.

Perhaps the most important implication is that the professional must in general follow the lead of the family by understanding the ways they construe events and not attempt to impose a system of constructs on them. Indeed, such an attempt would probably fail, since what may occur is a paradigm clash (Heifetz, 1980), as a result of the professional and parent not sharing similar assumptions. Such a clash would inevitably lead to an unproductive relationship. To do this, above all, requires respect for the views of the family. It means tolerating their explorations, no matter how irrational they might be in crises, and it means actively listening.

Since there is no absolute understanding of why children fail to develop or how they should be educated, then it is of value to construe the situation as an experiment. The professional's task is therefore to help the parents to elaborate their theories about themselves and their child in ways that enable them to decide upon methods of experimenting. The results of the experiments can then be evaluated, perhaps clarifying their situation and enabling them to experiment further.

The professional may at an appropriate time, offer the parents an explanation or a way of construing their situation. This may be a behavioural framework, or even personal construct theory itself. Whatever is offered, the effect is the result of a negotiation process with the family in ultimate control. In practice, as Kelly says, this requires enthusiasm, ingenuity and opportunism. It certainly means providing accurate and honest answers wherever possible to questions no matter how many times they are asked.

Negotiation, by definition, assumes an interactive process, and this process will be strongly influenced by the set of constructs the negotiators hold. If the professional construed her/himself in the role of transplanting his/her own skills onto the parent so that the parent acts as an assistant to the professional, then the interaction is likely to be one-sided, rather artificial and disrespectful of the parents. Compliance is also likely to be low. Alternatively, if the professional adopts a collaborative partnership model, then the negotiations may be more realistic, two-sided and much more productive. The possibility of explicit or unacknowledged clashes will be reduced and compliance will be increased. The risk of denying the parents their parental role is reduced, and such a model is more likely to foster self-efficacy in the parents and to decrease dependence on the professional.

What must be concluded from this is that it is important for the professional to have a clear understanding of her/his own models. As Heifetz (1980) has said

> professionals cannot work truly effectively with parents unless they are acutely aware of their own conceptual framework, understand the broad outline and finer detail of each parent's framework and begin to anticipate the manner in which the two frameworks interact as the parent – professional relationship evolves. (p. 350)

Personal construct theory gives not only a way of thinking about this, but also the means of assessing it.

The Parents

As the way the professional construes him/herself in relation to the parents, so the way the parents view the professional will determine the relationship that is established and the ultimate efficacy of their endeavours. In line with the importance of respect, personal construct theory assumes the fundamental importance of the parents' view both about the professional, and, of course, about the child. Given that parents are the most effective resource available for helping a child with mental handicap and given that their behaviour will be determined by their constructs of themselves and the child, the focus of intervention must be to facilitate their development of an effective construct system, beginning at the point of diagnosis.

Parental reactions to the disclosure of a severe organic disability have been variously described (Burden, 1978). Such reactions have been put into chronological sequence, and stages of shock, denial, emotional reaction, adaptation and orientation have been identified (e.g. Cunningham, 1979). Such descriptions are of obvious value, though in order to provide the most effective help, an understanding of the processes by which parents work through the stages is needed.

Solnit and Stark (1961) have attempted this from a psychoanalytic stance, and their discussion includes valuable insights. Yet its utility is limited by untestable assumptions and rather ill-defined concepts, such that it is not easily used and understood. It does not translate into direct suggestions for intervention.

Alternatively, the focus of personal construct theory is on the process of change, rather than on the specification of the content of intrapsychic processes. When faced with pregnancy, prospective parents begin to formulate constructs about children, and the role of parents. At birth, these constructs are available to anticipate interaction with the child, but the system develops more rapidly once the experience with a specific child has begun. Successful parenting may then be a function of elaborating a predictive model and changing it as necessary to anticipate the rapid changes that occur in the child.

Where the child is handicapped, the disclosure of the diagnosis may be assumed to invalidate, massively and suddenly, these developing constructs about normal parenting and children. As a result the parents will have no way of anticipating either immediate events (what is wrong with the child; what are the causes; should they consent to an operation), or the future (will the child live, walk, talk, etc.). It is this state that has been described as shock or emotional confusion. It is an extreme example of anxiety, since frequent parent comments like 'I didn't know what was happening' or 'I couldn't understand' indicate that the events with which they are confronted lie mostly outside the range of convenience of their construct system.

Subsequent reactions are strategies to cope with this anxiety by attempting to formulate a new construct system. Even denial can be seen as such a strategy since it provides a framework by reverting to the construct system used prior to the diagnosis. It may be associated with hostility or the individual's attempt to extort evidence in favour of the constructs invalidated by the diagnosis. A father's comment that 'He can't be handicapped because he is so beautiful looking' was followed by a statement describing the paediatrician as incompetent.

These and other reactions may be viewed as experiments exploring the situation, with constructs being adopted, perhaps inconsistently and for short periods, as strategies to provide at least a partial framework. Parents may explore the implications of killing the child, or rejecting her. These are temporary hypotheses to be tested. From other perspectives these may be seen as indicating pathological emotional states. Construct theory, however, portrays them as positive indications of change. Rather than chastising a parent's denial as unwillingness to accept the diagnosis, the professional should construe the parents as exploring their situation in order to achieve, at a particular time, one of a number of possible adaptations. As McCoy (1977) has said, emotions are defined as they are by Kelly, not in order to classify and treat but '. . . to enable a therapist to construe another's behaviour in a therapeutically useful manner' (p. 97).

The need, therefore, is to do more than recognise reactions, but to seek to understand them and the relationship between them. For example, the reaction described as low self-esteem may be closely related to the extreme reaction of parents to the diagnosis being withheld from them. Kelly's use of the notion of 'threat', as the awareness of an imminent comprehensive change in 'core' structures may make this meaningful. Whether or not they can cope is a major question with which parents are confronted, and withholding the diagnosis is easily interpreted by them as evidence of the physician's doubt. As we have said it is important for people to feel they are effective, so that anything a professional does to invalidate this must constitute a considerable threat and may evoke hostility and anger.

In this crisis parents are involved in what Kelly has called the CPC cycle (Circumspection, Pre-emption and Control). They consider many aspects of their situation (Circumspection) before they focus upon selected issues (Pre-emption) and then follow particular courses of action (Control). In models that have described stages, the phase of emotional reaction may equate to circumspection or the searching discussed above. The stages of adaptation and orientation, on the other hand, may be seen as pre-emption and control, where parents limit their exploration and seek answers to what can realistically be done in their situation. They can be seen as having a relative acceptance of the problems; they have achieved a relative adaptation or adjustment. The explorations allow the foundations of a new system of constructs to be laid and gradually a workable model. Parents may be said to be reoriented at this point and in a position to control events by pursuing particular courses of action anticipated as being of value to the child.

Although a general outline has been given here, nevertheless, specific parental characteristics, actions and reactions can be made meaningful. The content of parental construct systems has not been discussed and is not determined by the framework. Parents will begin with different constructs, will employ a variety of strategies and reconstruct different systems. Such variations will interact with the different ways in which the diagnosis is communicated, the nature of the handicap, the quality and the quantity of support services and the environment in which the family live (Cunningham and Davis, 1984b). It is, however, the unique construct systems of each parent that will determine how (or even whether) they interact from moment to moment with the child.

Parents who are in difficulty with their children may be those who are unable to construe their behaviour meaningfully and usefully. It may even be suggested that parent training programmes are effective, not because of principles of reinforcement, but because the parent is provided with constructs that are more appropriate than those held previously. Such constructs may be effective by making the child's behaviour more meaningful in relation to its context and, therefore, reducing parental anxiety. This may have the effect of either changing the parents' behaviour in ways that change the child's, or altering the parents' perception such that the child's behaviour is no longer seen as problematic. Fraiberg (1970) for example, emphasised successful outcomes resulting from helping parents of blind babies to observe, interpret and respond to the infant's behavioural cues. Such events in turn may alter the ways in which the parents construe themselves, in that they may see themselves as more in control, more effective, or better than they thought, and all of these have implications for subsequent amelioration of their situation.

The major implications here are that when attempting to help parents to change the behaviour of their children, their understanding of the child's behaviour should be explored. Once their constructs are clear, then they are in a position to evaluate them in terms of their usefulness in deciding what is best to do. For example, parents who construed their child's soiling as a disease of the stomach were aided by observation to reconstrue the problem as a fear of the toilet, which was isolated, cold, dark and noisy. This reconstruction suggested remedial actions, of changing the heating and lighting and accompanying the child; and these were indeed successful. The disease construction, on the other hand, suggested no action, because they had already been attending a paediatric clinic for months without effect. It is this kind of process that is the basis of the parent training approach described by Mancuso and Handin (1980). Parents' views are given significance. They are involved actively in exploring their ideas and developing new ideas and if successful they must take the credit and construe themselves more positively.

The Person With Mental Handicap

The fact that the professional construes people with mental handicap as actively involved in making sense of their world, is not only more respectful and more positive, but also this assumption in itself may help parents. This is because the professional will then be looking at the child in ways more similar to those of the parents, to whom syndromes and IQs have little useful significance.

We have discussed the parents' attempts to understand the child. This can mean to construe the child without reference to the way the child construes events him/herself. However, we have found it of considerable value to help parents experiment in order to establish what are the child's own constructs. It is easy for professionals and parents to make inferences that are erroneous and unhelpful about another person's constructions. The construct of attention-seeking may be one example. Unstructured or structured observation in a variety of situations often enables parents to see things they had not noticed before (i.e. to reconstrue). One child's attempts to touch boiling saucepans, construed originally as 'getting at me for not taking notice of her', became reconstrued as attempts to help, because similar actions and facial expressions were observed when mother was cleaning or ironing. Setting up a pretend stove in the kitchen solved the problem.

The understanding of another's constructions is made easier when the person is verbal. The situation, of course, is much more difficult when the person is preverbal. Nevertheless, by skilful experiment, requiring careful observation, time and patience, clarification can be gained. For example, a child's sudden groaning whilst watching television was initially construed as boredom, but the parents then noticed that it happened only when a channel was changed. They also noticed a pattern of looking that they construed as an attempt to restore the original programme. She looked fiercely at the television, then at the adult, groaned, then looked at the television again. This was construed as a high level of communication in a child who had been previously viewed as incapable of communicating. In another child, by careful observation and discussion, the meaning of 'bizarre' blowing behaviour was traced from his imitation of his father blowing a mobile, to signifying things suspended from the ceiling (including lights), to being a semi-vocal gesture indicating any light source.

Such constructions of the child's constructions have more than descriptive significance. For example, parents who had previously construed hand-flapping as a 'stereotypy', reconstrued it as communicating excitement. They were then able to use the same action to communicate their own feelings to the child. The general educational significance is that, instead of chasing developmental milestones, attempts may be made to understand what constructs are already available to the person and then to devise ways of elaborating them as necessary. The research quoted earlier has shown the usefulness of grids for this purpose and has suggested that the construct system of people with mental handicap may be undifferentiated and relatively simple in structure. As a result, the person may fail to discriminate important aspects of situations and might over-generalise.

To change this, an attempt should be made to help the child or adult discriminate more effectively, rather than providing extra stimulation, as parents may naturally do (e.g. Davis and Oliver, 1980), and professionals may advise. This might involve simplifying the environment and marking the significance of those aspects of the environment that are important. The prediction is given some support in that normal infants' language learning may be enhanced by the simplified and exaggerated language to which they are exposed (Snow, 1972). It is further supported by the conclusion that severely impaired people benefit more by structured experience and that incidental learning is not very effective (Clarke and Clarke, 1974b). It might also be the case that behavioural methods are effective, not because responses are followed by reinforcements, but because systematic and consistent contingency management presents the child or adult with very clear signals that facilitate effective communication of appropriate discriminations to be made. Certainly, a more general theory is needed to explain why, for example, one family were able to eliminate severely disruptive mealtime behaviour by simply switching off the previously ever present sound of their radio. Why may parents, trained to observe reliably and accurately, often have beneficial effects on their children without recourse to other methods? Why does a warm, supportive relationship not infrequently produce desired changes within a family? These are examples of questions that occur in clinical practice and to which personal construct theory may begin to provide answers.

Conclusion

In the area of mental handicap, intervention in many forms is beginning to be beneficial. However, the stage has now been reached when a comprehensive psychological framework is required if sense is to be made of the findings, evaluation studies planned and a rational, effective and economic approach to these problems developed. Such a framework must be prescriptive, as well as descriptive, and useful to a wide variety of professions working in this field. Personal construct theory is a potentially useful framework in this respect because it has application not only to the people designated mentally handicapped, but to the people, parents or professionals, working with them.

13 PHYSICAL ILLNESS: A GUIDEBOOK FOR THE KINGDOM OF THE SICK

Linda L. Viney

> Illness is the night side of life, a more onerous citizenship. Everyone who is born holds dual citzenship in the kingdom of the well and the kingdom of the sick. Although we all prefer to use only the good passport, sooner or later each of us is obliged, at least for a spell, to identify ourselves as citizens of that other place (Sontag, 1977, p. 3).

This account of the experiences of the healthy and the ill makes several points which are central to this personal construct account of physical illness. First, people who are ill (or, as we have come to call them, 'patients'), function psychologically much as healthy people do. They may appear to be distressed or even to act in self-defeating ways, but in most cases they are sane, fully functioning people reacting to severe stress from a variety of sources. Secondly, when people become patients, that role, together with their attendant pain and fears for the future, seems to remove them so far from people who are well that they might be in another country. To a large extent, patients become alienated from those around them. Thirdly, it is because of this tendency for patients to become alienated that it is important that well visitors to the kingdom of the ill — medical practitioners, nurses and other hospital staff — can understand what that other kingdom is like. A personal construct psychology guidebook for that kingdom can help to achieve that purpose. Fourthly, such a guidebook can aid the patients themselves to escape from that kingdom, experientially at least and sometimes even physically.

The guidebook provided here is a personal construct psychology model of patients' reactions to physical illness. It initially takes the form of a set of general propositions about people who are ill. Then follows a subset of more specific propositions concerning the construction processes of patients. Their emotions are considered, as are the social interactions in which they participate. This model will be presented in the next section of this chapter. The evidence supporting the model will be reviewed. Then I shall draw out some of the practical implications of the model for those responsible to and for people who are physically ill. Finally, I shall examine the value of this model as a guidebook for the kingdom of the sick.

A Personal Construct Psychology Model of Patients' Reactions to Physical Illness

General Propositions

1. All patients *try to make sense* of what is happening to them. Be it illness, injury, or hospitalisation, they try to establish some meaning in these events. For this purpose they develop interpretations of their current experience in terms of their past experience. These intellectual and emotional interpretations, or constructs, also enable patients to anticipate effectively their future experiences.

2. Such anticipation in terms of a construct system of already proven effectiveness may not be possible for seriously ill patients who are under considerable *threat* of pain, bodily mutilation or death, so that old constructs do not work well. It may also not be possible if illness-associated *events are new* to patients, so that new constructs are needed. Many of the events hospitalised patients experience are new to them, however familiar they may be to hospital staff.

3. The anticipations or constructs which patients hold concerning their illness may appear incomplete or inaccurate to others, yet they *determine how patients act.* They influence their reactions to all aspects of their care, including their following of treatment regimes. Alternative accounts of failures to follow drug regimes have emphasised cognitive factors alone: yet emotional factors are equally important.

The Construction Processes of Patients

4. Patients develop their constructs by *interpreting their own past experiences.* For adults seeking back for illness-related constructs, this often means that their most relevant set of constructs may have been developed when they were children. When they try them out, the evidence they carry of earlier stages of intel-

lectual and emotional development is apparent. Patients are then often described as undergoing regression by staff of a psychoanalytical persuasion.

5. Patients *differ in how they construe current experience* because of the different past experiences which have led to their different construct systems. No two patients can be assumed to be using the same constructs, even if they are facing the same illness or surgical procedure. The content and structure of the construct systems of each of them must be assessed.

6. Patients differ in the *permeability* of their construct systems, that is, the extent to which they can use them to make sense of new events such as new information about their illness or a new 'sick role' for themselves.

7. Patients may also have *constructs that are too loose* or make too many general predictions to be useful. They may also be too *tight* or too restrictive in their predictions. A construct such as 'Hospitals are strange places' will prove too loose for effective prediction, while one like 'I am a person who is *never* ill' will be too tight.

8. Patients can *change their constructs* by successfully reinterpreting their experience (and not necessarily by having new experiences). They can do this for themselves, but they may find it difficult in the restricting context of the hospital. Relatives and health professionals such as nurses and medical practitioners can help them do so: but sometimes a professional counsellor is necessary.

The Emotions of Patients

9. Broadly speaking, when patients' construct systems enable them to interpret and anticipate what is happening to them effectively, they experience positive emotions: when their systems are not effective they experience negative emotions. Two examples follow.

10. Patients become *anxious* when the events they experience are beyond the range of convenience of their construct system, that is, when they cannot make sense of them. They will become appropriately anxious, therefore, when they cannot meaningfully interpret a new piece of diagnostic information or when they are asked to make a decision about a painful or risky treatment with insufficient information.

11. Patients become *angry* when they are trying to secure vali-

dation for a construct which has failed them in their attempts at prediction. When constructs such as 'I can cope by myself' or 'I can understand everything that happens to me' are tested and found wanting by patients, recognition of their inadequacy leads to anxiety. Attempts to gain more support for them by bluff or argument, however, are expressed in anger. The frustration-related anger, which is also appropriate, should be expressed directly. Often, however, because of patients' constructs about themselves in the context of hospital, their anger is expressed only indirectly. In this way, the anger is perpetuated rather than put to good psychological use. The other way in which patients may deal with their anger is to turn it on themselves, a process which eventually imprisons them within their own self-blaming construct system.

12. *Expressions of these appropriate emotions* such as anxiety and anger, should thus occur for all patients. Counsellors can help with this process, not to inhibit it as they are sometimes asked by staff to do but to encourage it. They can also help when the constructs of patients are too loose or too tight. Yet another indication of a need for counselling may be seen in patients who use a construct consistently in the face of evidence which invalidates it, as when patients with advanced cancer maintain: 'That growth is not cancerous'. Psychoanalytic theory has accounted for such a reaction by describing it as denial, but this personal construct account opens up new avenues for the counselling of such patients.

The Social Interactions of Patients

13. Staff working with patients can *relate to them meaningfully* only if they understand their ways of making sense of the world. This ability of professional staff to be able to construe effectively the constructs of their patients is very important. Of course, the reciprocal of the proposition is also true. Patients can only relate to staff if they understand something of their construct systems. Here is an area of much miscommunication in hospitals.

14. Such miscommunication is more vital to patients than to staff because patients are dependent on staff to *validate their construct systems*. Patients are therefore very vulnerable to the attitudes, role expectations and misunderstandings of the professional staff. If they do not experience validation from them, they become alienated and socially isolated.

15. Even when good communication between patients and staff occurs, it is often the case that *some constructs will receive more validation* from them than others. Constructs of helplessness receive more validation from staff for patients, for example, than those of competence. Such constructs may prevent effective rehabilitation and preclude patients from eventually taking responsibility for their long-term health care. Counselling of hospitalised patients may be needed so that these iatrogenic outcomes of professional care may be avoided.

Support for the Personal Construct Model from the Literature

Now that the personal construct model of patients' psychological reactions to illness has been described, it is appropriate to consider if support for it is available in the literature of observation and research dealing with the physically ill. In this analysis of the literature, I shall deal with each proposition of the model, examining the most general propositions first. The propositions describing the search of patients for meaning and the frustration of that search by threat or uncertainty will be considered in some detail. However, the proposition that patients' actions are determined by the way they structure their experiences will not be discussed because useful but lengthy arguments for its validity for people in general are available elsewhere (Kelly, 1955; Giorgi, 1970). The evidence for the five propositions concerning the construction processes of patients will then be examined, as will that for the propositions regarding patients' major emotional reactions of anxiety and anger. Finally, the observations and other data collections relating to the social interactions of patients, especially as they lead to alienation and foster constructs of helplessness will be examined before turning to the practical implications which can be drawn from the model.

The search by patients who are ill for meaningful interpretations of what is happening to them has been reported by observers from many theoretical persuasions other than personal construct psychology (Benoliel, 1974; Mechanic, 1977). They view their illness as an enemy or a challenge, a punishment or a relief (Lipowski, 1960). Cardiac patients, for example, have been shown to strive hard, even in a weakened post-coronary state, to provide interpretations of their symptoms and their causes (Cowie, 1976; Koslowsky, Kroog and La Voie, 1978). This process has been described as a 'normalising' of the symptoms by which a social sharing and ordering takes place (Straus, 1975). The constructs patients develop in this way are apparent in the language with which they choose to express themselves (Warner, 1976-77), as are their anticipations of possible outcomes of their illness (Blumberg, Flaherty and Lewis, 1980). However, the threat constituted by pain may interfere with such anticipations (Melzak, 1980), as can fear of bodily mutilation (Viney and Westbrook, 1982a; Viney, in press,b) or death (Epting and Neimeyer, 1983; Rowe, 1982). However, it is possible for seriously ill patients to anticipate even death effectively (Viney and Westbrook, 1983; Viney in press, a). While events which are new to patients may seem initially less disruptive than these sources of physical threat, the uncertainty and planlessness that arise from illness and hospitalisation and the subsequent need to process much new information efficiently and quickly may constitute one of the most important blocks to interpretation and anticipation by patients at both the intellectual and the emotional levels (Leventhal, 1975). This general proposition, like the first, has received support from the research of psychologists, sociologists and psychiatrists.

The five propositions about the construction processes of patients are next considered. The foundation of illness-related constructs in patients' experience of much earlier events has been observed, not only in the emotional expression of patients, but in the child-like logic they sometimes employ (Cassell, 1976). If earlier constructs of illness-related events are not available, metaphors or constructs accounting for similar but in no way identical events may be used by patients. These attempts at anticipation can be effective (Mair, 1977a): they can also, when applied to illness, lead to misinterpretations which lay the ground work for unnecessary threat, unwanted anxiety and avoidable frustration-generated anger (Sontag, 1977).

The different constructs which individual patients use, as a result of their different pasts, are apparent in differences as simple as those between paraplegics who blame themselves for the accidents which have caused their disabling injuries and those who blame others (Bulman and Wortman, 1977). However, the intellectual and the emotional implications of constructs can be highly complex (Viney, 1983b). While patients differ in the permeability of their constructs before illness, if they have lost much mobility their constructs may become even less permeable. Several observers have noted the 'shrinkage' of the experienced world which seems to occur for many bedridden patients (Cassell, 1976; Van Den Berg, 1980). The proposition concerning permeability, together with those describing loose and tight constructs and the capacity of patients to change their constructs, all have to do with the adaptability of patients. More psychologically adaptable patients have been observed to adjust to illness better (Achterberg, Matthews-Simonton and Simonton, 1977) and to survive life-threatening illness for longer (Worden and Sobel, 1978). Such adaptability has also been linked with the maintenance of health (Antonovsky, 1979).

The distinction between negative and positive emotions in terms of the relative effectiveness of application of the construct system has proved a useful one (McCoy, 1981). Illness, injury and hospitalisation, together with many forms of treatment bring inherently with them enough disconfirming and invalidating experiences to lead to the prediction that anxiety and anger will form part of a common pattern of reaction to illness. These predictions have received considerable support (Lewis and Bloom, 1978-79; Rodda, Miller and Bruhn, 1971; Viney and Westbrook, 1982a). One study found early expression of anxiety to be associated with good rehabilitation later (Viney and Westbrook, 1982b). The same study showed support for the hypothesis that patients who express their anger directly will fare better than those who express their anger indirectly and passively. The imprisoning effects of turning anger in on oneself in the form of depression and self-blame have been described elsewhere (Rowe, 1978): in patients dealing with physical illness, the more they are imprisoned by illness-related disability, the more their anger is likely to be translated into self-blame (Viney and Westbrook, 1981).

The social interactions of patients are determined much as they are for people who are well. It is only in so far as staff can understand the constructs of patients and patients can understand the constructs of staff that they can communicate meaningfully (Stringer and Bannister, 1979a). Much miscommunication does occur in hospitals (Plutchik, Jerrett, Karasu and Skodol, 1979; Straus, 1975). Staff can always draw on other relationships outside the ward for the validation of their constructs. It is the hospitalised patients who, isolated from family and friends, are dependent on the staff whom they see as having higher status than themselves for such support (Janis and Rodin, 1979). If it is not available, then a sense of alienation develops from both staff (Leventhal, 1975; Van Den Berg, 1980) and family (Blumberg *et al.*, 1980; (Wortman and Dunkel-Schetter, 1979). Even when communication is good between patients and staff, it may lead to some constructs receiving more validation than others (Kelly, 1955). Patients' descriptions of themselves contain many references to helplessness and few to competence (Raps, Peterson, Jonas and Seligman, 1982; Westbrook and Viney, 1982). When they are lying motionless in bed and communicating with mobile staff and family their very lying position conveys helplessness (Van den Berg, 1980). Several observers have argued that the dominance of this helplessness construct for hospitalised patients is the result of interactions with hospital staff (Anderson, 1981; Taylor, 1979). Unfortunately, its use by patients has been linked with poor rehabilitation (Viney and Westbrook, 1982b). More participation by patients in decisions relating to their own care while they are in hospital would do much to reduce the dominance of this construct for patients, as well as to increase the likelihood that they will take responsibility for their own health in the long term (Clarke and Viney, 1984).

Practical Implications of the Personal Construct Model

I shall now consider the implications for the care of medical and surgical patients which can be drawn from this personal construct psychology model. The implications of the general propositions will be discussed first and then those concerning the patients' construction processes. Then implications based on this account of the patients' emotions and social interactions will be examined. Several case studies describing individual patients will be reported.

If all alert patients try to make sense of current illness-related events in order to anticipate those in the future, then it is important to keep even restricted, bed-bound or otherwise disabled patients moving forward psychologically in this way. Helping them to leave the prison they have formed with their own construct systems has been found to achieve this goal. When patients recognise their own role as the creators of their illness-related constructs, they are freed psychologically from the prison of illness-based disability because they can choose to alter these constructs at any time (Viney, 1983b). A number of psychological therapies, for cancer for example, have relied on changing the content of key patient constructs (Simonton,

Matthews-Simonton and Creighton, 1978).

Blocking of effective anticipations in patients can be relieved by a number of techniques, depending on whether it is caused by threats or the need to deal with many new events. Threat of bodily mutilation, for example, can be reconstrued as in stress inoculation (Girodo, 1977). Its implications can also be reappraised (Langer, Janis and Wolfer, 1975). If death is the threat, patients can be helped to deal with their impending loss of family and friends, not by taking them through a series of stages of bereavement which has been proposed from within another theoretical framework, but by fostering adaptive rather than dislocative changes in their construct systems (Woodfield and Viney, in press). If too much new information with which the construct system cannot deal causes the block, then allowing patients to work with that new information at their own pace is necessary, whether the information be about impending death or the need for surgery. There is evidence that psychological preparation for surgery improves both the psychological and the physical outcomes of that surgery (Schmitt and Wooldridge, 1973; Vernon and Bigelow, 1974).

The practical implications stemming from this account of construction processes at work in patients — how they develop their constructs, how their content differs and how their construct systems differ in their adaptability — are many. However, the most important of these is the need to assess the construction processes of each patient to answer these questions. What is the content of his or her illness-related constructs? What are their implications for illness-related action by the patient? What past events provided the basis for the development of such constructs? Do these constructs help the patient to understand current illness-related events and to anticipate effectively likely outcomes? Are they too tight or too loose? Can the patient change his or her constructs? A description of a particular case may make the need for such assessment clearer. Shirley G. at 45 years of age showed an unusual degree of distress while she was waiting in her bed on the ward for relatively minor surgery to be carried out. Nor was she cooperating well with the staff. Assessment of her most salient construct revealed why: 'My mother died in this bed. I will die in it too.' Her mother had been 94 years old and very ill when she died. Shirley's construct was too tight for effective anticipation. It was also linked with other constructs to do with losing loved ones, with which she could not immediately cope. She was moved to another bed so that the surgical procedures could take place. After surgery she was helped to reinterpret some of her experiences of loss by modifying her constructs at her own pace. She recovered from her surgery with no complications.

The emotions generated by the failure of patients' constructs to anticipate what is about to happen which are most distressing to them appear to be anxiety and anger. A number of self-monitoring techniques are available to patients to help them deal with these emotions (Rudestam, 1980). However, professional counselling of anxious or angry patients is sometimes necessary because of the rigid constructs of staff who wish to work with only 'good patients' who have a 'stiff upper lip' or are 'always polite'. A set of counselling programmes for use in hospitals has been developed (Viney and Benjamin, in press) and their outcomes evaluated (Viney, Clarke, Bunn and Teoh, 1983). Both anxiety and indirectly expressed anger were found to be reduced for the counselled patients when they were compared on discharge with the patients who were not counselled. This crisis intervention counselling of patients while they were in hospital also led to them maintaining these gains a year later in the community. Humour can also help in dealing with these emotions. A description of another case is appropriate here. Paul T. at 50 years of age, was anxious and frustrated because of the long time it was taking for his leg ulcer to heal. He would talk to neither his wife nor most of the staff about his feelings. However he liked to have one senior nurse do his dressing. They shared a history in the army about which they often joked. The nurse was able to turn this empathic humour from the army to Paul's current plight. She enabled Paul to take a new perspective on his cherished constructs which he could no longer employ effectively: 'A strong man needs help from no-one' and 'My wife will only love me if I'm a strong man.' He was soon confiding his fears and frustrations to his wife. Their relationship improved and so did his ulcer.

Social interactions for hospitalised patients are often less than ideal. When meaningful communication does occur between staff and patients, it is likely to be concerned with events of central importance to the patients such as bodily mutilation and death. It is important, therefore, that staff be aware of the constructs which they themselves employ to deal with these threatening events before they are ready to listen to those of patients. More often, such social interactions are not taking place and patients are alientated. Their resulting isolation can sometimes be broken down by family members (Viney, 1983b), although professional counselling may be needed. Such isolation may not occur at all in hospitals in which patients groups are encouraged. These groups may be run by staff (Ferlic, Colman and Kennedy, 1979; Wellisch, 1981) or by the patients themselves (Gartner and Riessman, 1977).

The latter, self-directed groups often prove the more successful means of providing validations of constructs other than 'I am helpless'. The hospital-based counselling programme which I described above reduced such helplessness in the short term but not in the long term (Viney *et al.*, 1983). This was unfortunate because this construct is particularly dominant for people dealing with illness which is chronic rather than acute in nature (Viney, 1983a). A third case will illustrate this. Janice H. had been suddenly hospitalised in her twenties with diabetes mellitus. She understood little about her illness, its treatment, its course or her rights to information about them. As a result she was experiencing much anxiety. Her dominant constructs were 'I'm so silly. I wouldn't understand if they told me. When I'm ill, I just give up'. The counsellor structured her interaction with Janice so as to provide validation of rival but related constructs, such as: 'I mightn't understand when they first tell me but I'll get the hang of it soon enough'. This reinterpretation of her own ability, which occurred at her own pace, led her finally to participate, not only in monitoring her own insulin levels while in hospital but in planning the future management of her disease.

Toward a Guidebook for the Kingdom of the Sick

I have presented this personal construct approach to physical illness as a set of propositions which together form a model. The model has been tested here in two ways: by a survey of the relevant literature for support and refutation and by a description of some of the practical implications of care for patients hospitalised in general hospitals. Is the guidebook it provides for the kingdom of the sick necessary or can we travel in the kingdom of the sick without it?

The propositions which make up the model are, in fact, testable hypotheses. Most of them, however, have not yet been tested using the logic of the experiment. The main type of relevant data which has been available has been observations by both health professionals and researchers. Their observations have provided some support for the model. The results of some naturally occurring experiments have been monitored. It is only recently, however, with the drawing of practical implications from the model, that some of these hypotheses could be fully tested.

Of course the implications for patient care which have been drawn from the model are also evidence of its value. A model of patients' psychological reactions to illness which led to no recommendations for practice with patients would be of little use. Some of these recommendations involve the use of specific techniques, such as the psychological assessment of general hospital patients, psychological preparation of them for surgery, stress inoculation and crisis intervention counselling. Others have been more general. Shirley, with her single dominant and tight construct. Paul, whose construct system made it difficult for him to relate to his wife when his ulcer did not heal, and Janice, whose constructions of herself as helpless stood in the way of her coping with her diabetes, all showed the need for patients to understand their own illness-related constructs. This was apparent, not only in relation to the treatment of their current symptoms of illness but in terms of maintaining their health in the future. Equally important is the need for staff working with patients to understand their construct systems. Each medical practitioner, nurse, social worker and occupational therapist needs a guidebook for the kingdom of the sick. I hope that this chapter goes some way towards providing it.

PART THREE

CHANGE

In this final part of the book, we return to a more general level. Having spelt out in Part Two some practical guidelines when faced with specific problems, we describe approaches to helping people irrespective of the presenting problem. One of the things that should become evident is that construct therapy is not restricted to a narrow set of methods. In fact, as Hugh Koch will argue, construct theory can offer an approach to understanding the processes in other forms of psychotherapy, such as 'cognitive therapy' or 'group analysis'. Finally, it is suggested that construct theory has implications for change 'beyond the clinical context', at the level of society and institution.

14   INDIVIDUAL PSYCHOTHERAPY

Fay Fransella

The Nature of Personal Construct Psychotherapy

> The psychology of personal constructs and the philosophy of constructive alternativism upon which it is based lead one to view psychotherapy as a reconstruing process. (Kelly, 1955, p. 937)

So says Kelly, thereby placing psychotherapy firmly in the centre of his stage. He also states the basic theme of his theory as being *the psychological reconstruction of life*.

> We even considered using the term *reconstruction* instead of *therapy*. If it had not been such a mouth-filling word we might have gone ahead with the idea. Perhaps later we may! (Kelly, 1955, p. 187)

The philosophy of constructive alternativism with its emphasis on a personal, internal, reality rather than a universal reality 'out there', means that an individual's interpretations are neither truly right nor wrong. There are always alternative ways of construing any event. Therefore, the 'as if' approach takes on particular significance in the therapeutic setting. The client is invited to play with ideas, to look at some mighty serious aspect of life 'as if' it were something different. Looking at it from a different perspective may enable the client to start behaving, experimentally at first, in a different way. The use of this 'as if' approach to behaviour is nowhere more in evidence than in 'fixed role therapy' to be described later.

Advantages and Disadvantages of a Content-Free Theory of Therapy

One great advantage of working with such a very abstract theory is that the therapist has no limiting structures to impose on the client. There are no rights and wrongs in his or her problematic ways of construing the world. The therapist has no specific oedipal complexes or transference neuroses to resolve, no special resistances to overcome nor peak experiences to strive for. Personal construct theory is virtually empty of content. Each person's ways of construing are the best they have available for experimenting with the world at the present time.

Some find it a great disadvantage using a content-free theory, for it means that the therapist and client have to work closely together to build a unique structure for understanding the problem. This structure has to be built *from scratch and couched in the client's own terms*. To achieve this, the therapist listens in such a way that she can 'subsume' the client's construing system within her own. The task is made even more difficult because, in so subsuming, the therapist needs to 'suspend' her own personal constructs — as far as is humanly possible — and use only those professional and theoretical constructs that Kelly provides.

Since values only exist in the eye of the construer, the content-free nature of the theory is one of its main attractions to those who have chosen to work within its framework.

In place of content, Kelly provides a blue-print of how we may continually strive to elaborate and define our construing system and, thereby, increase our ability to predict events. It is we who have created ourselves as we successively construe events through life and flesh-out the actual being that is 'me'.

With only a blue-print describing how we go about building ourselves, and with no details of the style and form and passions and weaknesses that each one of us has uniquely created, the therapist *can* only work with the person in the person's own terms. The therapist *can* have no answers. It is the client who has the answers. All the therapist can do is try to understand the client's views of the world, and thereby the problem, and so go hand-in-hand with the client exploring possible alternative ways of viewing the world, which will ultimately lead to reconstruction and a more useful slant on the problem area.

Skills of the Therapist

The professional skills of the therapist, as well as much of his repertory as an experienced human being, are brought into the transaction. He offers as much of both as he thinks can be used. But it is the client who weaves them into the fabric of his own experience. (Kelly, 1980, p. 21)

Some General Skills

Kelly provides a formidable list of skills the personal construct therapist should acquire. It includes the need to be an acute observer of all events pertaining to the client, for construing can be seen in behaviours as well as heard aurally. The therapist must be skilled verbally, for he has to learn to talk the language of the client. The therapist needs to be adventurous in experimenting along with the client. The therapist must be creative, with creativity meaning 'trying out one's unverbalised hunches'.

> Creation is therefore an act of daring, an act of daring through which the creator abandons those literal defenses behind which he might hide if his act is questioned or its results proven invalid. The psychotherapist who dares not try anything he cannot verbally defend is likely to be sterile in a psychotherapeutic relationship. (Kelly, 1955, p. 601)

Some Specific Skills

The Credulous Approach. The therapist must be able to adopt the credulous approach. This fundamentally means taking everything the client says at face value. If the client says something that looks like a definite lie, it is believed because the client is lying for some good reason. The clinician asks herself what the client is trying to communicate by that lie.

Being credulous means listening to the meanings that lie behind the words. The clinician does not interpret what the client says into his own language, he makes no value judgements. Rather he strives to learn the language of the client — both what is expressed verbally and non-verbally.

Subsuming and Suspending. However, the ability to subsume the client's construction system is probably the first and foremost skill a personal construct psychotherapist must possess. Without it he or she cannot start.

Subsuming starts with the therapist playing a role in relation to the client. He attempts to understand the constructions the client is placing upon events. Next the therapist must suspend his own personal construction system — particularly those constructions to do with values. The therapist's personal view of the world is put literally 'out of mind'.

Yet, to suspend one's own personal construction system, however imperfectly, without something to take its place, would leave an awe-inspiring vacuum. To take its place Kelly describes a system of professional constructs within which the therapist may subsume the client's system. This means that the therapist should be able to say:

> Since all clients have their own personal systems my system should be *a system of approach* by means of which I can quickly come to understand and subsume the widely varying systems which my clients can be expected to present. (Kelly, 1955, p. 595)

As he 'gets inside' his client's construing of the world, the therapist may, for short periods of time, get so immersed within that person's world that the distance between them seems to vanish.

The Subsuming Construct System

All the time the therapist has been listening creduously to the construing of the client through his conversation and non-verbal deliberations, she has been trying out the professional constructs for fit. Her own construing system has been suspended and she begins to subsume her client's system.

Basically, the professional constructs can be divided into those that describe types of construct, types of construing, and those relating to the awareness of change. These have already been discussed in more detail in the opening chapter; here we are concerned with how they may be used to give an understanding of where the client now stands and the possible avenues open to him along which he may travel to change.

Types of Construct

Superordinate and Subordinate Constructions. Throughout his early sessions Roger referred to his passionate concern for *justice* and his hatred of *injustice* of every kind. Almost everything boiled down to this issue — his past employers' treatment of him, the government, or partners in a marriage. But when asked for a specific example of injustice as he experienced it at the moment, he could only think of someone pushing in front of him in a bar. It seemed that, for him, his construct *justice – injustice* was very superordinate with a very wide range of convenience.

The therapeutic task was to fill in some of the subordinate structure so that he did not continually have to leap from the highest diving-board into the deep end only to find he could not swim.

In therapy, a current situation was examined in detail to see how he now dealt with it, and alternative ways of handling it were role-played. This had the effect of 'detaching' the incident from the superordinate issue of *justice* and bringing it down to a more manageable level of *manners*.

Regnant Constructs. John was constantly looking for 'the norm'. Recurring themes were 'Surely all normal women expect . . . '; or 'Surely any normal man would insist . . . '. Regnant constructs are those governing a whole constellation of constructs, commonly seen in the use of stereotypes.

Valerie, for instance, appeared to have put a lot of her personal anger with her parents into militant feminist notions. She tended to see sexist behaviour in men in every encounter. For her, *men* was regnant over *sexist*. With such simplistic thinking, she never had to question the pros and cons of sexism nor whether men can have attributes other than sexist ones.

She was encouraged to observe the men with whom she worked more closely. She was soon able to see that they did have some attributes that were indeed non-sexist. She found ways of reconstruing men without having to abandon that very powerful construct altogether.

A very clear example of a regnant construct with a very wide range of convenience is provided by Luke. During the second session he was discussing how he could ask for something like a packet of fruit pastilles without stammering. In that specific situation he said he had predicted he would be fluent because:

> fruit pastilles are quite easy things to ask for um they were not what I shall call *a status-loaded object* . . . I've been thinking about the reason why there are some things I find it difficult to ask for and some things I find easy and I have decided that my mind works in this sort of odd way. It attaches to the objects being asked for a certain status. (Fransella, 1972, p. 162)

Luke came to see that he classified all objects according to the extent to which they carried status. The importance for him of this psychologically cumbersome system was that it determined whether or not he would stammer and even its degree of severity.

Core Versus Peripheral Constructs. Core constructs are those which give us our identity and justify our existence. For many people seeking psychotherapy, the complaint has become part of the person's core role' construing. Nowhere is this better demonstrated than with those who stammer. Luke spells out the implications of having a core role construct centred on the problem in response to my asking whether he knows when he is going to stammer badly:

> I think I do — I think there is a feeling almost that *I am a stammerer* — and therefore I should stammer . . . It's in every sort of situation. I — as a matter of fact, this was something that I was waiting for an opportunity to mention. Even now, at this very instant, I'm talking pretty fluently — I have been for about five minutes — I feel it's wrong — I can feel this in me. I feel "I'm talking fluently but I shouldn't be". (Fransella, 1972, p. 179)

Types of Construing

Constriction Versus Dilation. In the normal course of events as we go through life there are times when it is an advantage to narrow or constrict the breadth of the world in which we live and, at other times, to expand or dilate it. But occasionally we take up an extreme position and then find it difficult to carry out our daily life activities. Both strategies can be seen as attempts to deal with incompatibilities.

When dilating their construing, a person starts jumping from topic to topic, lumps past and present together. Everything suddenly becomes relevant to, say, their problem or to the fact that they are a clever chap. In psychiatric terms this is commonly called 'mania'.

The opposite way of dealing with incompatibilities is to retrench. To draw in one's boundaries. To live in a smaller and yet smaller world. This process may be called 'depression' if it continues. In her study of the treatment of a group of people who were depressed, Sheehan (1984) found that the amount of 'conflict' in their construing system did, indeed, increase as they moved toward being less depressed.

Tight Versus Loose Construing

> The loose construction is like a rough sketch which may be preliminary to a carefully drafted design. The sketch permits flexible interpretation. This or that feature is not precisely placed. The design is somewhat ambiguous. (Kelly, 1955, p. 484)

Roland loved loose construing to the point that he sometimes had difficulty in extricating himself from it (indicative of schizophrenia in medical circles). For instance, during the laddering (see pages 294–5) of the construct *masculine* versus *nopt masculine*, he explained that masculine people are weak and aggressive whereas not masculine people personify strength:

> I think they have a kind of solidity um, being er I mean I actually can't point — a lot of the sort of usual things about being in touch, but you know in this one (points to a construct on the paper) in a more primitive kind of way. I think about being in something about one's feet being on the ground and almost sort of certainty, I mean it's funny, funny thing actually, there are whole notions in there I find a bit strange to take . . . I'm thinking about it much much more primitive, physical and um, in a sense down to earth in another way I don't know that I find myself today reacting against it "as it is" — too primitive and too um, can't quite think of the word um, it's kind of very rigid, kind of stereotypes, I don't feel very much fluidity about . . .

Luke demonstrates that it is not the laddering process itself that gives rise to loose construing. When laddering his *status* construct he came up with the idea that those with status are not likely to be refused.

> It is like this. If one has status or is respected, which are the same thing, then if someone is infinitely respected they would say what they want to a person who would immediately rush off and do it. If a person commanded zero respect and they said to someone "I want so and so", their reply would be "go and do it yourself". And so everybody lies somewhere between these two — but I suppose the majority of people would be happy about having people refuse to help them or having people downright rude to

them. (Fransella, 1972, p. 168)

I will leave comments on that piece of construing until later. Suffice it for the moment to serve as an example of a tight piece of construing.

Levels of Awareness. Instead of unconscious processes, Kelly preferred to use the more elaborate construct of 'levels of cognitive awareness'. Constructs can be 'suspended', or have one pole 'submerged' or be 'preverbal'. All of these can be said to be at below the conscious level of cognitive awareness. As with many other forms of psychotherapy, it is often the aim to make the client more cognitively aware of what is going on at other levels of their system — particularly the preverbal.

Here we enter the realms of dependency, core construing, and psychosomatics. Preverbal construing takes places as the infant begins to discriminate between elements in his or her environment. These are often to do with the infant's dependency. Sometimes adults continue to use the constructions they developed as infants when depending on others for survival. Such construing may have an overlay of great verbal fluency. At first sight this verbal fluency in a client may be seen as a good prognostic sign: anyone who is so adept with words and who is able to rationalise her problems so well would seem to be a very promising person for psychotherapy. Alas, this could be a faulty assessment. As you wade through the words you realise that it is extremely difficult to get to grip on those underlying constructs.

Maria was a person whose preverbal, dependency construing got seriously in the way of her forming satisfying relationships and interfered with her climb up the managerial ladder at work.

She believed that her mother hated her, and had even hated her as a young child. Using the professional construct of 'preverbal construing' in subsuming Maria's world, one can only imagine the desperation of the child as she struggled to get the warmth and love she so passionately sought. This struggle against rejection was never resolved. She became hostile — in Kelly's sense — by refusing to accept the invalidation of her construing that mother did, actually, love her. She never elaborated and 'up-dated' her construing of relationships as she grew up.

In adult life Maria constantly sought 'loving mums'. Anyone would do. Any friend became the best, the most wonderful person in the world and gave Maria the most wonderful relationship. Any man who showed an interest in her became devoured as she fought for the nourishment she so greatly yearned for. All the relationships soon foundered.

Preverbal construing can also show itself in physical complaints. Roland's presenting complaint was vomiting in times of stress; Maria had severe headaches that interfered with her doing her job properly. With no words to act as anchors for the constructs, the client can only 'behave' them or 'act them out'.

At first sight there is not much difference between this description of preverbal construing and Freud's idea of unconscious processes. However, the similarity is only skin deep. For in construct theory there is no psychic energy. That is, there is no energy invested in the unconscious (non-verbalised) ideas that continually 'pushes' to get them into consciousness. In construct theory constructs are bi-polar discriminations which we 'bring out' and place over the events with which we are confronted. It is only then that the dynamic of emotional feeling comes into play.

The Emotions of Construing

As Button has been at pains to emphasise in Chapter 1, feeling, thinking and behaving all combine to form what we call construing. Part of the personal construct psychotherapist's professional system of subsuming constructs concerns the identification of the threats, anxieties, guilts and hostilities that may help or hinder the client's progress.

For example, too rapid an 'improvement' can become over threatening to the client and lead to its opposite — relapse. Luke spells this out himself.

> I think I may stammer more because I . . . probably haven't had the fact that one day I would be a fluent speaker brought home to me with a bang . . . I suddenly sort of began to say "Ah yes, — I'm going to be a fluent speaker". (Fransella, 1972, p. 193)

The threat had come in the previous week in which he had said 'A few weeks ago you asked me if I could imagine what it would be like to be fluent. And I said that I wouldn't *like* to imagine it because I was not confident that I would ever become fluent. But now I am pretty confident.' He became aware that, if he continued on along the road he was travelling, he would be faced with comprehensive change in his core construing (threat) and he was not ready yet.

Such a client might now become hostile and produce ample evidence for the therapist that he has not 'really' changed at all. Kelly says that where there is hostility the therapist should look for guilt. In Luke's case, the guilt lies in the awareness that he has been dislodged from his core role construing — that is, he is a stutterer.

Likewise, too rapid a dilation of a depressed client's construing, premature loosening in a client who fears letting go of control, may lead to anxiety, for both face a world relatively unconstruable.

In personal construct terms, none of these ways of construing are 'bad' in themselves. In fact, Kelly argues that some level of anxiety accompanies any change as we push ourselves into the unknown; hostility is a way we have of protecting ourselves when we do not seem able to deal with changes appearing on the road ahead and so forth.

The Client and the Therapist

'Psychotherapy takes place when one person makes constructive use of another who has offered himself for that purpose.' (Kelly, 1980, p. 21).

Kelly likened the relationship to that between a research student and supervisor. Although this is not a common relationship, what Kelly was getting at was that the client, like the student, has considerable knowledge about and interest in a particular problem; that supervisors and clinicians have experience in the sorts of difficulties students and clients may get themselves into; and that they have some skills at designing experiments clients or students may find worth conducting. But, most important of all, client and clinician, student and supervisor, are in it together.

Commitment on the part of both parties is required. The client accepts that the therapist has no answers, that he has to search for them himself, and that he must be willing to commit himself to the struggle involved in reconstruing. It rarely comes easily. The client also takes on the commitment of carrying out a considerable amount of 'homework' between sessions — since most of the 'work' is done away from the consulting laboratory.

Likewise the therapist must be committed to the cause of the client and be prepared to work equally hard at understanding that client and her problems.

Much as one would like to say that client and clinician are equal partners, this is obviously not true. The client has come to the clinician for a specific purpose and, although client and clinician may well design new experiments together, it is the client who tries them out. It is never the client who designs experiments for the clinician to carry out — at least, not the experiments they design together.

The therapist does not play himself. He does not talk to the client as an equal — if that were ever possible in this highly institutionalised setting. In personal construct psychotherapy *the therapist is the validator of the client's experimental ventures*.

This is not as cold-blooded as it sounds and does not take place at a conscious level — or only rarely so. For instance, when Luke expressed his view that most people (by which he meant people who did not stammer) do not mind when others are rude or refuse to help (see page 283), my response was to invalidate him. I gave an example in which I was quite at a loss to know how to react to a person's refusal to help me. When he had got over his amazement and shock he said: 'That is a very interesting thing, because I feel that *fluent people can deal with any situation and that if I was fluent I would be able to.*' The aim of the therapist is to help the client design and conduct some new experiments and, in so doing, find alternative ways of seeing things — that is, to reconstrue.

The Goals of Therapy

Starting from the notion that a person with a problem is someone who, for the moment, cannot find any alternative way of dealing with it, then the goal must be to help the client *find* those alternatives. It must be to help the client get 'unstuck'. As Kelly puts it: 'Man may not now choose his past but he may select his future.' (Kelly, 1955, p. 833)

There is no goal of 'mental health' to strive toward, for Kelly adamantly rejected the medical model (Chapter 1, pp. 28–30). He preferred the concept of 'functioning'. Optimum functioning is when our predictions are, for the most part, validated. We are correct in our interpretations more often than we are wrong. This gives us reasonable control over our world. When we *are* wrong, when our predictions *are* invalidated, we deal with this by reconstruing or by repeating the experiment and not by being 'hostile' and setting out to fix the outcome so as to prove ourselves right.

Although the goal at the start of therapy may include the removal of the problem, this very often changes as reconstruction progresses. New issues emerge and old ones lose their importance. For instance, Roland's life-long problem of vomiting at times of stress took a back seat as he reconstrued his problem during the first three sessions. He wrote about it thus: ' . . . he hasn't got it right yet. He has to begin to make his world and he doesn't quite know how. So now I would describe him as "a *grown-up child* who doesn't know how to go on." '

Understanding the Client's World

It must always be borne in mind that the personal construct psychotherapist is not tool-bound. There are no standard tests to be used. The all-important thing is to discover how the client construes himself and his world and the identification of avenues available for movement. Kelly emphasises it thus:

> Unlike most personality theories, the psychology of personal constructs does not limit itself to any pet psychotherapeutic techniques. More than any other theory, it calls for an orchestration of many techniques according to the therapist's awareness of the variety and nature of the psychological processes by which man works towards his ends (Kelly, 1980, p. 21).

The first step in the psychotherapeutic process is to get a glimpse inside that person's world and to subsume it within the system of professional constructs. Only then can hypotheses about the nature of the problem be formulated and a treatment plan prepared.

Although standard tests are not used, there are several techniques coming directly from personal construct theory and practice to aid enquiry. But you may use none or all or any others that you think may better serve the inquiry in hand.

The techniques of construct elicitation and repertory grid technique have already been described by Button (Chapter 2). These may be used at any stage in therapy, but have been found particularly useful in the first few sessions when the therapist struggles to arrive at some ideas of why the client may be psychologically 'stuck'. On the basis of these findings, treatment can be planned. There are some other techniques which often play a major part in personal construct psychotherapy; these include some other methods of eliciting constructs and the use of role play and enactment.

Eliciting Constructs From the Client

There are many ways of asking the client to give a sample of her constructs. Non-systematic methods, such as allowing the client to talk about her experiences and problems, allow the therapist to gain a glimpse into her construing system. But the elicitation of constructs in relatively standard ways enables the therapist to gain greater insight into the meanings that may lie behind the words used. For instance, for one person not being successful may mean failing whereas for Roland it was 'not yet successful', a very different meaning indeed. Button has already described Kelly's triadic method of elicitation and so other methods will be described here. One of these is by the use of the 'self characterisation'.

The Self Characterisation. Kelly's first principle runs: If you don't know what is wrong with someone, ask him: he may tell you. The self characterisation is an example of this principle and the credulous approach in action. The carefully worded instructions invite the person to tell one about himself.

> I want you to write a character sketch of (for example) Harry Brown, just as if he were the principal character in a play. Write it as it might be written by a friend who knew him very *intimately* and very *sympathetically*, perhaps better than anyone ever really could know him. Be sure to write it in the third person. For example, start out by saying, 'Harry Brown is . . . ' (Kelly, 1955, pp. 332–6).

Writing in the third person minimises anxieties and threats and the lack of specific instructions about length, content and so forth provides maximum room for the client to choose what it is that the therapist is going to be privileged to share.

It is often useful both for the client and the therapist in the early stages of the sessions to ask the client to write about themselves as they are now and then as they will be when their problem has been eliminated. Thus, Rosemary wrote first about herself now:

> Rosemary regards herself as a shy person. She has made herself a quiet reserved type because of her stammer. Due to the fact that

she may stammer and cause a mess of a conversation, she often refrains from speaking expect for the usual daily greetings. Perhaps she may be considered somewhat rude — however unintentionally — as she usually avoids asking of one's health or how a holiday was spent. She may be considered unfriendly but it is only to avoid embarrasement.

However, she is usually granted on her good sense of humor This she does to hide all her embarassment. If, a conversation was full of blocks and hesitated pauses, she may often crack a joke at the end to hide her uneasy feeling or to distract their attention. This often is quite successful.

On the whole she is far from a nervous person. She has no fears regarding, for example, darkness, lifts, travelling and she is usually quiet calm in areas of emergency. However, all her nerves begin to get into action before she opens her mouth and begins to speak. This is due to the fear of stammering & making a fool of herself — so obviously in this state of mind, the speaking is vastly more hesitated.

According to the opinion of her parents and proved by various I.Q. or examinations, she appears to be over average in the degree of cleverness. However, in school years she never proved this in class, due to her stammering. In order to avoid the embarrassment of answering a question in French oral and making a complete mess of the class rhythm, she would often pretend that she was ignorant of that context, & allow another child to go ahead with the correct answer, but had to put on an act as though she was completely vague of the subject matter. This led to a stage when she rejected the homework as she considered it worthless to study hard & the next day pretend as if she were completely ignorant. This happened with few subjects. However, subjects without any oral work she tried to do well.

Meeting strangers is really an ordeal to her. This is due to considering what their impression would be on her. By hestitating greatly in a conversation could put the person off her.

When she is upset about something she tends to stammer more than usual.

Rosemary appears to be giving a picture of someone who sees her whole personality in terms of her effect on others. She sees her stammer as having 'made her' into this shy, quiet person since childhood. She points out that she is not a nervous person except when she is about to open her mouth. There are several references to her giving a false impression of herself to others.

The therapist might reasonably ask himself whether Rosemary is giving a false impression of herself to him; particularly in relation to her being above average in intelligence since the grammar and spelling suggest this may possibly not be the case. But Rosemary is giving a particular impression of herself, and the therapist accepts this as 'true' — at least for the time being, perhaps coming back later to explore the issue further.

The therapist might also be interested in finding out what Rosemary would be like in her view if she were her 'true' self and not dominated by her stammer. To gain some insight into this she was asked to write about her potential future self:

Rosemary is a keen worker. She is an efficient typist and is able to tackle her share in the office world. She is capable and responsible. She can easily discuss a topic with another. She is friendly and likes meeting and speaking with people. She is popular at work and with friends.

However, occaisionally she tends to be somewhat selfish and thoughtless with regards to other people. She may refuse to go shopping for another member of staff or reject doing the low jobs in the office. This appears to be for no apparent reason except for the possibility of pride.*

(*P.S. This sort of behaviour was practiced often while I had the stutter. Because I couldn't speak sophisticatedly, and first impressions of strangers were not always so high of me due to my stammer, I needed respect greatly. To me respect was everything. I often refused minor office routine jobs because I thought they were taking advantage of my speech, and judged me to be the person like the way I spoke. I had to be perfect or else I would loose my respect. If I made an error in typing I would be upset for a large percentage of the day, as I imagined I was loosing the respect I had).

Occaisionally she may appear to be quite arrogant. She tends to show her feelings of like and dislike openly and is more friendly with clever and lively girls.

She is enthusiastic to learn, and enjoys taking evening classes in interesting subjects. Her social life is good. She enjoys parties and is usually in the centre of crowds. She has a keen sense of humor. She is fun to have around the place.

In Kelly's words, the self characterisation is 'nature babbling to herself'. Here we have a girl who is given the opportunity to think out loud about herself from two different perspectives. In some ways they seem like descriptions of two different people. The therapist has to find a way of enabling Rosemary to move from the stammering self to the fluent self — which may well involve a re-creating of the latter.

Rosemary has provided some valuable data about herself. Particularly important for therapy may be her strengths; she is capable, responsible and enthusiastic to learn. The therapist would need to ensure he offers her obvious respect — perhaps trying to encourage the idea that people can be respected even though they are not perfect. But such treatment planning would only come when all the data have been collected.

Laddering of Constructs. Constructs elicited by the self characterisation, the triadic method, or any other way, may be 'laddered'. Their pathway into more and more abstract areas is traced step by step (Hinkle, 1965).

Roland's constructs were laddered to elicit the increasingly superordinate or abstract constructs. In this process you first ask the client which pole of the construct he would prefer to be — Roland said he would prefer to be *not masculine* as opposed to *masculine*. He was then asked to specify why he had this preference; why it was more important for him to be not masculine rather than masculine. After considerable thought he replied that not masculine people could just '*be*', *without strings* whereas masculine people were *aggressive children*. The questioning is always formulated in the context of 'why'. In response to the further question focusing on the advantages, for him, of being someone who had no strings attached to them, he replied that you could live *without a mask* whereas those who were *aggressive children* always had to *wear masks*.

Roland's ladder for the construct *successful* versus *not yet successful*, with his preference on the *not yet successful* pole, showed that successful people were *committed to one course of action for life* and thus were *feeling in a constant state of tension* whereas those who were not yet successful had *more possibilities open to them* and so were *more relaxed*. Being successful had clear penalties such that it was better to remain the potential (the not yet successful) genius.

Laddering in this way is a form of structured interviewing and therefore not similar to free association. The client is kept within the confines of the network of implications for each particular construct.

As can be seen from these two examples, considerable insight can be gained into the construing system of the client in a relatively short period of time. But it is not only the therapist who gains insight. Roland commented at the end of the *masculine* versus *not masculine* ladder saying that there was something wrong. It was not that he felt the construct inappropriate, he was 'sure it is right'. It was rather that he came to a realisation that there was 'something claustrophobic about it'. This procedure for collecting data was therefore also something he found useful and it indeed seemed to be the start of the reconstruing process itself for him.

Pyramiding. This has been described by Landfield (1971) as a means for exploring the more subordinate or concrete levels of the construing system. Whereas laddering basically asks 'why', pyramiding asks 'how' or 'what'.

The initial instructions are 'think of a person with whom you feel most comfortable and whose company you enjoy. Do not tell me who it is, but let me know if it is male or female. Now give me an important characteristic of that person.' The reply might be 'sympathetic'. What kind of person is not sympathetic?' 'An egocentric person'. The questioning continues in this vein asking for a description of the kind of person who is described by the construct pole and its opposite elicited.

This can be particularly useful for those who have difficulty in tightening their construing.

The ABC Procedure. Tschudi (1977) extended Hinkle's (1965) notion of 'implicative dilemmas' by describing a method for pinpointing reasons why some clients are unable or unwilling to change. The client is asked to specify the advantages and disadvantages of both poles of a construct. This is particularly useful when carried out with constructs in the 'problem' area. Very often the dilemma can be spotted in a few minutes.

Tom was having problems at work. He had done well to achieve a managerial position while quite young, but was increasingly getting irritable and not doing his work as well as he knew he was able. His construct was *doing something useful* versus *being a free rider*. The advantage of doing something useful is that you are *better rewarded and achieve more*, and the disadvantages of being a free rider are that you *value yourself less and people see you as a cheat*. However, when asked for the disadvantages of being better rewarded and achieving more he replied that it is *time-consuming, boring and dull*, whereas the advantages of being a free rider are that there is *more time for other interests and you can be creative*. Tom had isolated the nature of his dilemma and set about resolving it.

The Bases of Psychological Movement

Psychological movement in personal construct psychotherapy centres around the cycles of creativity, experience and decision-making. Change, or reconstruction, takes place either by moving the self from one pole of a construct to the other ('slot change'), or by elaborating and reorganising the construing system in a systematic way, or by developing new constructs.

The Cycles of Movement

The Creativity Cycle. As has been detailed in Chapter 1, to be creative one has to be able to move from tight to loose and then to tight construing. 'The loosening releases facts, long taken as self-evident, from their rigid conceptual moorings. Once so freed, they may be seen in new aspects hitherto unsuspected, and the creative cycle may get under way.' (Kelly, 1955, p. 1031).

The ability to loosen one's construing is often one of the first lessons the client has to learn. But this is useless without the ability to tighten once some new aspect has been sighted. Bannister sees the person with the type of 'thought disorder' found in some schizophrenic patients as being someone who is unable to complete the creativity cycle (see Bannister and Fransella, 1980 for an account of Bannister's theory).

The Decision Making or CPC Cycle. When needing to come to a decision, we first circumspect (C) the alternatives available — there are all sorts of ways of dealing with the issue. Eventually one construct has to be selected or 'pre-empted' (P), and then one pole of that construct chosen (C). The Choice Corollary states that the pole chosen will be the one which provides the better opportunity for further elaboration of the construing system. It is this choice that precipitates you into action.

Hilda had a decision to make about how to deal with the advances of men. She eventually pre-empted the construct *relate to them all* versus *be selective*. She chose to *be selective*. In therapy she had elaborated her construing sufficiently to feel that being selective would be the more likely to provide her with the greater possibility for increasing her ability to deal with the world.

The Cycle of Experience. In Kelly's theoretical system experience is about reconstruing. We have experience as we successively construe events. The whole of psychotherapy can therefore be seen in terms of human experience rather than as treatment. As Kelly puts it:

> psychotherapy needs to be understood as an experience, and experience, in turn, understood as a process that reflects human vitality. Thus to define psychotherapy as a form of treatment — something that one person does to another — is misleading. (Kelly, 1980, p.21)

In his *The Psychology of the Unknown* Kelly (1977) talks about the cycle of experience starting, as does all construing, with *anticipation*. In fact our processes as human beings are psychologically 'channellised' by the ways in which we anticipate events. Coupled with anticipation we need to have commitment. We need to stick our neck out and get involved with events. But even this is not enough:

> Only by adding *reconstruing* to the sequence of psychological processes can the full cycle of human experience be completed and man freed from his Sisyphean labours. The cycle of human experience remains incomplete unless it terminates in fresh hopes never before envisioned. This, as I see it, is no less true for the puzzled scientist than for the distraught person who seeks psychotherapeutic escape from the psychological redundancies that he has allowed to encompass him, or, for that matter, for the experienced sinner who finds in repentance, not reincapsulation within a dogmatic system, but the full restoration of his initiative. (Kelly, 1977, p. 9)

The Reconstruing Process

There are three basic types of movement Kelly sees as being in-volved in the reconstruing process. Sometimes a form of movement is observed in the client which, while being superficial, can produce some devastating results. The client can '*slot rattle*'. He can shuffle from one pole of a construct to the other and back again, repeating this sequence *ad nauseam*. In some sense this is not reconstruing at all, for the client is merely moving an element, himself, from one pole of the construct to the other. One week he can be as gentle as can be, the next he is renowned for his aggression.

Some clients show this when they are changing in other ways. For instance, a woman may lose a stone in weight and slot rattle from seeing herself as all things weak and undesirable to all things she would like to be. When events show her that she has not become like her ideal self just because she has lost a substantial amount of weight, she slots herself back into her old familiar niche — along with putting the weight back on.

A more comprehensive form of reconstruction is when constructs are reorganised and elaborated but not essentially revised. *Controlled elaboration* of this sort can be seen in Luke as he found out more and more about his superordinate constructs *respect* and *status*. He tightened up on them and made them more internally consistent. He learned what they were actually meaning for him and so he was better able to use them successfully. However, he did not form new constructs to take their place.

The third, and most difficult, type of change involves the creation of *new constructs*. By the careful introduction of new elements into the client's experience, old constructs may become so modified in the struggle to incorporate new elements that the meanings they have for the client actually change.

It was the second and third forms of change that Kelly referred to in the following:

> Psychotherapeutic movement can thus be said to get underway when a man starts questioning for himself what his immediate objectives may be and is thus led to initiate actions that challenge whatever previous notions he may have held as to what his limitations were. This is the first step in redefining his poten-tialities. He sets out to be what he is not. (Kelly, 1980, p. 20)

Ways of Encouraging Change

Almost everything that has been written about so far in this chapter could equally well have been subsumed under this heading — they are all ways of helping a client change.

Techniques for Construing Exploration as Vehicles for Change

For example, controlled elaboration was being used with Luke as he was encouraged to explore how he related fruit pastilles to status and respect.

Roland used writing varieties of self characterisation as his main therapeutic tool (Fransella, 1981). In one piece, written towards the end of therapy, he discusses the role it played:

> A further question which needs to be explored is whether writing of this kind is a masturbatory self indulgence, or whether it plays a tougher, more active part in how he conducts his life.
>
> Again my feeling is that the evidence suggests that it is not masturbatory self indulgence. Roland does seem to be becoming more involved with other people. He gives much more of himself than he has in the past. Of course, there is still a certain reserve and some of the reserve is a hangover from his past, but there is a new component which could be described as a realistic reserve, a recognition that the reflection and thought which seems to be necessary for him may not be necessary for others.

It is noteworthy that his construing is now much less 'loose' than it was in the excerpt given on page 285: he is able to pin issues and arguments down much more precisely.

Equally, the elicitation, laddering, pyramiding of constructs, the use of the ABC method for exploring constructs, the completion of repertory grids are all used as means whereby the client is encouraged to explore his or her own construing system and thereby start on the road of reconstruction.

Role Play and Enactment

Kelly was particularly interested in role play and enactment having been influenced by Moreno's work on psychodrama. For instance, if it is agreed that a person's feelings be explored more fully, an appropriate technique is selected. A man who feels he might kill someone if he ever lost his temper may be encouraged to talk to a cushion in a Gestalt-like fashion 'as if' it were his father. The consulting room is a laboratory where experiments can safely be carried out and their results examined. Finding that losing his temper did not result in murder — only a battered cushion — allows these feelings to be explored.

His use of role enactments is closely linked with his theoretical construct of role:

> The function of enactment procedures is to provide for elabora-tion of the client's personal construct system, to provide for experimentation within the laboratory of the interview room, to protect the client from involving core structures before he is ready to consider abandoning them, to free the client from pre-emptive constructions too tightly tied to actual events and to persons, and to enable the client to see himself and problems in perspective. (Kelly, 1955, pp. 1145-6)

Whenever role play is used, Kelly suggests it is valuable to reverse the roles. Not only does this give the client at least two perspectives on the problem, but sometimes provides the therapist with valuable further insights into the client's construing world. This can be particularly effective if the client–therapist roles are reversed.

Landfield (1980b) gives the example of Dr Tom whose wife said he had a drink problem but who insisted that the few drinks he did take 'wasn't really drinking!' With roles reversed, Landfield repeated Dr Tom's statements back to him and asked what he, in the role of therapist thought. After a few moments of perplexity, Dr Tom blurted out, 'I'd say that you are a god-damned alcoholic!' Such enactments often need last no more than one or two minutes to be effective. Sometimes, indeed, they turn out to be powerful medicine.

Kelly does describe one form of therapeutic method which he called *fixed role therapy*. But he was concerned that it should not be thought to be THE procedure for the personal construct therapist, but was given as an example of how the theory can be applied in the psychotherapeutic context. He says:

> Let us hope I have not focused so sharply upon fixed role therapy as to leave the impression that it is the only therapeutic method to be derived from personal construct theory. There are so many other implications of the theory it would be a pity if this parti-

cular method I happen to have used in no more than ten per cent of my therapeutic efforts over the years were to be regarded as the definitive explication of personal construct psychotherapeutics. (Kelly, 1973).

An important idea is embedded in fixed role therapy. There we find the idea that we have created ourselves and, having become dissatisfied with the current model, that we can create a new one.

Fixed role therapy uses the self characterisation as its starting point. The client writes one and then the therapist writes a second version. The aim is that it should offer the client some workable ways of being that are neither the opposite to what they are now — no-one willingly stands life on its head — nor a simple replica of the first. For instance, instead of seeing men as either always being about to pounce because of her irresistibility or shunning her because of her unattractive fatness, Hilda tried deciding whether or not *she* liked *them*.

A whole character sketch is written in this way and then discussed with the client. It is modified until the client feels that she can 'get inside' that person and feels comfortable there. For she is now asked to live that role for a week or two. She must eat, dress and behave just as she thinks this other person would do. During this adventure she will have constant access to the therapist.

In taking on this alternative role, the person behaves in alternative ways and finds others respond to this new behaviour differently. She may find that some of these new ways are useful to her and can be explored further while others have unpleasing consequences. It is with the therapist that she will discuss these successes and failures and will test out yet others in the safety of the consulting room. Together they make predictions about future happenings, and struggle to put new experiences into words.

Fixed role therapy is based on the ideas that we might all usefully be seen as scientists and on Kelly's notion of role. Fundamentally, it is about creation.

Man understands his world by finding out what he can do with it. And he understands himself in the same way — by finding out what he can make of himself. Man is what he becomes. What he becomes is a product of what he undertakes — expected or by surprise. The peculiar genius of psychology, if it has one, is to see man in this perspective — as what the continuing effort of living can make of him. (Kelly, 1973).

Reasons for Resisting Change

Since the person is regarded as a form of motion — we are alive and therefore we move — Kelly's approach does not require any additional concept of 'motivation' or of 'forces' to explain why we move. With no 'force' there is nothing to defend ourselves against and therefore no need to 'resist' in the psychoanalytic meaning of the term. Kelly states it thus: 'Since we do not employ a defensive theory of human motivation, the term does not have the important meaning it must necessarily assume for the psychoanalysts. Instead, we recognise necessary limitations of various persons' construct systems.' (Kelly, 1955, p. 1101).

There is now considerable evidence that clients who are currently construing the world in certain ways decide to resist change (Fransella, 1984). For instance, a client who is construing events from a very well-organised, tightly-knit standpoint will see any substantial movement as threatening and anxiety-making and will rightly resist attempts to push them toward reconstruing; so will the client who perceives that the therapist is implicitly asking them to change their core construing; or who suddenly becomes aware that reconstruction has already gone further than they had imagined.

All are behaving perfectly reasonably *from their own perspective*. It is the therapist who is doing a poor job of subsuming the client's construing if they merely see the client's behaviour as resistance — and therefore something to be overcome.

Recognising When the Goal Has Been Reached

It is common practice for personal construct psychotherapy to be faded out. Clients are given increasingly long intervals between sessions up to four weeks. By this time the client is clearly conducting his or her own experiments and actively creating a new life for themselves. When the client and the therapist wonder why they are spending time together — it is time to call a halt. The client is truly on the move again:

> . . . the task of psychotherapy is not to produce behaviour, but rather to enable the client, as well as the therapist, to utilize behaviour for asking important questions. In fact, the task of

psychotherapy is to get the human process going again so that life may go on and on from where psychotherapy left off. (Kelly, 1969h, p.223).

15 GROUP PSYCHOTHERAPY

Hugh Koch

My motivation for writing this chapter is to discuss what personal construct theory, research and practice has to contribute to the understanding and running of therapeutic small groups. In most psychiatric or community services these days, both for reasons of economic necessity and theoretical stance, the group therapy modality is widely used. Although it is possible to find one type of group approach being exclusively practised, it is more frequent to find several approaches being utilised with different client groups. Most group therapists express the following dilemmas in setting up a therapy group:

1. What are the main aims in group therapy?

2. What are the main therapeutic processes which facilitate realising these aims?

3. What are relevant measures meaningful to both patient and therapist, to assess progress?

I have chosen to organise this chapter around a number of considerations, which include these questions, and which I consider important in understanding therapy groups and the group therapeutic process. I will not present a comprehensive review of all theoretical approaches to group therapy, nor a systematic review of any single theory, but will assume some basic knowledge of the different group approaches.

One of the major problems facing the 'student in group interaction' is the perplexing array of complex theories, often expressed in idiosyncratic language associated with the authors' own background and often only loosely related to the practical techniques advocated. To aid clarity, Bascue (1978) presented a conceptual model of the different group therapies (see Figure 15.1) which is a good place to start.

For the purpose of this chapter the main group therapy

Figure 15.1: Conceptual Model of Group Therapy (Bascue, 1978)

Therapeutic Dimensions

	TEMPORAL	
Past	_____	Future
External	SPATIAL _____	Internal
Cognitive	VOLITIONAL _____	Affective
Verbal	ACTIONAL _____	Behavioural
Individual	SYSTEMIC _____	Group
Leader Activity	FOCAL _____	Member Activity
Manifest Meaning	SYMBOLIC _____	Latent Meaning
Problem-Solving	JURISDICTIONAL _____	Personality Change

approaches are taken as being Group-Analytic, Interpersonal and Cognitive-Behavioural. For a description of each and an historical perspective, the reader is referred to Cobb (1979). Each of the main group therapy approaches could be differentiated by their relative positions on Bascue's therapeutic dimensions. Group therapy is clearly not a uniform approach to treatment, and covers a wide range of techniques, each having its own basic assumptions. However, there is increasing general recognition of the importance of social experience and process within the group setting. I shall, therefore, first consider a personal construct view of interpersonal relationships and well-being. Subsequent sections will cover assessment for group therapy, therapist and patient views of group interaction, serial changes in group therapy and finally a personal construct approach to group therapy.

Interpersonal Relationships and Construct Theory

According to Kelly (1955), the elaborative potential of a given relationship is governed by: 1. the level of 'commonality', providing validation, and security; 2. the level of understanding, or more precisely 'sociality', providing extension and elaboration. Commonality and sociality are inadequate predictors of success or failure in a social setting when taken alone. Both are important.

The *commonality corollary* indicates that while each individual group member is unique, individuals can share common under-standings. This commonality provides some consensual validation for the individual's views. Such validation is 'reinforcing'. It secures current structures, tightening relationships among constructs in the system and provides some assurance of the workability of present structures. This psychological security can enable the individual to consider the validity of new, alternative constructions.

The *sociality corollary* implies that relationships in a group setting are limited by the degree of understanding, i.e. the interactants' ability to subsume one another's constructions of experience. Thus a major factor in limiting the development of interpersonal rela-tionships is the level of understanding between interactants. By subsuming another person's constructions, an individual adds the perspectives of the other person to his or her own understandings. One is in a better position to look at a group situation if one is able to bring more than one set of related constructs to bear. One is also more able to see others' points of view. This understanding enables the extension of the system.

Validation and elaboration are primary objectives of relationship formation and maintenance within groups. Long-term successful relationships are characterised by a recurring pattern of validation and elaboration. Reid (1979) endorsed the importance of cyclical patterns of construing processes, recognising three necessary modes: *Pre-emption/circumspection* (exclusion or inclusion of more than one construction of a single event), *constriction/dilation* (exclusion or inclusion of more than one event on which to base an interpretation or impression) and *choice*, which is central to the explanation of action. These three modes are how feelings of control are maintained. An example clarifying this: A woman comes to work and quarrels with her boss. She feels that purely on the basis of this bad quarrel (constriction), her relationship with him is useless (pre-emption) and the only thing left to do is avoid him (choice/decision). An alternative approach would be to consider other events which may have a bearing on the quarrel (dilation) and consider alternative interpretations of the quarrel situation (cir-cumspection) like a frank exchange of views, momentary loss of tempers which might be better dealt with by a positive and sym-pathetic approach or letting things blow over (choice). Thus in the course of a social encounter a person might follow a sequence of construction involving, in succession, circumspection, pre-emption and control, leading to a choice of action (Kelly, 1955, p. 515).

According to Landfield (1980b), psychological health and well-being is associated with moderate relationships between three major modalities: *feelings*, *values* and *behaviour*. The healthy person can take a 'perspective' view by relating feelings to values to behaviours and simultaneously discriminate between them. For example, a sexual feeling may (or may not) lead to developing social and sexual intimacy and action. Similarly an angry feeling about someone may (or may not) imply something about one's worth as a partner. Landfield felt that moderate relating of feelings, values and behaviour enabled a person to experience feelings without being confused or overwhelmed by them. Support for this comes from Leitner (1981b) who differentiated between students and psychiatric patients in terms of perspectivism.

The alternatives to 'Perspectivism' as described above are 'Literalism', and 'Chaotic Fragmentalism'. Literalism is defined as 'a way of thinking, feeling or doing which implies the restricted and absolute interpretation of an event or a relationship' (Landfield, 1980b, p. 315). A literal person will be unable to discriminate between feelings, values and actions. For example, having sexual feelings for others means the same as *being* adulterous (behaviour) and implies being a bad spouse (values). As a result this person might choose between not acknowledging the feeling or impulsively acting on it. Literalism has been shown to be associated with psychopathology by Leitner (1981 a, b). Chaotic Fragmentalism is defined as 'an unorganised complexity of thinking, feeling and doing which implies an unrestricted, loose, undirected, and shifting interpretation of an event or relationship' (Landfield, 1980b, p. 316). For example, even though, a husband is aggressive and abusive to his wife (behaviour), he feels he loves her. Feelings, values and behaviour are not systematically related to one another. This has, again, been shown to be empirically linked to severe psychopathology (Leitner, 1981 a, b).

In summary, then, 'psychological well-being' (Button, 1983a) may lie in the following areas:

a. The ability to experience and provide commonality and validation.

b. The ability to experience and provide understanding and hence extension and elaboration.

   c. The ability to experience recurring cycles of commonality and understanding.

   d. Cyclical patterns of pre-emption/circumspection, constriction/dilation and choice.

   e. The ability to take 'perspectivist' views rather than 'Literal' or 'Fragmented' views, in relating Feelings, Values and Behaviours.

Breakdown or restriction in relationship building and maintenance occurs when the above processes are not available or inadequately developed. These ideas provide a theory of individuality and interpersonal activity, and offer an important model for understanding the development of a therapeutic group process.

Problem Formulation and Assessment for Group Therapy

Personal construct theory offers a promising approach to defining therapy focus and a number of studies of group therapy will be described which utilise this approach. Such studies are based on the conviction that the essential problems or issues brought to therapy and changed by therapy are best described by defining and elaborating the client's personal construct system, where the aim is to identify, in a shared language with the client, the constructions underlying the client's presenting problem and inability to change, and to relate treatment and the evaluation of its effectiveness to those constructions. It is also important that treatment foci encompass more than one modality (Lazarus, 1976; Leitner, 1981a). Many measures have been derived from the data obtained from grid elicitation prior to therapy. These range from simple target problem indices and ratings thereof, e.g. relaxed – tense; depressed – happy; to indices of 'unconscious splitting' (Ryle, 1975) or 'chaotic fragmentalism' (Leitner, 1981a). In summarising these varied derived measures, it is hoped to illustrate the variety of indices for construing problems and assessing changes in these problems as a result of group therapy.

Target Problem Ratings

In early meetings with the client via non-directive discussion, the therapist identifies, in the client's terms, what the goals of therapy are. These can be embodied in straightforward target problem rating scales (Candy *et al.*, 1972) on which progress can be monitored by successive ratings. The therapist may also offer his own formulation of the client's problems and suggest additional target problems, e.g. 'prone to anxiety', 'restricted social life', 'lack of sexual confidence'. These formulations by client and therapist may be extended through more direct enquiry, or through the mutual interpretation of data derived from repertory grid inquiry. Repertory grid data, in particular may reveal areas of difficulty in, for example, ways in which the client can only conceive of a limited range of potential modes of relating to others (Ryle, 1975; Ryle and Lipshitz, 1976b). The utility of making individualised predictions for therapeutic change in group therapy assessment has been well illustrated (Koch, 1983a).

Element and Construct Relationships

Numerous derived measures are available from repertory grids elicited from clients. These include: self-significant other isolation/ closeness, parental identification, parental evaluation (ideal-self – parent distance), sexual identification, self isolation, polarisation and splitting in self-others construing, meaningfulness of symptom, and self-esteem. Further detailed information can be found in Koch (1983a). Elaboration of certain construct relationship assessment leads to the following.

Dilemmas, Traps and Snags

Ryle has suggested that a client's inability to change is best conceptualised in terms of 'Dilemmas', 'Traps' and 'Snags'. While the client can only see possible action in terms of his dilemmas, while his interactions with others are mutually maintained in terms of traps, or while change has, or is felt to have, snags, the possibility of change is slight (Ryle, 1979a). Once the client's Dilemmas, Traps and Snags (DTS) can be identified, therapy can be usefully related to these underlying formulations which if consensually identified by therapist and client will have extensive explanatory power. The resolution of the D, T and S becomes the goal of therapy and the basis of a further target problem rating. Ryle (1979a) identified six main groups of interpersonal problems most commonly found:

1. Distance or 'in danger' dilemmas; either isolated or at risk.

Emotional closeness provokes fear of loss of self or damage to self.

2. Dyadic control dilemmas: either controlled or controlling; either powerfully giving or helplessly receiving.

3. (a) Must/won't dilemmas: obligations are responded to by resentful compliance with a loss of free will.
   (b) Problem of feelings and control: either tightly controlled or chaotic emotionality.

4. 'Sex-role' dilemmas: either strong or sensitive; either logical or emotional.

5. Traps: acting out of one dilemma with partner who plays the complementary role in the dilemma, e.g. 'I'm always logical, she's always emotional'.

6. Snags: feared consequences of certain thoughts, feelings and actions (which are aimed at resolving or confronting a dilemma).

These DTS situations can be elicited and measured via construct correlations arising from a repertory grid, e.g. constructs 'looks after' and 'gives in to' highly correlated illustrating the snag of 'if caring, then submitting'.

The use of the 'dyad grid' in assessment has increased in recent years. As we have seen in Chapters 2 and 10 the dyad grid (Ryle and Lunghi, 1970) incorporates elements as relationships of one person to another. The constructs therefore become descriptive of inter-actions and the client's implicit theory of relationships. The value of conceptualising some neurotic problems as relationship dilemmas involving issues of dependency, control and care-given and the value of the dyad grid in identifying a particular client's dilemmas have been well established (Ryle, 1979a).

A variation in the use of dyad grids in multi-person systems has been suggested by Watson and Karastergon–Katsika (J.P. Watson, personal communication) in their family relationship grid. Family members used supplied constructs to each describe family relationships. These elements were sorted to form a consensus grid so that each member's view of one particular relationship could be viewed from different viewpoints, compared and contrasted. This is clearly translatable into group therapy terms, where it could be possible to look at a member's relationship with another member or therapist as seen by all the group members.

More than two dyad grids with similar elements and constructs (supplied) can be collated via the 'Series' programme (Slater, 1964) in such a way as to provide a 'CONSENSUS' grid which is representative of the group of grids. For example, the dyadic relationships of each group member with other members, therapist and family members can be investigated to produce 'group' predictions of beneficial change, along, for instance, group-analytic theory.

Literalism, Fragmentalism and Perspectivism

Leitner formulated ways of measuring the types of relationships between the emotional, evaluative and behavioural implication of traditional constructs via his concepts and measures of literalism, chaotic fragmentalism and perspectivism (Leitner, 1981a).

Unconscious Processes

Ryle (1975) suggested that grid data provide access to unconscious mental processes such as 'splitting' and mental conflict. Splitting arises from the client resolving ambivalence by separating opposing qualities between different people. The principal component analysis indicating the magnitude of first factor variance and mean construct variation allows an approximate guide to a client's splitting process. 'Oedipal' patterns are reflected by the sexual identification measures described earlier, whether these are obtained via grids with individuals or dyadic relationships as elements. 'Repression/denial' can be suggested from the non-use of certain constructs, e.g. with an emotional implication, or from a lack of discrimination on constructs which are negatively loaded, e.g. sexuality, aggression. Of all the so-called unconscious processes, perhaps most research has centred on 'transference' (Koch, 1983a; Ben-Tovim and Greenup, 1983). The recognition, assessment and utilisation of transference phenomena have assumed a place of central importance in analytical group therapy and the effects of transference interpretations have been discussed by Malan (1979) and Koch (1983a) who found them to be important ingredients in successful short-term individual and group psychotherapy respectively.

Construing Group Interaction: Therapists' and Patients' Views

Several attempts have been made to clarify dimensions of inter-personal interaction in group sessions. Such attempts have been largely based on non-therapy groups, and fall into one of the following three types of categorisations:

a. 1. Aiding attainment by the group; 2. Individual prominence and achievement; 3. Sociability (Bales 1956; Carter, 1954; Mann, 1961).

b. 1. Control; 2. Affection; 3. Inclusion (Schutz, 1958).

c. 1. Dominance – submission; 2. Love – hostility (Foa 1961; Leary, 1957).

These were largely theoretically defined. Some empirical support has been forthcoming from studies by Giedt (1956), Mann (1961) and Chance (1966).

An alternative approach to the identification of group interaction dimensions is to explore what ideas experienced group participants or observers normally use when construing 'the group'. McPherson and Walton (1970) asked seven experienced clinicians to observe a therapy group and describe the intra-group interactions of the participants, via repertory grid elicitation. A principal components analysis of the combined grids isolated three independent dimensions differentiating group members who are (1) assertive and dominant from those who are passive and submissive, (2) emotionally sensitive to others from those who are insensitive and (3) aiding the attainment of group goals rather than hindering them. These dimensions are approximately similar to those in previous studies and may therefore represent the major ways in which the interpersonal interactions of people differ.

It is interesting to note that the language used by these experienced therapists in the study cited above involved words to describe constructs which are well-known to most, if not all, therapists but are either too superordinate or, equally possibly, too far removed from what 'actually occurs' within the group sessions and might be of doubtful relevance to the participants themselves. It was to test out this possibility that a study was recently carried out by the author which attempted to elicit from participants of two types of therapy groups the constructs used to understand and make sense of the group sessions they attended. The two groups studied were:

1. *Short-term Anxiety Management Training (AMT) Group.* This consisted of four members plus one therapist and involved a high level of didactic information giving, plus sharing of views and practical difficulties about anxiety control, relaxation and home practice. The repertory grid elicitation took place after the fourth and final session.

2. *Long-term Group-Analytic Group.* This consisted of six members and two therapists. It involved procedures and assumptions encompassed by the Foulkes and Anthony (1957) group analytic approach. There was free and open discussion, little overt direction from the therapists, and a group goal of understanding thoughts, feelings and behaviour via the group process. Repertory grid elicitation was carried out after the group had been meeting for approximately nine months.

The repertory grid elicitation followed the procedure described by Leitner (1981a), with modification suggested by Watson (1970b) and Koch (1983a) for the investigation of group members perceptions. Each member was interviewed by the investigator (myself) and elements under discussion were the member him/herself, and other members of the group he/she attended, including the therapist(s). Nine 'traditional' constructs were elicited via Kelly's (1955) triadic method. Although each member only had experience of other members named in the list of elements via the group experience, it was stressed that group-related constructions were of predominant interest.

Each construct was then taken and, via the procedure described by Leitner (1981a), the emotional, behavioural and evaluative implications of this construct were elicited. For example, beginning with the more positively rated pole of the first construct, the subject was asked, 'what might a——(construct pole) person in the group feel (do, value) in the group?' The emotional, behavioural, and evaluational constructs were placed on three new repertory grids resulting in a total of four grids, including the 'traditional construct' repertory grid. The members were then asked to complete the ratings on each grid using a 1 – 100 rating scale.

Initially, the four individual grids from the AMT group were combined into a single grid having five elements and 36 constructs (the nine traditional constructs elicited from each member). The grid was analysed by the method of principal component analysis described by Slater (1964). The three largest components extracted accounted for 51.38 per cent 23.05 per cent and 14.49 per cent respectively. Those constructs which had the highest loadings on each component (with corresponding low loadings on the remaining components) are shown in Table 15.1 along with the rater who used them. A notional label is given to each component, i.e. one which encompasses as many of the constructs as possible.

Table 15.1: AMT Group Traditional Constructs: Constructs with Highest Loadings

Component I: 'Relaxing Activity — Tense Passivity' (51.38%)

Group Member	Construct		Loading
A	Shows the way in the group	— Led by others	1.91
B	Brings up topics	— Disinterested	1.80
	Relaxed	— Tense	1.89
C	Discusses important things	— Talks about trivial things	2.00
D	Able to relax	— Tightens up	1.99
	Helps bring others out of shell	— Leaves others alone	1.86

Component II: Verbalisation — Silence' (23.05%)

Group Member	Construct		Loading
A	Chatterbox	— Not free to talk	1.75
B	Talks about how to solve problems	— Not constructive	1.50
C	Talkative	— Quiet	2.00

Component III: 'Social — Unsociable' (14.49%)

Group Member	Construct		Loading
A	Easy to get on with	— Difficult to get on with	1.49
B	Gets on well with others	— Gets on badly with others	1.50
C	Easy to talk to	— Difficult to talk to	1.24

The implication grids (behavioural, emotional and evaluative) were then combined into a single grid for the AMT group consisting of five elements and 108 constructs and factor-analysed. The three largest components extracted accounted for 52.72 per cent, 22.84 per cent and 11.65 per cent respectively. Table 15.2. gives the main constructs representing each of the components. Labelling these components was more difficult as each label had to encompass behavioural, emotional and evaluative aspects of construing.

Table 15.2: AMT Group Implication Constructs: Constructs with Highest Loading

Component I: 'Competence – Helplessness (in social interaction)' (52.72%)

Group Member		Construct	Loading
A	Feels able to conquer problems	— Feels powerless	1.91
	Feels things go well	— Feels things go badly	1.97
B	Gets to know people	— Keeps others at a distance	1.95
C	Helps create easy atmosphere	— Creates difficult atmosphere	1.94
D	Gives ideas to others	— Keeps ideas to self	1.95
	Feels knowledgeable	— Feels stupid	1.95
	Feels helpful	— Feels unhelpful	1.96

Component II: 'Closeness — Distance' (22.84%)

Group Member		Construct	Loading
A	Opens up to others	— Keeps a distance from others	1.74
B	Likes others	— Dislikes others	1.82
	Feels it is important to need people	Feels it is unimportant	1.95
C	Discusses worries openly	— Keeps things to self	1.73

Component III: 'Positive Social Behaviour – Negative Social Behaviour' (11.65%)

Group Member		Construct	Loading
A	Socially uninhibited	— Socially inhibited	1.38
B	Smiles at others	— Looks disgruntled	1.15

Following this, the six individual grids from the analytical group were combined into one single grid having eight elements and 54 constructs. The three largest components extracted from the analysis accounted for 39.37 per cent, 21.12 per cent and 15.77 per cent respectively. Table 15.3. gives the main constructs representing each of the components. The implication grids were then combined and analysed as in the previous group and the three main components accounted for 35.38 per cent, 18.69 per cent and 12.38

per cent respectively and are described in Table 15.4.

Table 15.3: Analytical Group Traditional Constructs: Constructs with Highest Loadings

Component I: 'Assertive Group Facilitation – Anxious Group Avoidance' (39.37%)

Group Member		Construct	Loading
A	Tries to sort out problems	— Talks about good things only	2.53
B	Doesn't 'pull punches'	— 'Walks on egg shells'	1.86
	Leads group	— Doesn't take a stand	1.62
C	Gives answers	— Unable to give answers	2.39
D	Frightened of others	— Doesn't care what he/she says	2.59
E	Brings problems up in the group	— Keeps things concealed	2.13
F	Suggests solutions	— Unconstructive	1.84

Component II: 'Self-Expression – Inhibition' (21.12%)

Group Member		Construct	Loading
B	Listens	— Talks	2.41
	Active	Quiet	2.11
C	Talks in group	— Silent	2.07
D	Keeps things to self	— Tells others things	2.19
E	Expresses himself	— Says little	2.00

Component III: 'Positive Social Reinforcer – Negative Social Reinforcer' (15.77%)

Group Member		Construct	Loading
B	Relaxing towards others	— Uptight with others	2.17
C	Friendly	— Argumentative	1.90
E	Sympathetic	— Dissenting	2.15
F	Follows up on what is said	— Changes the subject	1.98

As already stated, this study elicited ideas from the group participants themselves, not from the experimenter or the therapists, and these ideas were expressed in their own words. I do not feel it is very productive to fit the component labels agilely and neatly into those arrived at by previous researchers although this would not largely be too difficult. Dimensions of activity-passivity' in relation to 'general social behaviour', 'social problem solving 'and' group

Table 15.4: Analytical Group Implication Constructs; Constructs with Highest Loadings

---

Component I: 'Emotional Comfort and Sociability – Emotional Discomfort and Unsociability' (35.38%)

Group Member	Construct		Loading
A Confident	—	Embarrassed	2.57
Happy	—	Sad	2.58
Discusses problems with group	—	Keeps problems to self	2.53
B Feels good	—	Feels bad	1.77
C Gives answers	—	Holds back comments	2.43
D Talks easily	—	Talks with difficulty	2.02
E Expresses happy thoughts	—	Keeps thoughts to self	1.78
F Makes suggestions	—	Keeps ideas to self	2.25
Talks about positive things	—	Talks about 'black side'	2.30

Component II: 'Reciprocal Relationship Building – Relationship Avoidance' (18.69%)

Group Member	Construct		Loading
A Listens more to others	—	Talks but doesn't listen	2.57
Feels being on the same level as others is important	—	Feels being on the same level as others is unimportant	2.25
B Puts helpful ideas forward	—	Doesn't help	1.33
D Able to talk to others	—	Tends to withdraw	2.40
Open emotionally	—	Defensive	2.42
F Feels it is important to make a positive contribution	—	Feels it is unimportant to make a positive contribution	1.93
Feels it is important to get on better with others	—	Feels it is unimportant to get on better with others	1.41

Component III: 'Develops Intimacy – Avoids Intimacy' (12.38*)

Group Member	Construct		Loading
C Feels it is important to pay people back for their help	—	Feels this is unimportant	2.17
D Easy going	—	Hostile	2.20
E Feels it is important to feel like other people	—	Feels this is unimportant	1.37

	Feels it is important to be at one with others	—	Feels this is unimportant	2.01
F	Feels it is important to help others		Feels this is unimportant	1.91

goal facilitation' were all present, with the dimension of 'intimacy-distance' also being personally relevant to group members. Further research could be done to define these dimensions more precisely and tie them more specifically to the explicit therapeutic aims of each group, and look at how group goals are reached. What was of great interest in this study, and different from previous studies of group interaction and therapy, was the elicitation of different types of implication constructs. For instance, in the analytical group, the avoidance' was contributed to by behavioural constructs such as 'Listens more to others – talks but doesn't listen', emotional constructs such as 'open emotionally – defensive' as well as evaluative constructs such as 'I feel being on the same level as others is important.' Using the personal construct approach to measurement, this method devised by Leitner (1981a) perhaps offers one of the next important steps in following changing perceptions of group members of group interaction.

Serial Change in Group Therapy

Depending on the orientation of the group approach, much theoretical activity has centred on identifying successive developmental phases which occur, or are thought to occur, during the group process. Some studies have attempted to follow serial changes during the life of the group. Developmental models have been provided by group theorists, e.g. Hill, Murray and Thorley, (1979), Tuckman (1965). Many are of interest but couched in rather vague terms and definitions. Bach (1954) described the psychotherapy group passing through the following stages: initial situation testing — leader dependence — pairing and competing — fantasy and play — work group. Views of development which emphasise phasing have to contend with the fact that phases are seldom, if ever, clear cut, that mixed and transitional phases occur, and that behaviour assumed to be a primary characteristic of one phase also appears in others. Coffey, Friedham, Leary and Ossema (1950) suggested a developmental task approach to the problem of defining group movement. They saw any group as being confronted with certain basic issues:

1. Problems of consensus (development of emotional support).
2. Problems of conflict (dealing with differences within the group).
3. The relationship of the individual to the group (preserving individuality yet accomplishing the group's work).
4. Problems of authority (coming to terms with the relationship to the leader).

He suggested that there was no one particular sequence — the implication being that the group deals repeatedly with these issues.

Many of the variables discussed in earlier sections of this chapter which emerge from personal construct theory can be usefully measured serially to obtain an idea of what phasic changes occur in personal construing of members participating in some form of group therapy. Watson (1970b; 1972) and Fransella and Joyston – Bechal (1971) studied aspects of process and outcome chiefly by the use of group measures (e.g. 'intensity', 'consistency') rather than individual measures of change in the repeated administration of supplied grids. Serial change was monitored by Winter and Trippett (1977) in studying a 2-year psychotherapy group of Kleinian orientation. Constructs which because of consistently high construct means, were indicative of being most descriptive of group members, were 'intelligent', 'caring', 'anxious', 'able to accept self' and 'depressed'. Agreement on the meaning of 'depressed' was initially low but increased considerably, while the reverse was true for 'angry'. This latter construct may have been rather 'impermeable' initially, and this perhaps changed and became more open or permeable to difference in application, with more behavioural elements being subsumed within its range of convenience. The similarity of patients' and therapist grids increased during treatment with a convergence in their use of constructs suggesting partly, that the patients 'learnt the language' of the therapists.

Koch (1983a) monitored changes in self-esteem and subjective anxiety as measured by monthly repertory grid ratings throughout the duration of three nine-month group-analytic groups and related these changes to changes in other self-perceptual variables (parental and group member 'identification' and 'transference') in attempts to validate empirically, using control groups, the theoretical positions of Yalom (1970) and Malan (1979). In all these therapy groups, there were significant increases in perceived relatedness between self, group members (including therapist) and parents. In particular, there was a significant relationship between increased transference relationship involving the 'mother figure' and improvement. These results provided some support for Yalom's (1970) curative factors in group psychotherapy, namely 1. universality — the sharing of personal information and the consequent identification between the sharers; 2. social learning — use of imitation process; and 3. recapitulation of family group experience, with the possibility that the relationships involving the maternal figure are of greater importance. Process analysis indicated that the variance in the changes in improvement variables which could be accounted for by the self-perceptual variables varied between anxiety, some aspect of change in perceived similarity between self, family member and group member (including therapist) was associated with improvement. The results are consistent with part of Malan's (1979) description of a 'Triangle of Person' (p. 80) with the addition of further therapeutic linkages in terms of identification of self with other, therapist and group members, and parents. Figure 15.2 indicates the usefulness of highlighting linkages in terms of 1. how a person identifies himself with another person, i.e. the degree to which he ascribes to that person the qualities he also ascribes to himself; and 2. generalisations or transference of perceptual attributes from parents to those in the group. These concepts are similar to concepts of modelling and imitation (Bandura, 1965) and 'genetic insight', 'transference' and 'translation' (Yalom, 1970). The therapeutic value of linking the past with the present by identifying similarities between parents and others has received further empirical support from individual psychotherapy process researchers (Malan, 1976; Marziali and Sullivan, 1980).

Recently, studies have attempted to clarify the relationships between repertory grid data on group process and other kinds of information about these groups and their members (Ben-Tovim and Greenup, 1983; Caplan *et al.*, 1975; Koch, 1983b). The usefulness of the repertory grid approach to serial measurement would be questionable if the data it provided had little association with other kinds of information.

Caplan *et al.* (1975) elicited grid data (elf-esteem, parental identification) on a monthly basis from members of a 13-month

Figure 15.2: Modified Triangle of Person with Therapeutic
Links

OTHER (O)   O/T and O/GR Links   THERAPIST (T)
                                                        GROUP MEMBERS (Gr)

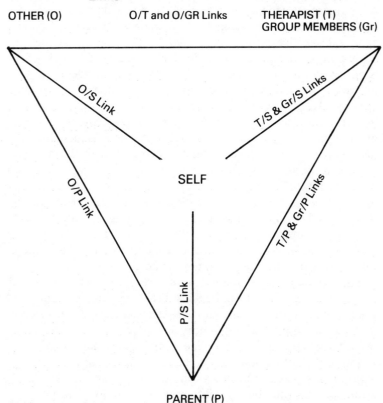

PARENT (P)

psychotherapy group and related these data to measures of verbal
behaviour during group sessions. The patients' level of identification with their fathers was positively related to the number of topics
raised, especially about family members. Self-esteem tended to
decrease when they talked about sex and increase when talking
about other relatives. They, thus, found evidence that for group
members, speaking, being spoken to and introducing several kinds
of topic into the group were significantly associated with grid variations, such as self-esteem and pattern of parental identification.

Koch (1983b) followed this line of inquiry by investigating change
in verbal affective expression (hostility, affection, anxiety, depression, self-esteem) within sessions of two psychotherapy groups run
along group analytical lines, and the relationship between changes

in affective expression and personal construing derived from group members' repertory grids (described in Koch, 1983a). Correlates of self-perceptual changes in terms of affective expression were expressions of hostility (Group A), expression of affection (Group B) and total affective expression (Group A). The analysis of data from both groups and groups combined indicated that expression of hostility was a good predictor of change in self-esteem and that overall verbalisation was a good predictor of change in subjective anxiety. Overall verbalisation, a reliable predictor of improvement, includes self-disclosure which is a prerequisite for the formation of meaningful interpersonal relationships. As verbalisation and self-disclosures increase, the membership increases its involvement and mutual responsibility. This is consonant with Peres (1947) who demonstrated that successfully treated patients in group therapy made twice as many self-disclosing personal statements during therapy as those unsuccessfully treated. Although carried out in the individual therapy field, Ben-Tovim and Greenup's (1983) study investigating how grid measures of transference related to therapist's interventions is important to cite here.

The research designs of studies summarised here, with their search for group processes of predictive value, have, despite their good points, ignored the relationship between curative factors, stages of therapy and individual differences. Factors of considerable importance to each patient may be salient at different stages in therapy for different patients. For example, the relevance of emotional expression for 'restricted individuals' who seldom experience or express strong affect would be quite different from those with problems of impulse control and considerable emotional lability.

A Personal Construct Approach to Group Therapy

It is apparent that a group therapist must have an underlying model which is theoretically consistent while, at the same time, permitting technical eclecticism. The former helps to integrate and make sense of the group members' experiences and also to understand the strengths and weaknesses of particular therapeutic schools. The latter allows for technical diversity. A Personal Construct approach satisfies these two criteria.

In general terms, the group therapist's role is to construe as accurately as possible the outlooks of other group members. In reflecting back these outlooks, he tries to encourage them within a system which is broader, more abstract than, and somewhat different from that of the other group members. Personal change amongst group members occurs when the therapist accepts the group members, is genuinely interested in the group members and can be empathic and understanding of them. In this way, 'literalisms' such as certain feelings and action being unacceptable to a person or the group's values (feeling-value and behaviour-value literalising) can be challenged and modified. For example, the self-condemnation for having and experiencing certain feelings can be modified by the therapist's genuine acceptance and positive regard for the group members. With repeated experiences of this sort whether it be in structured role-plays, dyadic experiments or unstructured discussion, usually centred on the here-and-now, members begin to differentiate between feelings, values and action and move towards a more perspectivist position.

In the initial stages of any therapeutic group's life, special attention is given to the initial acquaintanceships characterised by searching for commonality and validation by the group members, with little attempt to elaborate their construct systems by seeking out differences betweem themselves and others. The search for commonality is of paramount importance, endorsing Yalom's (1970) curative factor of 'universality'. At this time, the ground rule of most group therapies is endorsed, i.e. taking responsibility for the consequences of his/her action. This avoids fragmentalism of responsibility. This stage results in the development of personal/ social support within the group which can either be construed as facilitating other therapeutic factors or can be seen as therapeutic in itself.

Following this stage, group members move from this position of relative psychological security to clarify and discuss differences in construction which enable the elaboration of systems of understanding (Duck, 1979a). As relationships within the group develop, reciprocal elaboration becomes more critical, with each person contributing to the extension and definition of other members' systems of understanding. Recurring patterns of validation and elaboration are encouraged: prolonged, exclusive validation is avoided as this stagnates the group process. Grossly asymmetrical elaboration is avoided as this leaves members anxious or threatened.

Two major stages occur in most groups in addition to the two phases mentioned. These involve basic issues relating to (a) the relationship of the individual to the group and the need to preserve individuality yet still accomplish the group's 'tasks', and (b) the relationship of group members to the leader/therapist, i.e. the issue of authority. These two major issues are explored in some way via the clarification and modification of the cyclical processes of pre-emption/circumspection, constriction/dilation and choice, and the clarification and modification of 'dilemmas, traps and snags' (Ryle, 1979a) and whether they operate in 'literal, fragmented or perspectivist' ways (Leitner, 1981a, b).

To illustrate some of these processes, three types of therapy group will be described and discussed. The first of these, the Interpersonal Transaction Group was explicitly developed along personal construct theory lines. The other two (cognitive therapy for depressives and group analytic therapy) do not derive from construct theory but I have chosen to interpret the methods and processes involved in terms of construct theory language.

Interpersonal Transaction Group (IT)

Landfield (1979) devised the IT group to study and facilitate the interpersonal process. It focuses on dyadic interactions among persons, emphasising sharing and listening, and generally aimed at the first of the stages mentioned, namely the development of support and increased sociality. According to Landfield, small groups are preferable to large groups, as the larger group offers a greater possibility for disengaging from interactions which are becoming too threatening. Intense anxiety and hostility may promote unwillingness to share, listen and understand. Conversely, he argues that exclusive, face-to-face, dyadic interaction provides more information about how group members construe their world.

The IT group develops within the context of many brief (4-8 minutes) dyadic encounters. These self-disclosure dyads involve the discussion of assigned topics, e.g. 'things I value', 'ways people commonly misunderstand me', 'difficulties at home'.

After the first dyadic interaction, individual group members take different partners. This serial rotation continues until each member has discussed every topic with every other member. This direction by the therapist controls the frequency, duration and content of interaction.

Three superordinate constructs are provided and discussed by the therapist at the outset and throughout the group's life. These constructs are 'listening versus not listening', 'sharing versus not sharing', and 'respecting versus not respecting'. The preferred or desirable poles were 'listening carefully', 'sharing, but not to the point of great discomfort', and 'trying to understand without invalidating the other person's points of view' (respect). It was felt that these constructions would help group members bridge the gaps between their own construct systems and those of other group members, and therefore increase 'sociality'. Although not overtly part of the programme, it can be seen that, as part of the brief dyadic discussions, members could be encouraged via the eliciting and sharing of each other's views, to move from 'pre-emptive' to more 'circumspect' strategies, and from constricted to more 'dilated' strategies, as well as developing more 'perspectivist' views.

Cognitive Therapy Group for Depressives

The cognitive therapist aims to communicate two key assumptions to members of the group. These are 1. interpretations of reality are not identical to reality, but are inherently fallible, and 2. beliefs are hypotheses which are subject to disconfirmation and modification (Bedrosian and Beck, 1980). In particular, the therapist attempts to clarify how the major cycles of construing involving Pre-emption and Constriction interact with and reduce the choices of the group members.

Cognitive therapy groups are conducted along lines suggested by Beck (1976). They progress from a discussion of the principles of cognitive therapy to training group members to monitor relationships between events, their interpretation of events and their resulting moods. Finally, members are instructed how to appraise the validity of their constructions by examining them for cognitive distortions and by collecting confirmatory or disconfirmatory evidence through the use of day to day behavioural 'experiments'.

Group members often communicate faulty, irrational assumptions which are held in conjunction with negative views of self, the world, or the future. These assumptions often clearly contain certain literalisms which predict failure and depression unless clarified and modified. For example, group member A cites the behaviour — feeling literalism 'if my husband disagrees with me, it must mean he doesn't love me.' Member B cites the behaviour — value literalism 'if I make a mistake at work, it shows what a totally inept person I am'. Member C cites the feeling — value literalism 'if my wife doesn't love me anymore and wants to leave me, then it must mean I'm a worthless person and unlovable'. Using thought diaries, behavioural assignments, feedback and group discussion, the therapist encourages members to test out these assumptions, to gather data outside the group and 'shape-up' more perspectivist thoughts to conteract these literalisms. For example, a more perspectivist response to situation (A) might be 'well, we do agree on other things', or 'I can't expect him to agree with me all the time'. Although Leitner (1981a) argues that cognitive therapy does not challenge fragmentalism, perhaps in one way it does by challenging the belief held by many chronically depressed clients that current feelings cannot be modified by manipulating their values or actions (i.e. feelings – behaviour and feeling – values fragmentalism). Additionally, the use of homework assignments in some way addresses the fragmenting of values and behaviour in that it encourages the group members to act on a newly discovered value, e.g. 'practising generating positive thoughts is good for me' (Covi, Roth and Lipman, 1982).

Group Analytic Psychotherapy Group

Group-analytic technique commences with the encouragement of loosening construing in the direction of speculative and varying predictions away from concrete, exact and unvarying predictors. Techniques equated with loosening are encouraging free-association and fantasy dream association via non-directive reflection. Later in therapy, stages of encouraging tighter construction via Interpretation, and the introduction of the therapist's frame of reference repeatedly complete cycles of construing and reconstruction.

Issues of developing support and trust, and tolerating conflict are accompanied by discussion of authority and separation. Such discussions encourage the clarification of dilemmas well described by Ryle (1979a) in which anxiety concerning separation/closeness is expressed, e.g. 'if I get too close to my husband, I feel overwhelmed, but if he's not around, I feel abandoned'. Other dilemmas such as the sex-role dilemma, e.g. 'I am either too logical or over-emotional' are typically expressed. Individual dilemmas become marital traps in which both partners' dilemmas form a dysfunctional match. These marital traps may 'transfer' into the group and a similar match be formed by two group members with each other.

In many ways, the analytical approaches to group therapy

attempt to deal with both literalism and chaotic fragmentalism. Members are invited to explore and consider any action they have taken or might take in the future (via free association). This increases the chance that feelings and impulses, previously hidden, may in fact be expressed, i.e. on the one hand modifying fragmenting between thoughts, feelings and behaviour, but on the other hand discouraging the literalism between feelings and actions whereby a feeling automatically leads on to 'acting out'. Resistance is dealt with by, on the one hand, adopting a condemning negativistic response to clients' difficulties and difficult behaviours (thereby challenging the literal equating of behaviour and value as a person) but invites the clients to take responsibility for the consequences of actions (thereby challenging the fragmenting of behaviour and value).

When dealing with the various types of transference within the group, the clients are encouraged to explore and understand their intense within-the-group feelings towards each other and the therapist without necessarily acting upon them, confronting the feeling — behaviour literalism. In the same vein, members may express intense negative feelings without condemnation by the therapist or the group, modifying feeling — value literalism.

From the analytic point of view, problematic feelings and impulses (supposedly originating in the id) are not related or integrated with values (originating in the superego) or with behaviour (from the ego). The two main analytical interventions of confrontation and interpretation are two important techniques aimed at modifying these chaotic fragmentalisms. Additionally, excessively 'permissive' superego responses leading to acting out feelings without any negative connotation being placed on these actions (behaviour – value and feeling – value fragmentalisms) can be modified by confrontation as well as the opposite superego response of excessive 'harshness' which punishes actions, however minor (feeling – value and behaviour – value literalisms).

Considering Bion's (1961) 'basic assumption' groups, a perspectivist approach involves eliciting the literalist relationship between feelings of dependency, aggression and sexuality/affection within the group and the positive values attached to each of these 'basic assumptions', e.g. 'being a good and successful group member means I should rely on the therapist for all my needs', and then by frustrating this relationship, modifying this literalism.

Foulkes' notion of 'group analyst' encourages the group member, as discussed in the cognitive approach, to modify the fragmented relationship between feelings and actions, and feelings and values, by taking more responsibility for their own learning and growth. Whitaker and Lieberman's (1965) 'focal conflict' approach, like Bion's 'basic assumptions' therapy attempts to modify the literalist relationship between disturbing motives and reactive motives (feelings), on the one hand, and shared solutions to these conflicts (behaviour) on the other hand, which are inappropriate attempts to maximise gratification of the disturbing motive.

Conclusion

It can be seen by the discussion of these three types of group approach that the personal construct approach has great applicability. Although many would go further and elaborate it into a form of therapy in its own right, this does not appear to have as great an advantage as suggesting it as an approach which could be used to encompass and understand many therapeutic approaches. It offers an approach with which to understand at a greater and more personal depth the way in which members of therapeutic groups construe, function and change as a result of their group experience. I would like to end with comments made by a member of the analytical group described earlier in this chapter. She said that for her group therapy offered the opportunity to reveal to herself and others aspects of herself which she had always kept hidden. It also allowed her to learn how to listen more to others and feel good about this. Both these opportunities led her to feel and behave differently outside group meetings. This group member, like Kelly himself, saw herself as an 'experimenter' in this case in group therapy, the purpose of which was liberation from relying on a deficient 'map' in an 'unfamiliar country' and movement towards a clearer outlook on her interaction with others via processes of validation, elaboration and increasing perspectivism.

16　A CONSTRUCT APPROACH TO FAMILY THERAPY AND SYSTEMS INTERVENTION

Harry Procter

Introduction

Many different approaches to family therapy have been devised over the years, most relying on the idea that families have systemic properties (e.g. Palazzoli, Boscolo, Cecchivi and Prata, 1978; Watzlawick, Beavin and Jackson, 1967). How a group of people living together come to exhibit these properties remains a mystery however. Construct theory can provide a very elegant model of family functioning with immediate relevance for what to do in therapy.

This chapter develops further ideas contained in Procter (1978; 1981). Although the *family* and *family therapy* are the focus of convenience of these writings, the ideas are intended to apply just as well to other groups — work and friendship groups, organisations and even transient acquaintanceships. Perhaps the terms *social construct* and *social construct system* should be used instead of 'family construct' and 'family construct system'. An example of intervening in organisations other than the family can be found in 'Developing Family Therapy in the Day Hospital' (Procter and Stephens, 1984).

The Family Construct System

Kelly has argued that people evolve for themselves a certain unique way of construing and understanding the world which I will here refer to as their *position*. When regarded as a single entity, the gestalt or jigsaw of the positions of a group of people relating together has a life and identity of its own. It may demonstrate a dynamic equilibrium, or balance. It will show momentum, growth and elaboration. Changes will occur within it, such as people moving together around or swapping their positions, vacating or competing for them. It may oscillate regularly from one overall configuration to another. Over time gradual changes will occur and occasionally a sudden discontinuous change may come about, in which the pattern flips into a new configuration.

It is very difficult to describe these rich and complex processes in ordinary language. Also if you are present in a family situation it is very easy to be swept along by it and become absorbed in the content of the moment. So we will have to build up a picture of the situation slowly.

One way of doing this is to start by just considering two people in relation. In order to begin to understand interaction, I think it is necessary to consider the processes at two levels of analysis; a superordinate level (each person's construct or frame) and a subordinate level — their actions, choices — what they *do* in relation to each other.

Figure 16.1: The Construing Process of Louise and Mother

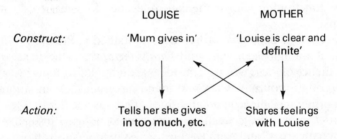

	LOUISE	MOTHER
Construct:	'Mum gives in'	'Louise is clear and definite'
Action:	Tells her she gives in too much, etc.	Shares feelings with Louise

Consider 26 year old Louise (Figure 16.1) engaged to a quiet and likeable man and living at home with her mother, father, two brothers and sister. Louise thinks her mum gives in too much with Jonathan who is 19 and has recently emerged from a catatonic psychosis. Louise tells her mum what she thinks when her mother is cross with Jonathan for spending too much money or going out too often. Mother is feeling a bit sad and weak and confides in Louise who has clear and definite opinions.

The constructs govern and channellise their actions (downwards arrows) and each one's action validates, more or less, the other's construct (diagonal arrows). The two positions maintain each other in what we might call a circularity or 'loop'. Each anticipates the other's responses and tends to evoke such a response if it is not forthcoming. The process is continuous and circular although we have to 'punctuate' it, to use Bateson's (1972) term, in order to describe it.

Jonathan, (Figure 16.2) young and impetuous, had been spending money and borrowing several hundred pounds from his mother for his MG and social life. Mother, with Louise present, complains to him about his irresponsibility.

Figure 16.2: The Construing Process of Mother and Jonathan

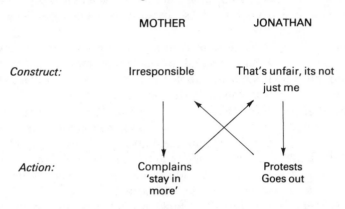

This dyad, although they are close, tends to 'go into runaway' (Bateson, 1972) or to escalate symmetrically pulling others in, especially Louise and the other brother, Mark. Thus we see in considering both these dyads the process of 'triangulation' (Haley, 1959b; Bowen, 1960). Jonathan is the main topic of the conversation between Louise and her mum. With his mum, Jonathan invokes his brother Mark — 'it's not just me, Mark does the same things.' The rows between mother and Jonathan bring in both the elder siblings. Mother, Louise and Mark join together in their view of Jonathan as irresponsible, and roundly criticise him. He responds in a way which validates their shared view of him. His reaction now is to leave home as soon as possible, making that desperate contrast reconstruction of independence':

HP	. . . who gets the most upset of the five of you?
Jonathan	We all get upset, actually.
Louise	Me, I think.
HP	Who gets the saddest?
Louise	I don't know about sad.
Mother	I do, I think.
Louise	Yeh, and I hear it from Mum, you see, and she tells me . . .

HP	Yeh? What does she say to you? What makes you say that you hear it from her?
Louise	Well, she just says, oh well, whether she's feeling at the time, she'll tell *me*, if she's feeling narked because he's spending money again like he hasn't got, or he won't stay in or something, she tells me.
HP	And what does Louise suggest to you in the way of advice?
Mother	Well, Louise is always saying I give in too much. Jonathan has always had his own way.
Jonathan	It's not just Jonathan is it, you know, I don't know why you're picking on me.
Mother	It *is*. It is, Jonathan. It's you.
Mark	And another thing. Jonathan thinks everybody's picking on him. He thinks everybody's against him.
Jonathan	Yeh well, when I can go and earn my own money I can lead my own life again. That's what I want. The sooner I can do that the better.
Mother	But Jonathan thinks it's better for him to get away from home. (Disparaging tone).
Jonathan	It is!

This comes from the third session of a brief course of therapy, which will be examined in more detail later.

It is fairly easy to see how two positions regulate and sustain each other in Figures 16.1 and 16.2. We can go on to build these diagrams up into triads and multi-person systems (see Figure 16.3). The positions of all the family members fit together in an analogue way except, of course, with more people each one will be tending to construe the *interactions between* others as well as the others' actions towards the perceiver. For example, Jonathan's perception of the others' coalition against him was probably a factor in his bid to leave the field, to want out.

I think the idea of a family construct system — this interlocking set of the different family members' positions — is a useful one. Similarity and difference are the engines which generate and regulate it. Perceived similarities and differences between family members are of central interest in people's lives. They refer to each other in taking up their positions. They have a choice to align themselves or to refrain from taking sides. Mother and Louise agree about Jonathan, and Mark joins them in their view. Children may emulate their older siblings and their parents or define themselves as different. As the children of a family grow, they often differentiate and go off in various directions. For example, a pair of identical twins carved out different territories for themselves, one becoming sociable and extrovert and choosing Science 'A' levels whilst the other did arts subjects and became more inward looking.

Figure 16.3: Construing in the Therapeutic System in Jonathan's Family

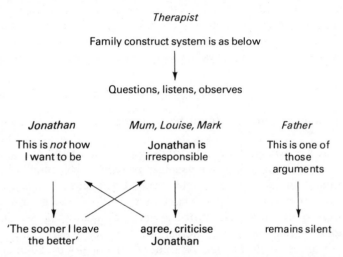

We can emphasise the construct as something in the individual's psychology, in his or her behaviour or thinking, something that channellises the person's life, 'a way in which some things are construed as being alike and yet different from others' (Kelly, 1955, p.105). Or one can emphasise constructs as actual similarities and differences or rather reflections of them. The truth is, of course, that these views are not contradictory and that they complement each other in a circular and dialectical way. I think that when Kelly defined a construct in terms of *three* elements or triads, he stumbled upon the same thing that the family therapists described in terms of *triangles* and *triangulation* (e.g. Bowen, 1960; Haley, 1959b). We could say that a construct is actually born out of the interactions between three people.

If our personal construct systems or 'positions' really are so interdependent, it has wide implications for psychology, in particular a personal psychology. Kelly formulated the choice corollary as a reaction against narrow hedonistic formulations of motivation. But I think we need to think in terms of broadening it again. For when we make a choice, it may well be that it is to extend, define or elaborate not just a personal construct system but a wider, shared system. Bateson (1972) argued for an ecological view of mind. When we become accustomed to driving a car or a lorry, somehow our body image expands to encompass the entire vehicle allowing us to manoeuvre around obstacles with exquisite precision. We may need to make the same kind of change in our psychological thinking. I think the family therapist Boszormenyi-Nagy was arguing a similar point in his ethical theory of family relations (Boszormenyi-Nagy and Spark, 1973). We are connected together by a web of invisible loyalties which permeate our choices and actions.

The Family in Context: How to be in Therapy

Just as we can see how individuals operate in a family or social context, the family or group itself can be seen in the context of the extended family, village, neighbourhood, religious or ethnic sub-culture or whatever the relevant network is. These groups are sources of the family's constructs and the family reality is daily shaped in the members' interactions with people in them. The family tends to select certain reference figures or groups (Shibutani, 1955). These can be postively valued — a grandfather, teacher, a political or artistic figure who epitomises the idea of the right or good way to live. There may be negative figures too, against whom members define themselves by contrast — certain neighbours, 'hippies', communists, or a rebellious person at school with whom the teenage child defiantly identifies. Both sets of figures are external validators for the family's constructs.

The way the family selects external validating figures and the constructs used are particularly important both in understanding how problems are formed and in the process of therapy. I can think of the woman (Figure 16.4) suffering from puerperal depression whose husband told me that various colleagues at work had told him that he should confront her and get her to 'snap out of it'. He said he had not done so, but spoke approvingly of the idea.

The external figures give authority to and stabilise a view of her (which she may well share too) that she is lazy or incompetent. In this case, the husband's mother also held this view. It turned out that *her husband* was also 'prone to depression' and that she and her son behaved in the same efficient and competent way with him. There was a tradition of construing and relating in this way which was reappearing in the next generation.

Figure 16.4: The Construing Process in a Marriage

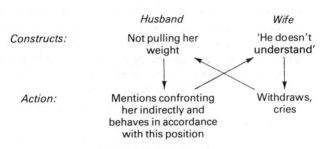

	Husband	*Wife*
Constructs:	Not pulling her weight	'He doesn't understand'
Action:	Mentions confronting her indirectly and behaves in accordance with this position	Withdraws, cries

So, if it had been simply dyadic, the process in Figure 16.4 would probably have been fairly transient and flexible, but it is arbitrary to isolate these two from what is actually a wider group reality. It has been caught in a web of perceived similarities and differences, or in the language of family therapy a network of interlocking triangles and coalitions.

It is difficult to understand psychological problems whilst ignoring this kind of process. Of course, we ourselves as therapists hoping to help our clients can be unwittingly maintaining a problem through exactly the same process. External figures can come into a situation and make an arbitrary *punctuation* of what is basically a circular continuous process. The wife is to *blame*, it is her fault, she had a difficult childhood, she is *ill* and needs some tablets, she is sinful. It is so hard for the poor husband. He is coping so *well*. Nowadays, with the pervasiveness of medical understandings of psychological problems, it is the well-ill construct that is usually placed over the situation, by family and professionals alike. In previous centuries it might have been a good-bad construct that was more commonly applied. Sometimes both these constructs are applied simultaneously.

This is not to say that these kinds of constructions cannot sometimes lead to resolutions of difficulties. But if they do not, a *polarisation* tends to occur. The husband amplifies his position as the wife gets more depressed and vice versa. The mother-in-law visits more to help with the children. This kind of process has been most eloquently described by Watzlawick, Weakland and Fisch in their book *Change* (1974), with their: 'when the attempted solution becomes the problem'. One of the important corollaries to this is that the apparent seriousness of a problem is not correlated with the difficulty of resolving it. It is commonly assumed for example that 'more serious psychopathology' like schizophrenia is 'deeper' and takes much longer to resolve. However, as we shall see later, the case with Jonathan shows that this is not necessarily so. One well-placed intervention basically neutralised the polarisation process. If the social conditions are right, one apparently insignificant pattern of positions can spiral off into the extremes of obsessional neurosis, chronic depression, child abuse, or any type of extreme deviant behaviour. We could see the task of therapy then as being to locate this core of the problem and deal with it.

In taking on a case like the woman with puerperal depression, we must be careful not to make *another* error. It is no good saying: 'well, there is a polarisation process going on here. If you two (husband and mother) would stop agreeing that Jill is ill and allow her to succeed in her new mother role . . . '. One or more of them would quite rightly come in and defend their construct. Who are *we* to go in and criticise the way people see things? Rather we make the basic Kellian assumption that people are doing things for good reason and that their choices are *elaborative* in some way. In this case, we make the assumption that *all* the people in a family or network are. It is a position of anthropological respect — Kelly was perhaps, above all, a first class anthropologist. These people are continuing to act in this way rather than make an alternative choice which in some way would be even *worse*. This could be many things and different for each of them — for example: marital conflict, or even breakdown, depression and loss of face in the mother, husband facing his own inadequacies and weakness compared to his wife or conflict between wife and her mother-in-law. Whichever, this pole is likely to be 'submerged', considered only with dread, or strongly repudiated by the family.

So, one works according to the principle of *acceptance*. Adopting the family or clients' reality and utilising their unique constructs, as emphasised by Kelly and M.H. Erickson, constitutes the basic therapeutic stance. Of course, accepting the clients' reality was a central tenet of Rogerian therapy. But it requires much more than simply reflecting or empathising with 'position'. This can become caught in a paradox. One can accurately emphasise with a 16-year-old boy, brought up in an army family who was referred for sadistic bullying. But it may be necessary to take a directive and authoritarian line with him, thereby thoroughly accepting his construct. I looked at him straight in the eye and said 'so you will be willing to take direction from me? . . . It will be necessary for you to perform the things I tell you to do with single-minded endurance if you are to become the fine soldier that you wish to be'. After saying this, his veneer of toughness began to melt away as he tearfully discussed his feelings about being adopted — material I chose apparently at this point to ignore. Accurately matching and utilising the client's constructs can result in rapid change and 'peeling of the onion' in this natural, spontaneous way. After this, the business of therapy will often consist of *protecting* the new seeds of improvement and helping the client nurture and grow them. Clearly these tender feelings about his real parents could quickly be swallowed up in his tough position again. This development only emerged *with me present*, taking the position that I was doing which could have been for him that of a future and respected trainer in the paratroopers. His tough position could return easily and probably would on the rugby pitch, covering and crushing his gentleness which is here emerging. So one takes the weight, as it were, by fully supporting the old position, and continuing to take a therapeutic position which complemented it. Too often, therapy flags or is prolonged because there is a failure to handle improvements with this kind of *care and attention* to detail.

Therapy carried out by the school doctor with this boy had become stuck in the way illustrated in Figure 16.5.

Figure 16.5: Construing Process Between a Boy and School Doctor

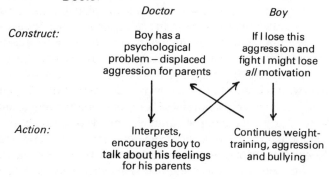

In my therapy with him, after some initial careful investigation, I started to take *his* position that there would be a danger of him losing his motivation which, he had told me, he used in his academic work as well. This was used as the basis for a simple task in which he was required to work himself up into his aggressive frame of mind for five minutes on the hour six times a day in order to learn to 'achieve precise mental control over his aggression'. I anticipate that this will support his system sufficiently to allow him safely to elaborate new alternatives, even as he began to do in the interview itself.

One will not know for a while what the family's or client's positions are and when one does, finding a way of relating to them in this accepting way may not be easy. Patience, creativity and hard work will be necessary. This takes time. In the meanwhile the principles of *manoeuvrability* (Fisch, Weakland and Segal, 1982) and *neutrality* (Palazzoli *et al.*, 1980) are extremely useful. These are both ways of avoiding being boxed in to a position prematurely by the family. Manoeuvrability — going slowly, qualifying one's statements, getting the clients to be specific and being hierarchically 'one-down' to the family — is a respectful and caring position to hold and it does the family no favours to allow any of one's choices to be closed out pre-emptively. Neutrality and not being drawn in to any one position or side within the family, is mainly achieved by the kind of questions one asks. However, it is important to remember that both acceptance and neutrality are communicated non-verbally or analogically especially through facial expression.

Of course, usually the different family members will not be agreeing in their positions and will not hold the external validating figures, either the positive or negative ones, in the same regard. Although part of the same shared family construct system and dialectically related, there will often be completely contradictory positions held within the same family. If necessary one should not hold back from seeing family members separately, helping each to elaborate their own position and using that position to undermine the circularity. Such an approach was used with a middle-aged woman with depression which was being maintained by the husband's zealous overhelpfulness. Conjoint interviewing resulted in fruitless arguing. Seen separately, she, within her religious understanding of her predicament was encouraged to pray. A psychological framework was used with the husband: 'people with depression have low self-esteem and it is important not to be too competent because it makes them feel even more inadequate in contrast to you. Can you find a way to make a mess of some small thing each day to show her you can be fallible?' A very productive 'flip' occurred in their relationship without him even needing to carry out the task that I had set.

Usually, however, it is not necessary to go to this extent. People often *think* that they have to agree and be consistent when in fact they do not have to be. One can say of two parents 'undermining' each other: 'Mother, your toughness is just what Jeremy needs at this time so that he can learn acceptable limits of behaviour. Father, your gentleness is also required so that he can feel safe whilst learning these limits. The toughness and the gentleness complement each other, they *fit together* very well'. This same approach is valuable in wards with an expectation that the nurses or shifts be in agreement.

A superordinate framework has been found under which the differing and apparently contradictory positions have been subsumed.

The Investigation: Questions

Questions form a vital part of most therapeutic approaches. Therapeutic questioning has been focused upon by the Mental Research Unit (MRI) and Milan groups (e.g. Herr and Weakland, 1979; Palazzoli *et al.*, 1980). Kelly also put stress on questioning and may have been one of the first writers to look at the matter. Questions about perceived similarities and differences form the basis of the repertory grid technique. He also provided seven basic questions with which to get started immediately:

1. Upon what problems do you wish help?
2. When were these problems first noticed?
3. Under what conditions did these problems first appear?
4. What corrective measures have been attempted?
5. What changes have come with treatment or the passing of time?
6. Under what conditions are the problems most noticeable?
7. Under what conditions are the problems least noticeable?

(Kelly 1955)

Another sort of question which Kelly emphasised comes from the basic definition of a construct: in what way are these two things similar that distinguishes them from this third thing? Or more simply, in what way are these two similar? In what way are the two of you different?

A single question of this kind can stimulate a fundamental revisior or nodal point in therapy. Erickson reports a case in which a wife had been having a series of affairs. The husband ostensibly did not know about them, although he related events which indicated her unfaithfulness. After several hours of interviewing the man he remarked:

> You know, if my wife were any other woman, I'd say she was having affairs. I asked: 'In what way does your wife differ from other women?' He said: 'My God, my wife *is* any other woman!' At this point he became quite upset, yelled, waved his arms, and proceeded to go over the same details again. The toothpaste in the bathroom, the razor blade, the breakfasts. He identified every detail in context. All afternoon I had been hoping he would say something that would allow me to ask that kind of question. That is why I let him repeat his story over and over again, looking for some little remark so that I could yank him outside that constricted configuration. Once he recognised that his wife was 'other women' there was nothing he could do about that new understanding.
> (Cited in Haley, 1973)

Kelly used the term 'transitive diagnosis':

> The term suggests that we are concerned with transitions in the client's life, that we are looking for bridges between the client's present and his future. Moreover, we expect to take an active part in helping him cross them safely. The client does not ordinarily sit cooped up in a nosological pigeonhole; he proceeds along his way. If the psychologist expects to help him he must get up off his chair and start moving along with him. (Kelly, 1955)

It is extremely useful to identify the individual or family's problem-goal constructs with their own particular verbal labels. One pole is often 'submerged'. Examples are tense-relaxed, naughty-mature, sick-cheerful. A great variety of idiosyncratic dichotomies will be encountered. In families a jumble of these constructs may exist with their implications contradicting each other, whilst the family members argue incessantly in their attempts to negotiate. Clarifying problems and goals can act like a powerful magnetic field in which the jumble of constructs becomes aligned into a set of parallel avenues along which the members can start moving.

One will want to know the validators, what will actually have to happen to indicate that the goal has been reached? What will convince the client that progress has been made? In going from superordinate to subordinate in this way the interview 'zig-zags' between the level of construct and action (Figures 16.1 to 16.5). Already a therapeutic shift in shared construing begins to occur, e.g. What do you make of him doing that? What makes you say he's irresponsible?

Another useful set of questions is derived from examining the constructs used to identify and distinguish the family or network members — a little bit like doing a live repertory grid with the elements sitting around assembled. Palazzoli and her team (1980) have stressed asking for *relative* rather than *absolute* questions (who gets *more* depressed, your mother or her mother? Who was *closest* to him of the three children?) They derive their theory from Bateson with his notion of *difference* (1972), an idea similar to that of Kelly's *construct* or the *bit* in information theory. One can see from the extract from Jonathan and his family (pages 329–30) the usefulness of asking 'who gets the saddest? Who gets the most upset?' These kinds of questions, utilising the family's *own* constructs, evoke a shower of information, producing a tendency for the family to start cross-checking meanings or for them to focus on internal images as they search their inner experience for validating evidence (Erickson and Rossi, 1979). The way in which families respond significantly to such questions lends weight to the notion of a family construct system.

It is also worth searching for *whole-figure constructs*. Family members steer their lives in comparison with others around them: in words as 'I am not like my father'. 'You remind me of my sister', 'Her baby is just like granny'. More often the same constructs guide action and interaction without the people being aware of the fact. As Scott and Ashworth wrote (1969) the family may be organised around an *ill-well* construct, but at first young Roddy may be construed and treated like his mad uncle before he is overtly labelled as crazy. Similarities and differences are articulated through the *actions* which they govern. We copy, imitate and develop the same interests or go for a contrasting activity.

Exploring the generations of a family reveals interesting repeated patterns of similarity and contrast, sometimes demonstrating like- nesses in alternating generations. Peter who was suffering from auditory hallucinations liked bell-ringing as had his dead grand- father. He was not only like his grandfather in his odd authoritative manner, he had stepped into his shoes and went to visit his granny every day dutifully. We pointed out quite rightly that if he was to start going out into the world and make a success of his life his granny would be lonely and would have to face her loss all by herself each day. In a way he *was* his grandfather in the family construct system. To develop an individual requires creativity on the part of the family.

Questioning guided by a consideration and exploration of the family construct system is a very useful therapeutic tool — in individual and family therapy. The same methods can be extended to work with organisations. It will give a good deal of data useful in deciding how to respond to them.

Intervention

The two-level diagram that we have hopefully been able to work out during the investigation will now serve as a useful tool in the intervention. In a dyad (for example see Figure 16.2) a change in any one of the four cells in the diagram can lead to a shift in the entire arrangement. This gives us four possible targets for inter- vention and of course we may choose to intervene with more than one simultaneously. In a triad, more difficult to represent in two dimensions, there will be six possible places to intervene.

Intervention, of course, does not necessarily mean active or precisely worked out procedures. It can mean *not* doing things, remaining silent, allowing the client or family to work, observing, listening or asking neutral questions. We inevitably and mutually influence each other.

Whether one chooses to concentrate more on the level of action and behaviour or more at the level of construing will depend on the particular case. The intervention should be created anew for each situation although good ideas from one's own and others' successful work are often helpful raw material, from which to start. New action or interaction can be suggested in the form of a task, a ritual or a post-hypnotic suggestion, or more simply an idea. It may be suggested directly or indirectly, for example in the form of a therapeutic metaphor or anecdote. It is best to introduce the prescription of new behaviour in terms of the client's or family's *own* constructs and frames, by appealing, for example, to *their* religious or aesthetic values.

So new action can be suggested within existing constructs. Conversely new constructs may be introduced in the context of existing interactions, as in many of the 'paradoxical' approaches to treatment (Haley, 1963; Watzlawick *et al.*, 1967, 1974). This basically consists of explaining to the family that what they are doing already is a good thing. As Kellians, of course, we make the assumption that people are doing things for what are to them basically good reasons; to extend, define or elaborate their construct systems. But they are not necessarily conscious of the reasons. In fact, we are usually unconscious of the wider elaborative implications of our actions even when profoundly motivated by them. But this is a benign and interpersonal view of the unconscious, different from an intrapsychic one seething with hedonic wishes So in this therapeutic approach one is helping the client or family get in touch with the elaborative superordinate value that is unconsciously governing their choices and experience. This, I believe, will only be properly grasped when the interpersonal construct system around the problem is sufficiently well understood. It is not therefore a 'manipulative procedure' though this is not to defend those who misuse it as such and believe that the naive prescribing of a paradoxical task or a 'positive reframe' constitutes the task of therapy.

We also have the two other options — to go for change at both levels and for no change (utilisation) at both levels. This is a very simple scheme and is designed to be. The rest is compassion and creativity.

Now Jonathan was a 19-year-old psychiatric patient, with all the symptoms of an acute catatonic schizophrenia. Whilst on a skiing holiday with his friend in Switzlerland, he started becoming incomprehensible, saying that he was Jesus and worrying about sin and religious ideas. He appeared to be experiencing auditory hallucinations. He was treated with heavy tranquillisers and sent back to a general hospital in England where he underwent various medical tests. He was becoming increasingly mute, with twitching of the face and catatonic rigidity. He was hardly breathing and had developed a chest infection.

I was asked to see him after everything usual had been tried except that ECT was considered too dangerous in his condition. All drugs had been withdrawn as he was only deteriorating with them (no further drugs were prescribed). I knew that he had thought he was Jesus and that he had actually been a carpenter. When I entered the dormitory where he was by now, in a psychiatric hospital, he was lying on the bed, a nurse trying to get him to drink, his hands and arms rigid in front of him in distorted gestures. Jonathan was quiet so I would be too. I said 'Hello Jonathan' quietly and sat down by the bed and breathed with him for twenty minutes. This method of 'pacing' may be the most basic way we have of validating another's choices. Then various suggestions were introduced in Ericksonian fashion: there were a lot of things about him that I did not know, but I did know that during his life he had learned a tremendous number of things. It was hard the first time he used a chisel, but as he continued it got easier to get an even shaving of wood — and learning to sharpen chisel and plane blades . . . Various aspects of carpentry were discussed and interspersed with suggestions to become increasingly relaxed and comfortable. Learning to read and write, to stand up, take steps and walk, to enjoy drinking beer were mentioned casually in the context of a consideration of memories of successfully learning the feel of a hammer, learning to use a screw-driver as a child, buttoning up clothes, sawing a plank of wood in the correct fashion. His breathing deepened a little but it was not possible to tell if he was registering anything. However, the next day he was reported to be more responsive and when I saw him in the evening he was shuffling around the ward with his neck craned forward, mumbling incomprehensibly.

The next step was to interview the parents without Jonathan. I explained to them what I had done and started the session with a detailed consideration of Jonathan's interests and abilities. He liked skiing of course and sports generally. He was keen on Duran Duran. Like his sister Louise he liked to make his own mind up, a bit bigheaded. Mother did most of the talking, interrupting Dad who said with tears in his eyes. 'He comes to his Mum with his little problems and the girls go to their Dad more'. He bought an MG sports car before he went on holiday and was several hundred pounds in debt to his mother. He went out quite a lot and generally spent money in a rather irresponsible way. There was conflict between Jonathan and his elder brother, Mark. Father joined in,

'Yes, Jonathan just says "I'll do what I want," when I try and tell him what to do'. When Jonathan was late to dinner Mark had come in saying 'You could have let Mum know', Jonathan replied 'Mind your own business and keep your pecker out of it'.

Mum had to do everything for him. She usually bought all the Christmas presents for Jonathan to give round the family, but had failed to do this last Christmas. He had been very upset and embarrassed opening all the presents that he received from the others. After another fight after Christmas Jonathan had actually packed his bags and left for two nights, staying at his girl friend's. But they thought that 'Mark should have been kicked out too'.

'Jonathan had a girl friend, they weren't living together but had slept together', the mother continued. She was very upset because it had emerged from Jonathan's friend that he had been sleeping with various girls in Switzerland before the trouble started. He had received several letters from girls he had met out there.

When he came home, Jonathan had been saying some strange things. Though he had never been religious before, he was preoccupied with sin, and said that he could speak any language. He could bring certain people back from the dead by twiddling his ring.

A general plan was outlined. I said I often found it helpful in such cases to meet with the family over a series of sessions. We could continue to have him in hospital but it was usually best for the patient to be cared for by the family, under our guidance, as they knew him much better than we ever could. However, this would have to be discussed with the consultant and the hospital team. We would wait until next week at the same time when we would have another meeting and decide then if Jonathan could go home.

Next Friday evening I met the parents again, this time with Jonathan. He had been home for the weekend and was refusing to walk, eat or wash. He spat out food like a baby and would not let anybody else do anything. He refused to come downstairs and had had no bowel motion, Mother told me. She thought that it was psychological, 'He seems to want to be treated like a two year old'. It was agreed he should go home with them that night. I said, 'It will be very difficult for you and all your resources will be stretched to the limit, but it will be an opportunity to assess your resources. Note carefully what happens so that we can discuss it in detail in our session at Southwood House on Thursday morning.' He would be on leave from the ward, so if it got too strenuous for them they could take him back at a moment's notice. In any event we would meet on

Thursday in the clinic where I work with a small team of colleagues who can observe and help with the session from another room. We would appreciate it if they could bring anyone around who seemed to be relevant. We often found it helpful to see other people in the family because they could give us useful information, and perhaps we would be able to come up with some useful guidance or ideas to help them in their management of Jonathan.

Before the session on Thursday morning, I explained to Richard Skinner, Helga Clark and other colleagues in the team what had happened so far. We examined the family tree and noted the family's position in the life-cycle, with four children (Louise 26, Mark 22, Jonathan 20 and Sarah 14) still at home. Louise had a steady boyfriend, Pete. Mother was still figuring closely in all of their lives, and we thought that Jonathan's impulsive bid for independence had resulted in too much threat and anxiety and had destabilised the family system. His psychotic regression had allowed a resumption of the mother's nurturing role. With the two older children leaving, Jonathan was carrying the weight for the remainder.

With these hypotheses and a rough plan I went into the session. Jonathan was led into the therapy room. He sat between his parents lolling over on to one or the other of their laps, they would then return him to the upright position. Louise, Peter, Sarah and Mary (Jonathan's girlfriend) were present, but Mark was unable to attend.

Care was taken in this interview to try and make a personal relationship with each of the family members. I thanked them for coming and explained again how, in dealing with problems such as this, we often find it helpful to meet with the rest of the family who will be working as a team to help the patient. The main polarisation that the family had made between Jonathan and the rest of them was thus accepted. I said that a little later in the session I would be asking them in detail how Jonathan had got on and what particular difficulties they had had, so that we could work out the best advice for them. But first, I continued, it would be useful to get some background information. There followed a slow and gentle exploration of the family constructs and positions — who had been working the hardest with Jonathan? — Mum then Dad, then Louise, Mark, Sarah and Mary least since she had only visited once. Mum, who referred to herself in the third person, had been most upset about it, but Louise had been very helpful in taking the pressure off her. With the children leaving home, Mum would miss Louise most. Nobody would particularly miss Mark, in fact, they had expected him to leave a long time ago. Jonathan, in general, seemed to be more like his father in his quietness and tendency to worry as opposed to Mum, Louise and Mark who were more sociable and talkative. Mark was the 'family jester' who kept them all amused.

The problems with Jonathan had centred around washing, eating and going to the toilet. Mother had been principally involved in this, in fact, he had not allowed anyone else to feed him. They asked if they should be more sympathetic or strict. The message given to the family after discussion with the team floated the idea of a course of therapy in which we would continue to give them help and guidance in their work with Jonathan. We said that it was most important that they work hard for him, it does not matter, though if they are sympathetic or strict. But if they were to stop working so hard he could get worse. We had had a lot of thoughts about particular relationships and we had a number of ideas. We felt that he had a deep unconscious fear that, with the family reaching that time of life when the children leave home, the family break-up will be a deeply traumatic event. I turned to Jonathan and said, 'Jonathan, don't try and make any changes until we can deal with the issues'. And to the family: 'you are concerned, keen and intelligent, you have it in you to do the work and to organise your resources as a team. We would like to see you again on 31 March at 11.15 am, and could you bring Mark next time because he could be very helpful to us.'

This intervention, fairly typical of the MRI or Milan approaches (Palazzoli *et al.*, 1978; Watzlawick *et al.*, 1974) is an appeal to the elaborative components of Jonathan's choices. It is a leap of faith really, in that Jonathan had not yet said anything, but we make the assumption that, however much suffering is apparently involved, the symptom-bearer is actually finding that choice preferable to what may be to an outsider a more apparently straightforward or 'normal' choice. We do not know yet, we may never know exactly what this involves. So we start looking for it in the contextual reality surrounding the problem. The hypothesis will be refined or revised in the light of what happens next.

The whole family, two parents and the four children, were present at the next session, with Louise's boyfriend but without Mary, Jonathan's girlfriend. Jonathan was still demonstrating slow fluid trance-like movements but seemed more alert. Throughout the session there was much eye contact between him and Louise. He was sitting between Louise and Mark. Sarah had taken his previous seat between the parents.

Mark was very much the central figure in this session. He related in a very animated way how he had taken Jonathan to a disco. The latter was obsessed with good and evil. Whenever he saw anything black he pointed out that it was evil and white things were 'good'. He said that the rest of the family, particularly Louise, was evil. He had been pointing out particular references to love in pop-song lyrics and saying that they were important and significant.

The family responded to this with rational argument, humouring and anger. Mark, although amused, said that it was getting on his nerves and had taken him to the local vicar. Father had got angry, Jonathan had called him a 'chicken' and a quarrel between them had resulted in a brief admission back to the psychiatric hospital. I asked who was the most religious member of the family. Mum was the most religious and Mark least.

A telephone conversation with the GP before the session revealed that he thought Jonathan had improved greatly although he was worried, with Easter coming up, that there could be trouble over the weekend. He would prefer to see him back in the ward in case this happened.

The following intervention was presented to the family:

> Thanks very much once again, for giving us such useful infor-
> mation. It's each time we meet you, we have the best picture so
> far of what the problems have been, how it works. You know,
> each time we get some information, we kind of make some
> revisions in our understanding of it, like obviously, the things we
> said to you last time, you know each time we can get a slightly
> deeper picture, slightly more accurate.
>
> Jonathan in doing what he's been doing has been keeping
> everyone involved. Jonathan, it's a natural response that you
> have and it's what he should be doing. Jonathan is going through
> a period of late adolescence where a great deal of work and
> learning has to be done concerning intimate relationships, about
> the implications of making close relationships, both within and
> outside the family. Testing out what other relationships you
> have, working out the pecking order, the hierarchy particularly
> with regard to mother and father. In being close to your mother
> and challenging father's authority. This is something a boy has to

work out with his father.

You (father) are right to be angry with him, to assert your authority and I want you to continue to do this, but don't expect him to go along with you at the moment but don't let that stop you saying what you want, don't hold back from being firm with him.

Now, the religious material. This is part of his work in making sense of the morality of making close sexual relationships. The way you've been handling it is very good. Mark, you have been taking a joking, humorous stance. Mother, you have been thinking about the religious side of it and father, you have shown him your impatience, making it clear again that your job is to show him the limits of acceptable behaviour. But the important thing is to remember it is part of the natural work he is doing.

So, any mention of religion or things like the lyrics of songs, listen carefully and note down the actual words so that we can look at it in detail next time.

As far as the eating is concerned, this is part of the relationship between Jonathan and his mother and this is a very important thing in working out when to leave the nest. A mother is there to provide the warmth, the father the direction. Mother, keep close to him, keep him under your wing.

Now about the hospital, we have made an arrangement with the ward. Jonathan is on extended leave. If things get too much for you, all you have to do is to give them a ring and take him in.

Now tomorrow is Good Friday. Now it's a strange and paradoxical thing, because although it's called Good Friday it was really an evil day. It was an evil thing that Jesus was put to death on Good Friday. This is likely to be a particularly difficult time.

Basically, you're doing very well but it will continue to be hard work. We've got a few questionmarks about things like going out to discos. It may be a bit soon for that and we would have the tendency to hold back and be cautious.

We'd like to see you again on 28 April at 11.15 am.

When I went down to the waiting room four weeks later to greet the family, it was quite a shock to find Jonathan without a trace of his catatonic symptoms. He was bright and breezy and shook my hand in a confident way, speaking to me for the first time. The structure of the family had changed significantly, with father now a spokesman and Mark much quieter and less central.

Father told us that Jonathan was back to normal now and there had been no further examples of the religious preoccupations. He was driving his car again and involving himself in sport activities. The GP had pronounced him fit for work and he was starting again the following Monday. The only thing was, his mother said, he was not responsible with money.

Jonathan said he could remember everything that had happened. He recalled being in hospital, in a lot of pain, and remembered me talking about woodwork and finding it relaxing.

After this, the session developed into an argument about money and Jonathan's independence, (see again the excerpts on pages 329–30 and Figures 16.1 and 16.2). Mother, Louise and Mark protested about his irresponsibility with Jonathan asserting his status as an independent adult. Mark was much less comfortable with Jonathan in this role, the joking and jesting that there had been in relation to his brother's symptoms being entirely absent. He said, rather desperately, 'Jonathan just won't accept that he is mentally ill', an attempt to reinstate the construct that had been polarising the family.

In the intervention we said how pleased we were with the progress, that it was excellent and they all deserved congratulations for the way things were going. In the matter of going back to work, the GP had said that he should. We didn't want them to get us wrong, but to remind them that we had arranged to meet for ten sessions. We would like to err on the side of caution, we don't want to work too fast. 'We are not saying don't go back, we are prepared to let you go ahead and try'.

Various constructs were offered to describe the way they had been in the session. The arguments about money were a sign that progress was being made in issues that need to be negotiated at this time of life. It was useful that father could remain objective as was mother's willingness to go straight in there and put her point of view across. We were pleased with the way Louise and Mark, as the oldest were still concerning themselves with these matters in the family. That was good, and in this day and age one did not often see it, the children often just go away and look after themselves.

Jonathan's work was seen as very important in this matter. 'You are the one with your eyes set on the goal, acting as vanguard, putting yourself in the hot seat. In learning to leave the nest, children have to go through these things, putting your head on the block. You're doing it for Mark.'

'You're doing good work. There will be ups and downs. We would like to see you again on 9 June.'

The improvement had been maintained at the next session. The problems they had had with Jonathan were no different from those of other people in the same situation, the father explained. We therefore discharged them with six sessions 'in the bank' to be used if further difficulties should arise which they could not deal with themselves.

A follow-up one year later revealed that the family were all well, Jonathan working and with a new girlfriend.

Conclusion

Thinking in terms of how people's constructs are connected together and how they evolve in relation to each other can be a very useful and clarifying exercise. It helps in understanding and making hypotheses about well-functioning organisations as well as situations involving problems. It gives a rationale for investigating situations and a clue about how to respond to them.

Some of the basic ideas have been spelt out in this chapter. These can be built up into more elaborate theoretical constructs and most cases will require and warrant this. There has not been space to give the matter of *contrast poles* of family constructs the attention they deserve.

A construct analysis which reflexively examines the professional dimensions or 'meta-constructs' used by systems theorists also bears fruit. The constructs of hierarchy (up/down), proximity (close/ distant) and boundary (in/out) can be found in many of the writers of family therapy literature. These can be used to classify family constructs. More on this will be found in Procter and Dallos (in press).

These ideas are useful in the area of research on the family. For example, Farrell (1984) has examined the different ways in which family therapists and student nurses construe hierarchy in Jonathan's family. He found that the hierarchy in the family could be rated reliably and that it changed systematically from the second family session, when the catatonic symptoms were still present to the third when they had disappeared. He looked at the way different raters' constructs were linked to this basic up/down construct. Research on the way the family members themselves construe these kinds of dimensions would also prove very interesting.

Finally, it should be said that conceptualising the family or social construct system in this way can be useful and indeed is often essential in individual therapy as well as in conjoint work. We should keep the shared social reality in mind and understand how it works, even if we decide to intervene through only one person.

17 SOCIETAL AND INSTITUTIONAL CHANGE: BEYOND THE CLINICAL CONTEXT

Eric Button

The primary focus of this book has been on the clinical context, with a particular emphasis on making use of theoretical perspectives and research derived from personal construct theory. I hope that we have been successful in spelling out some of the implications for practice in the mental health setting. As mental health workers, I believe there is much we can achieve in helping our clients and their families to open up meaningful directions in their lives. It is clear, however, that 'disorders' don't start and end with clinically designated 'patients' or 'clients'. Behaviour and experience which may be labelled disordered, emerges within, gets 'treated' within and may change within a social context. Patients, their families and their helpers all live in a shared world within which there are problems, possibilities, hopes and expectations. It is a commonly expressed cliché that we live in a stressful society. Furthermore, the prevailing ethos regarding health is that we should look to our own life styles as causing health and illness. Rather than exclusively relying on attempting to change the construing of the designated patients we should, perhaps, also be looking beyond the clinical context. This might be described as preventative mental health, in which we attempt to create optimal conditions for more 'healthy' development. Although there seems to be ample scope for such an approach, this kind of development has been limited up to now so that most of what I have to say will be speculative, but it is hoped it may stimulate dialogue if not action. I shall divide this discussion into a consideration of several contexts in which mental health may be facilitated.

Society

Like the individuals of whom they are composed, societies seem to me to be quite capable of being construed in terms of Kelly's corollaries and 'Dimensions of Diagnosis'. In particular, they construe things differently from each other and they change in the

351

light of experience. But like people, they may also resist change and, taking the analogy with the individual further, it would be quite easy to regard some societies as 'unhealthy' because, e.g. they were unable to complete 'cycles of construing' or were persistently engaging in Kellyian 'hostility'. Like with the individual patient, however, such labelling would be a construction which would not necessarily be shared by all concerned. Furthermore a society which at one point in time might be regarded as disordered may, at another point, be viewed as far-thinking or advanced. Much could be said, also, about why societies often clash with each other in their attempts to validate their respective positions. I shall restrict my attention here, however, to the relevance of societies for the creation of mental health and mental illness.

The interplay between the individual and society is clearly complex, but the process of 'socialisation' implies an effect of society on the individual. So when an individual does not match up to society's expectations, his deviance may represent a threat to society. In other words the behaviour of individuals may seem inconsistent with the values and goals of that society. For example the expression of the right to freedom of choice may seem inconsistent with some forms of socialism, whereas a claim for jobs for all may be inconsistent with a capitalist society. This might seem like a far cry from mental health, but of course the use of psychiatry to dispose of 'dissidents' is well recognised. The term 'inconsistency', of course, implies a social interpretation of a person, such that the concept of construing is clearly at work. In the same way that structural aspects of the construing process are at work with the individual, they may also be a feature of societal construing. For example, a society which construes in a 'pre-emptive' way may expect men to be *nothing but* bread-winners. 'Constellatory' construction might lead men also to have to be at all times fearless, rational and strong. The activities that men-folk participate in may be seen as part of their attempt to validate the shared construct system of society. A consequence of such limiting construing will be that 'elements' (in this case people) who are out of line with expectation may be bullied into conforming or else may have to be construed in terms of some other construct. The inconsistent man in our above example may for example, be goaded by the challenge 'What are you — a man or a mouse?' Alternatively it might be inferred that he's not really a man but is 'effeminate'. A society which construed in a more 'propositional' way, however, might have no problem over such behaviour. Being a man, or a woman, for that matter, would not place limits on a person in this way but would allow the person to be free to pursue a variety of things irrespective of his/her sex. I am suggesting, therefore that in the same way as Harry Procter has argued in the previous chapter that there may be a family construct system there may also be societal construct systems. Like some individuals and some families, some societies may be less open than others. Although it is difficult to conceive of societies being completely static, history would suggest that societies and civilisations that resist change may be doomed to eventual extinction (e.g. Roberts, 1980). In the language of Kelly's choice corollary, a society preoccupied with 'definition' at the expense of 'extension' may lead to a neat order and security in the short-term but would pose severe restriction on societal members and be ill-prepared for eventual inevitable and possibly catastrophic change in the longer term.

If you accept my premise that there are such constructional differences between societies then you may be asking yourself what implications there may be for mental health. Mental health workers can carry on playing an established role of construing and treating people as ill, but they also have the option to challenge this conception and aggressively offer an alternative philosophy which encourages the quest for meaning, exploration and understanding. A more person-oriented stance seems to me to be indeed the predominant ethos in mental handicap nowadays as vigorously advanced by Davis and Cunningham in Chapter 12. That which we call mental illness, however, seems to me to lag behind mental handicap. Despite the challenges of the likes of Laing and Szasz, the medical-biological model of mental illness seems to predominate. A notable exception, however, seems to be the recent Italian 'revolution' in mental health practice in which a fundamentally social view of mental health (and backed up by law) has taken over in many parts of the country from the traditional custodial and medical approach (Lacey, 1984). You might question the extent to which as individuals we can or should attempt to change the way society views mental health. First, I would contend that there is ample evidence that individuals can change social constructions: the converse, of course is also true and the power of societies to destroy the individual is all too evident. Change, however, is ultimately mediated by a minority of individuals who eventually become the majority. It is notable that in the Italian example above the change was substantially attributed to the efforts of one charismatic person, Franco Bassaglia a psychiatrist, horrified by what he found inside the traditional psychiatric institution. Secondly, whether we like it or not, as mental health professionals we are already involved in influencing people, i.e. our patients. Even the arguably more humane treatment, psychotherapy, has rightly been illustrated by Frank (1974) to be basically a form of persuasion. If we have the right to influence our fellow citizens who become patients I would argue that we have equal right to attempt to influence the broader social network from whence our patients come. In fact the medical profession is a very good example of this as evidenced, for example, by their ardent and relatively successful campaign against smoking. After all, the broader society is well capable of 'defending' its position and it is unlikely that any change in philosophy would come about unless it made sense to enough people. As part of the ever-progressing dialogue between individuals and social groups I suggest therefore that constructive alternativism has something to offer to society and that it is of limited value if kept to ourselves. I would like to elaborate then on some of the 'institutions' which may play a part in fostering mental health.

Education

Arguably, at least second to family, comes the educational system in influencing the development of the person. Pope and Keen (1981), however, in their book *Personal Construct Psychology and Education* point to the great diversity of viewpoints regarding what education is and should be. One narrow vision of education has seen it as about the transmission of information or knowledge, with the child simply required passively to soak up all he needs to know from his teachers. The 'Progressive Movement' (Dewey, 1938), however, seems more in keeping with a Kellyian model of development, given its emphasis on progressive cognitive development through the interaction of the person and his/her environment. Pope and Keen, however, don't favour any particular model and instead emphasise the value of personal construct theory in reconciling the existence of varying constructions of education. Kelly, however, was somewhat cynical about formal education and seemed to imply that schools could actually inhibit the process of enquiry that was the essence of his model of 'man the scientist'. Certainly this is a point of view which has been echoed repeatedly since in one form or another. There seem to me to be several implications for education if one adopts a personal construct theory stance. First, one would place the person at the centre of the stage. In other words one's starting point would be the pupil not the institution or the teacher. That is not to say that the teacher's construing should be ignored: far from it: but to recognise that the elaboration of the pupil's understandings was the primary aim of the exercise. Secondly, one would be interested in the kinds of question the pupil was asking rather than deciding what questions he/she should be asking. Thirdly, one would aim to offer a setting in which opportunity was provided for the person to get answers to his/her questions, thus permitting continuing elaboration of his construct system and not discouraging him from continuing this pursuit. A particularly important implication of this principle is that one would *expect* questions, 'mistakes' and misunderstandings rather than seeing them as a sign of failure or stupidity. Fourthly, one would address the meaningfulness question: rather than either being pleased with acceptance and displeased with rejection of 'the syllabus' one would try and help the pupil understand why subjects were regarded as important and particularly aim to illustrate where they may be meaningful to their goals. Finally, one would place the elaboration of 'person construing' high up on the agenda, rather than secondary to 'academic' subjects: an understanding of people is arguably the most important and most complex of all 'subjects' the individual will have to wrestle with in life. This should encompass the whole realm of personhood including the crucial issue of how we make sense of our feelings as we deal with transitions and other inevitable sources of 'disturbance'. Not being an educationalist myself, I cannot judge to what extent schooling follows such principles. I would suggest, however, that the incorporation of such principles may go some way towards preventing some of the mental ill-health which can stem from a failure to develop a creative commitment to the process of living. Someone who has learnt to feel safe to ask questions and expects people to take varying perspectives rather than assuming there are absolute rights and wrongs is surely less likely to fall victim to a socially unworkable system of constructs.

In case there is any room for misunderstanding let me be clear that this view of education is not limited to the child pupil. The concept of continuing education seems to me to be entirely consistent with the above aims. The recent introduction of health education classes on aspects of coping with life seems to me to be a positive step. In fact, as indicated in Chapter 1, there seems to be a good case for viewing health services as very much an educational venture. This is a concept which is finding increasing favour in the medical field and I certainly use this model in my clinical work with people in difficulty or distress. At the same time, however, I think there is a similar risk of the health educators being presented as experts and not placing the learner at the centre of the stage. In the same way as I have argued with children at schools, I would see health education as best being a medium in which a setting is created where people can test out some of the questions that may be meaningful to them. In spite of my above emphasis on the importance of continuing education throughout life it seems to me to be crucial to place a major emphasis on the development of construction in children: 'unlearning' in adulthood is notoriously difficult, as all mental health workers will doubtless testify.

The Family

In spite of a number of attacks over the years, the institution of the family is very much alive, although less certainly 'well'. Family therapy is very much a fashionable movement of our time and Procter has well demonstrated in the preceding chapter the potential of a personal construct approach to problems which emerge in families. My concern here, however, is not with the clinical treatment of designated family problems, but with the ways in which the family as an institution can promote or stifle development and psychological well-being. My basic question is 'Do families encourage constructive alternativism? More specifically, Do they practice what Landfield (1980a) has called 'perspectivism'? I suppose the simple answer to this is that some do and some don't. Family therapy concepts like 'enmeshment', overprotectiveness and rigidity sound like families which are more concerned with definition than extension, with the main aim to validate a view of their family and by implication what their family is not. Certain cultures are said to promote strong family ties and regard the family tradition as the most fundamental value to preserve. The Jewish culture perhaps epitomises this concept, although it seems to me that almost wherever one goes one is confronted with pressures to conform to the expectations of families. Clearly the family is an integral feature of a society's attempts to validate its position. So, are families by definition concerned primarily with the definition of a belief system? Or can they be consistent with the potential for growth, development or 'extension' as stated in the choice corollary? Rather than attempt to dismiss families as a reactionary force, perhaps we should recognise what their chief virtue is. From a construct theory perspective I would suggest that this is that they provide validation and hold back the forces of uncertainty. This is no trivial role: without some predictability and security we are unlikely to venture. When faced with the unknown or the threatening we can take comfort in the familiar, the well-construed. My one comfort when contemplating the nuclear holocaust is that I would hope to be with my family. Somehow being snuggled up together seems to preserve in the face of destruction. The comfort of one's nearest and dearest on impending death testifies to the fundamentality of this institution.

In the same way that families can validate so they can invalidate. Behaviour which is not deemed to be consistent with expectations can be stamped upon, criticised or dismissed. The extent to which families resist the novel will presumably be a function of the 'permeability' of their 'system', i.e. Can their system incorporate new behaviour etc? Although some degree of impermeability must presumably be a feature of any construct system, a totally impermeable family system can only repeat itself, continually going over and over the same routines with each generation a virtual carbon copy of the last. Although such a family may be a myth, some families seem to come close to it with only the most peripheral of modifications possible.

Doubtless the family will continue for a long time to be the centre of human life. Nor is it my aim fundamentally to challenge the family as an institution. I am arguing, however, that families whilst generally being health-promoting can in some modes of functioning be pathogenic and inhibitory of both personal and social development. One thing we can do, however, is to *question*, to be open to alternative constructions of what families might be and might become. Families, like societies, which can't anticipate or accept the possibility of other kinds of family or society may be on the path to the unenviable choice of destroying or being destroyed.

Work

At a time when unemployment is sky-high there is ample reason to question the institution of work. Work is clearly a variable quantity with varying potential for constructive alternativism. We are constantly being told that those firms who don't look ahead and change are the ones who are likely to 'go to the wall'. Industries rise and fall and with them come and go whole masses of people. If this is the case then surely the ability to take different points of view and to innovate should be welcome features of a worker. All too often, however, one hears of workers being bored, stifled and at worst like robots: as one of my friends once said to me 'a monkey could do it!' Clearly all work has a repetitive aspect to it, but if psychological research has concluded anything, the message is that too much predictability and insufficient novelty lower motivation and performance. Furthermore, adverse mental health has been shown to be associated with the foregoing work conditions (Kornhauser, 1965). That is not to say that novelty can somehow be provided but the need for it can be anticipated and positively encouraged. In the same way that monotony can be psychologically 'unhealthy', so can excessive pressure or 'stress'. The demands of production, competition and the desire for promotion can create a climate in which a person is unable to fulfil expectations. It seems to me that at the heart of this problem is often the absence of 'sociality'. Managers and supervisors may be solely concerned with *their* aims and fail to recognise that there are other considerations. In turn workers may fail to understand their 'bosses' and purely see them as trying to undermine them. The polarisations in work are no more aptly illustrated than in the ever-present union-management battles, where each side seems to be primarily concerned with validating their respective positions, with little evidence of shared understandings and aims. The concept of a 'cooperative' is indeed a welcome, albeit ironic development in industry, with the implication that cooperation is something special – a luxury.

If a work setting is to be consistent with mental health there is a dual challenge. First, it must allow for elaboration of people's lives. A healthy work setting is one which fosters the individuality of workers, recognising the need for work to both have meaning and be at least partly controllable. Secondly, it needs to allow for understanding and a commonality of purpose between workers at all levels.

Leisure

I suspect that for many people leisure is the most pleasurable and sometimes most meaningful aspect of their life. Whereas for economic reasons people generally feel they have to work, leisure may be something they want to do. Like children, we love to 'play'. Rather than perhaps exclusively advocating mass leisure, I would suggest that we take seriously this positive feature of leisure as a context within which personal choice seems maximal. Maybe rigid boundaries between work, education, family and leisure are unhelpful? Is it too much to hope that the personal meaningfulness and pleasure that come from leisure could be an integral part of our working, learning and family life? Certainly it seems that for some work is their hobby: they enjoy it, it's a challenge, a manifestation of their most cherished values, a path towards personal fulfilment. Similarly, whereas education can be tedious, some are 'turned on' by it. The enthusiasm of the 'mature student' is consistent with the view that it works best when it is a choice meaningful to that person and not something you do because you have to. Family life, whilst often difficult and stormy can also be the focal point of the adventure of life. When family members are in tune with each other, when there's a mutual interest and joy in each other's developments then doing things with family can be a truly meaningful manifestation of one's development. Perhaps it is too much to hope that people can pursue all their ventures equally meaningfully in all contexts. All too often, work can become a haven from family or family can become a haven from work. I would suggest, however, that running through all these contexts is the potential for health and by implication ill-health.

Conclusions

It would not be in the spirit of personal construct theory to end with a conclusion. With each end there is a beginning and the business of anticipation goes on. Like in the latter stages of psychotherapy, however there is an opportunity to take stock, to reflect on where we've been and in what direction we may wish to proceed. In contrasting ways, my fellow contributors and I have tried to communicate our view that construct theory can be and is being applied to a wide range of 'disorders' or problems which fall under the umbrella of mental health-illness. All of us to varying degrees are directly involved in the clinical context and have had experience of trying to help people in difficulty. In exploring the wider context in this chapter, however, I have becoms increasingly convinced that the message of construct theory for mental health should not remain the precious possession of a select band of psychologists. If you find the ideas exciting, I hope you will share them and boldly put them into practice in creating a world in which enquiry, tolerance of difference and awareness of the 'illusions of reality' (Smail, 1984) guide our endeavours.

REFERENCES

Achterberg, J., Matthews-Simonton, S. and Simonton, O.C. (1977) 'Psychology of the Exceptional Cancer Patient: A Description of Cancer Patients who Outlived Predicted Life Expectancies', *Psychotherapy, 14*, 416-22

Adams-Webber, J.R. (1970) 'Actual Structure and Potential Chaos' in D. Bannister (ed.), *Perspectives in Personal Construct Theory*, Academic Press, London

Adams-Webber, J.R. (1973) 'The Complexity of the Target as a Factor in Interpersonal Judgement', *Social Behaviour and Personality, 1*, 35-8

Adams-Webber, J.R. (1979a) 'Construing Persons in Social Contexts' in P. Stringer and D. Bannister (eds.) *Constructs of Sociality and Individuality*, Academic Press, London, pp. 195-220

Adams-Webber, J.R. (1979b) *Personal Construct Theory: Concepts and Applications*, Wiley, Chichester

Adams-Webber, J.R. (1981) 'Fixed Role Therapy' in R.J. Corsini (ed.) *Handbook of Innovative Psychotherapies*, Wiley, New York

Adams-Webber, J.R. and Rodney, Y. (1983) 'Relational Aspects of Temporarary Changes in Construing Self and Others', *Canadian Journal of Behavioural Science, 1*, 52-9

Agnew, J. and Peacey, M. (1982) 'The Magic Garden', Unpublished Manuscript

American Psychiatric Association (1980) *Diagnostic and Statistical Manual of Mental Disorders*, 3rd edn, Washington, DC

Anderson, N.D. (1981) 'Exclusion; A Study of Depersonalisation in Health Care', *Journal of Humanistic Psychology, 21*, 67-78

Andrews, G. (1981) 'A Prospective Study of Life Events and Psychological Symptoms', *Psychological Medicine, 11*, 795-801

Antonovsky, A. (1979) *Health, Stress and Coping*, Jossey Bass, San Francisco

Applebee, A.N. (1976) 'The Development of Children's Responses to Repertory Grids', *British Journal of Social and Clinical Psychology, 15*, 101-2

Applegate, J.L. (1983a) 'Constructs, Interaction Goals and Communication in Relationship Development', Paper Presented at the 5th International Congress on Personal Construct Psychology, Boston, Massachusetts

Applegate, J.L. (1983b) 'Construct System Development, Strategic Complexity and Impression Formation in Persuasive Communication' in J. Adams-Webber and J. Mancuso (eds.), *Applications of Personal Construct Theory*, Academic Press, Toronto, pp. 187-206

Arnkoff, D.B. and Glass, C.R. (1982) 'Clinical Cognitive Constructs' in P. Kendall (ed.), *Advances in Cognitive Behavioural Research and Therapy* (vol. 1), Academic Press, New York

Ashworth, C.M., Blackburn, I.M. and McPherson, F.M. (1982) 'The Performance of Depressed and Manic Patients on Some Repertory Grid Measures: A Cross-Sectional Study', *British Journal of Medical Psychology, 55*, 247-55

Auden, W.H. (1976) *Collected Poems*, Faber, London

Bach, G.R. (1954) *Intensive Group Psychotherapy*, Ronald Press Co., New York

Baillie-Grohman, R. (1975) 'The Use of a Modified Form of Repertory Grid Technique to Investigate the Extent to which Deaf School Leavers Tend to Use

361

Stereotypes', Unpublished MSc Dissertation, University of London

Bakan, D. (1967) *On Method*, Jossey Bass, San Francisco

Baker, R., Hall, J.N., Hutchinson, K. and Bridge, G. (1977) 'Symptom Changes in Schizophrenic Patients on a Token Economy: A Controlled Experiment', *British Journal of Psychiatry, 131*, 381-93

Bales, R.F. (1956) 'Task Status and Likeability as a Function of Talking and Listening in Decision-Making Groups' in L.D. White (ed.), *The State of the Social Sciences*, University of Chicago Press, Chicago

Bandura, A. (1965) 'Influences of Models' Reinforcement Contingencies on the Acquisition of Initiative Responses', *Journal of Personality and Social Psychology, 1*, 589-95

Bandura, A. (1977) 'Self-Efficacy: Towards a Unifying Theory of Behavioral Change', *Psychological Review, 84*, 191-215

Bannister, D. (1959) 'An Application of Personal Construct Theory (Kelly) to Schizoid Thinking', Unpublished PhD Thesis, University of London

Bannister, D. (1960) 'Conceptual Structure in Thought Disordered Schizophrenics, *Journal of Mental Science, 106*, 1230-49

Bannister, D. (1962) 'The Nature and Measurement of Schizophrenic Thought Disorder', *Journal of Mental Science, 108*, 825-42

Bannister, D. (1963) 'The Genesis of Schizophrenic Thought Disorder: A Serial Invalidation Hypothesis', *British Journal of Psychiatry, 109*, 680-6

Bannister, D. (1965a) 'The Genesis of Schizophrenic Thought Disorder: Retest of the Serial Invalidation Hypothesis', *British Journal of Psychiatry, 111*, 377-82

Bannister, D. (1965b) 'The Rationale and Clinical Relevance of Repertory Grid Technique', *British Journal of Psychiatry, 111*, 977-82

Bannister, D. (1983) 'Self in Personal Construct Theory' in J. Adams-Webber and J.C. Mancuso (eds.), *Applications of Personal Construct Theory*, Acadmic Press, Toronto

Bannister, D., Adams-Webber, J.R., Penn, W.I. and Radley, A.R. (1975) 'Reversing the Process of Thought Disorder: A Serial Validation Experiment', *British Journal of Social and Clinical Psychology, 14*, 169-80

Bannister D.and Agnew, J. (1977) 'The Child's Construing of Self' in A.W. Landfield (ed.) *1976 Nebraska Symposium on Motivation*, University of Nebraska Press, Lincoln, Nebraska, pp. 99-125

Bannister, D. and Bott, M. (1973) 'Evaluating the Person' in P. Kline (ed.), *New Approaches in Psychological Measurement*, Wiley, London

Bannister D. and Fransella, F. (1966) 'A Grid Test of Schizophrenic Thought Disorder', *British Journal of Social and Clinical Psychology, 5*, 95-102

Bannister, D. and Fransella, F. (1967) *Grid Test of Schizophrenic Thought Disorder: A Standard Clinical Test*, Psychological Test Publications, Barnstaple, Devon

Bannister, D. and Fransella, F. (1971) *Inquiring Man: The Theory of Personal Constructs*, Penguin, Harmondsworth. Also Second Edition 1980, Penguin, London and 1982, Kreiger, Malabar, Florida

Bannister, D., Fransella, F. and Agnew, J. (1971) 'Characteristics and Validity of the Grid Test of Thought Disorder', *British Journal of Social and Clinical Psychology, 10*, 144-51

Bannister, D. and Mair, J.M.M. (1968) *The Evaluation of Personal Constructs*, Academic Press, London and New York

Bannister, D. and Salmon, P. (1966) 'Schizophrenic Thought Disorder: Specific or

Diffuse?' *British Journal of Medical Psychology, 39*, 215-19

Barnes, B. (1983) 'Doubts and Certainties in Practising Psychotherapy' in D. Pilgrim (ed.), *Psychology and Psychotherapy: Current Trends and Issues*, Routledge and Kegan Paul, London

Barr, H.L., Langs, R.J., Holt, R.R., Goldberger, L. and Klein, G.S. (1972) *L.S.D: Personality and Experience*, Wiley, New York

Barratt, B. (1977) 'The Development of Peer Perception Systems in Childhood and Early Adolescence', *Social Behaviour and Personality, 5*, 351-60

Barton, E., Walton, T. and Rowe, D. (1976) 'Using Grid Technique with the Mentally Handicapped', in P. Slater (ed.), *The Measurement of Intrapersonal Space by Grid Technique'*, vol. 1, Wiley, Chichester

Bascue, L.O. (1978) 'A Conceptual Model for Training Group Therapists', *International Journal of Group Psychotherapy, 28*, 445-52

Bateson, G. (1972) *Steps to an Ecology of Mind*, Ballantine, New York

Bateson, G., Jackson, D.D., Haley, J. and Weakland, J. (1956) 'Towards a Theory of Schizophrenia', *Behavioural Science, 1*, 252-64

Beail, N. Repertory Grid Technique and Personal Constructs: Applications in Clinical and Educational Settings, Croom Helm, Beckenham, Kent

Beail, N. and Beail, S. (1982) 'Dependency and Personal Growth', *New Forum, 8*, 58-60

Beck, A.T. (1963) 'Thinking and Depression1: Idiosyncratic Content and Cognitive Distortion', *Archives of General Psychiatry, 9*, 325-33

Beck, A.T. (1973) *The Diagnosis and Management of Depression*, University of Pennsylvania Press, Philadelphia

Beck, A.T. (1976) *Cognitive Therapy and the Emotional Disorders*, International Universities Press, New York

Beck, A.T. and Rush, A.J. (1978) 'Cognitive Approaches to Depression and Suicide' in G. Serban (ed.), *Cognitive Deficits in the Development of Mental Illness,* Brunner/Mazel, New York

Beck, A.T., Rush, A.J., Shaw, B.F. and Emery, G. (1979) *Cognitive Therapy of Depression*, Guildford, New York

Becker, H.S. (1953) 'Becoming a Marijuana User', *American Journal of Sociology, 59*, 235-42

Bedrosian, R.C. and Beck, A.T. (1980) 'Principles of Cognitive Therapy' in M. Mahoney (ed.), *Psychotherapy Process*, Plenum, New York

Beech, H.R. and Liddell, A. (1974) 'Decision Making, Mood States and Ritualistic Behaviour Among Obsessional Patients' in H.R. Beech (ed.), *Obsessional States*, Methuen, London

Benoliel, J.Q. (1974) 'The Dying Patient and the Family' in S.B. Troup and W.A. Greene (eds.), *The Patient, Death and the Family*, Scribners, New York

Ben-Tovim, D.I. and Greenup, J. (1983) 'The Representation of Transference through Serial Grids: A Methodological Study', *British Journal of Medical Psychology, 56*, 255-61

Berger, M.M. (ed.) (1978) *Beyond the Double Bind*, Brunner/Mazel, New York

Berjerot, N. (1972) 'A Theory of Addiction as an Artificially Induced Drive', *American Journal of Psychiatry, 128*, 842-6

Beveridge, M. and Evans, P. (1978) 'Classroom Interaction: Two Studies of Severely Educationally Subnormal Children', *Research in Education, 19*, 39-49

Bieri, J. (1955) 'Cognitive Complexity-Simplicity and Predictive Behaviour',

Journal of Abnormal and Social Psychology, 51, 263-8

Bieri, J. (1966) 'Cognitive Complexity and Personality Development' in O.J. Harvey (ed.)' *Experience, Structure and Adaptability,* Springer, New York

Bion, W.R. (1961) *Experiences in Groups,* Tavistock Publications, London

Bleuler, E. (1950) *Dementia Praecox or the Group of Schizophrenias,* International Universities Press, New York (originally published in 1911)

Blum, S.B. (1980) 'Changes in Alcoholics' Self-Esteem in Relationship to Perceptions of Drinking and Sober Roles During Treatment', Unpublished Doctoral Dissertation, University of Nebraska-Lincoln, Lincoln, Nebraska

Blumberg, B., Flaherty, M. and Lewis, J. (eds.), (1980) *Coping with Cancer,* US Department of Health and Human Services, Washington DC

Bonarius, H. (1970) 'Fixed Role Therapy: A Double Paradox', *British Journal of Medical Psycholody, 43,* 213-19

Bonarius, H. (1977a) 'The Interactional Model of Communication: Through Experimental Research Towards Existential Relevance', in A.W. Landfield (ed.), *The Nebraska Symposium on Motivation 1976,* University of Nebraska Press, Lincoln, Nebraska

Bonarius, H. (1980) *Persoonlijke Psychologie, Deel 2, Ontwikkelingen in de Theorie en de Praktijk van Constructenpsychologie.* Van Loghum Staterus, Deventer

Bonarius, J.C. (1977b) 'The Interaction Model of Extreme Responding' in A.W. Landfield (ed.), *The Nebraska Symposium on Motivation 1976,* University of Nebraska Press, Lincoln, Nebraska, pp. 291-343

Bond, A. and Lader, M. (1976) 'Self Concepts in Anxiety States', *British Journal of Medical Psychology, 49,* 275-9

Book, T.L. (1976) 'Personal Construct Changes During Alcoholism Treatment', Unpublished Doctoral Dissertation, University of Nebraska-Lincoln, Lincoln, Nebraska

Boston, S. (1981) *Will My Son: The Life and Death of a Mongol Child,* Pluto Press, London

Boszormenyi-Nagy, I. and Spark, G. (1973) *Invisible Loyalties: Reciprocity in Intergenerational Family Therapy,* Harper Row, New York

Bowen, M. (1960) 'A Family Concept of Schizophrenia' in D. Jackson, *The Aetiology of Schizophrenia,* Basic Books, New York

Bronfenbrenner, U. (1975) 'Is Early Intervention Effective?' in M. Guttentag and E. Struening (eds.), *Handbook of Evaluation Research,* vol 2, Sage, Beverley Hills

Brown, G. and Desforges, C. (1977) 'Piagetian Psychology and Education', *British Journal of Education Psychology, 47,* 7-17

Bruch, H. (1974) *Eating Disorders: Obesity, Anorexia Nervosa and the Person Within,* Routledge and Kegan Paul, London

Bruch, H. (1978) *The Golden Cage: The Enigma of Anorexia Nervosa,* Routledge and Kegan Paul, London

Bulman, R.S. and Wortman, C.B. (1977) 'Attribution of Blame and Coping in the Real World: Severe Accident Victims React to their Lot', *Journal of Personality and Social Psychology, 35,* 351-63

Burden, R. (1978) 'An Approach to the Evaluation of Early Intervention Projects with Mothers of Severely Handicapped Children: the Attitude Dimension', *Child: Care, Health and Development, 4,* 171-81

Button, E.J. (1980) 'Construing and Clinical Outcome in Anorexia Nervosa', Unpublished PhD Thesis, University of London

Button, E.J. (1983a) 'Personal Construct Theory and Psychological Well-Being', *British Journal of Medical Psychology, 56*, 313-21

Button, E.J. (1983b) 'Construing the Anorexic' in J. Adams-Webber and J. Mancuso (eds.), *Applications of Personal Construct Theory*, Academic Press, Toronto

Button, E.J. and Whitehouse, A. (1981) 'Subclinical Anorexia Nervosa', *Psychological Medicine, 11*, 509-16

Caine, T.M., Smail, D.J., Wijesinghe, O.B.A. and Winter, D.A. (1982) *The Claybury Selection Battery Manual*, NFER-Nelson, Windsor

Caine, T.M., Wijesinghe, O.B.A. and Winter D.A. (1981) *Personal Styles in Neurosis: Implications for Small Group Psychotherapy and Behaviour Therapy*, Routledge and Kegan Paul, London

Cameron, N. (1964) 'Experimental Analysis of Schizophrenic Thinking' in J.S. Kasanin (ed.), *Language and Thought in Schizophrenia*, Norton, New York, pp. 50-64 (originally published in 1944)

Candy, J., Balfour, H.G., Cawley, R.H., Hildebrand, H.P., Malan, D.H., Marks, I.M. and Wilson, J. (1972) 'A Feasibility Study for the Controlled Trial of Psychotherapy, *Psychological Medicine, 2*, 345-50

Caplan, H.L., Rohde, P.D., Shapiro, D.A. and Watson, J.P. (1975) 'Some Correlates of Repertory Grid Measures Used to Study a Psychotherapy Group, *British Journal of Medical Psychology, 48*, 217-26

Carlin, A.S., Post, R.D., Bakker, C.B. and Halpern, L.M. (1974) 'The Role of Modelling and Previous Experience in the Facilitation of Marijuana Intoxication', *Journal of Nervous and Mental Disease, 159*, 275-81

Carroll, R.A. (1983) 'Cognitive Imbalance in Schizophrenia' in J.Adams-Webber and J. Mancuso (eds.), *Applications of Personal Construct Theory*, Academic Press, Toronto

Carter, L.F. (1954) 'Recording and Evaluating the Performance of Individuals as Members of Small Groups', *Personnel Psychology, 7*, 477-84

Cassell, E.J. (1976) *The Healer's Art*, Penguin

Chance, E. (1966 Content Analysis of Verbalisation about Interpersonal Experience' in L.A. Gottschalk and A.H. Auerbach (eds.), *Methods of Research in Psychotherapy*, Appleton-Century-Crofts, New York

Chapman, L.J. and Chapman, J. (1973) *Disordered Thought in Schizophrenia*. Prentice Hall, Englewood Cliffs, New Jersey

Chein, I., Gerard, D.L., Less, R.S. and Rosenfeld, E. (1964) *The Road to H: Narcotics, Delinquency and Social Policy*, Basic Books, New York

Chetwynd, J. (1977) 'The Psychological Meaning of Structural Measure Derived from Grids' in P. Slater (ed.), *Dimensions of Intrapersonal Space*, Wiley, London

Childs, D. and Hedges, R. (1980) 'The Analysis of Interpersonal Perceptions as a Repertory Grid', *British Journal of Medical Psychology, 53*, 127-36

Clark, D. (1974) 'Psychological Assessment in Mental Subnormality' in A.M. Clarke and A.D.B. Clarke (eds.), *Mental Deficiency: the Changing Outlook*, Methuen, London

Clarke, A.M. and Clarke, A.D.B. (1974a) 'Experimental Studies: an Overview' in A.M. Clarke and A.D.B. Clarke (eds.), *Mental Deficiency; the Changing Outlook*, Methuen, London

Clarke, A.M. and Clarke, A.D.B. (1974b) 'Severe Subnormality; Capacity and Performance' in A.M. Clarke and A.D.B. Clarke (eds.), *Mental Deficiency: the*

Changing Outlook, Methuen, London

Clarke, A.M. and Viney, L.L. (1984) 'Primary Prevention of Illness: Social Systems and Personal Power', *Australian Psychologist, 19*, 7-20

Cobb, J. (1979) 'Group Interaction' in P. Hill, R. Murray and A. Thurley (eds.), *Essentials of Post-Graduate Psychiatry*, Academic Press, London

Cochran, L. (1976) 'Categorisation and Change in Conceptual Relations', *Canadian Journal of Behavioural Science, 30*, 275-86

Cochran, L. (1977) 'Inconsistency and Change in Conceptual Organisation', *British Journal of Medical Psychology, 50*, 319-28

Coffey, H., Friedham, M., Leary, T. and Ossema, A. (1950) 'Results and Implications of the Group Psychotherapy Programme', *Journal of Social Issues, 6*, 37-44

Collier, H.O.S. (1972) 'Drug Dependence: A Pharmacological Analysis', *British Journal of the Addictions, 67*, 277-86

Cosijns, P., Peuskens, J. and Tilmans, B. (1977) 'Une Experience de "Token-Economy" chez les Jeunes Patients Schizophrenes', *Acta Psychiatrica Belgica, 77*, 174-93

Covi, L., Roth, D. and Lipman, R.S. (1982) 'Cognitive Group Psychotherapy of Depression: The Close-Ended Group', American Journal of Psychotherapy, 36, 459-69

Cowie, B. (1976) 'The Cardiac Patient's Perception of his Heart Attack', *Social Science and Medicine, 10*, 87-96

Craft, M. (1979) *Tredgold's Mental Retardation*, 12th edn, Bailliere-Tindall, London

Crisp, A.H. and Fransella, F. (1972) 'Conceptual Changes During Recovery from Anorexia Nervosa', *British Journal of Medical Psychology, 45*, 395-405

Crockett, W.H. (1965) 'Cognitive Complexity and Impression Formation' in B.A. Maher (ed.), *Progress in Experimental Personality Research'* vol. 2, Academic Press, New York

Crockett, W.H. (1983) 'Constructs, Impressions, Actions and Construct Change: A Model of Processes in Impression Formation', Paper Presented at the 5th International Conference of Personal Construct Psychology, Boston, Massachusetts

Crockett, W.H. and Meisel, P. (1974) 'Construct Connectedness, Strength of Disconfirmation and Impression Change', *Journal of Personality, 42*, 290–9.

Cromwell, R. (1963) 'A Social Learning Approach to Mental Retardation' in N. Ellis (ed.), *Handbook of Mental Deficiency*, McGraw-Hill, New York

Cummings, S. (1976) 'The Impact of the Child's Deficiency on the Father', *American Journal of Orthopsychiatry, 46*, 246-55

Cunningham, C.C. (1979) 'Parents' Counselling' in M. Craft (ed.), *Tredgold's Mental Retardation*, 12th edn, Bailliere-Tindall, London

Cunningham, C.C. (1983) 'Early Support and Intervention' in P. Mittler and H. McConachie (eds.), *Parents, Professionals and Mentally Handicapped People*, Croom Helm, Beckenham

Cunningham, C.C. and Davis H. (in press, a) *Working with Parents*, Open University Press, London

Cunningham, C.C. and Davis, H. (in press, b) 'Early Parent Counselling' in M. Craft (ed.), *Tedgold's Mental Retardation*, 13th edn., Bailliere-Tindall, London

Davidson, P. (1982) 'Issues in Patient Compliance' in T. Millon, C. Green and R. Meagher (eds.), *Handbook of Clinical Health Psychology*, Plenum, New York

Davis, H. (1983) 'Constructs of Handicap: Working with Parents and Children', *Changes, 1*, 37-9

Davis, H. (1984) 'Personal Construct Theory: A Possible Framework for Use', *Mental Handicap, 12,* 80-1

Davis, H. and Oliver B. (1980) 'A Comparison of Aspects of the Maternal Speech Environment of Retarded and Non-Retarded Children', *Child: Care, Health and Development, 6,* 135-45

Davis, H., Stroud, A. and Green, L. (1984) 'Parental Interaction and Children with Mental Handicap' (in preparation)

Dawes, A.R.L. (1979) 'A Personal Construct Theory Approach to Drug Dependence', Unpublished MSc Thesis, University of Cape Town

Dawes, A.R.L. (1981) 'Becoming Drug Dependent; An Exercise in Construct Elaboration', Paper Presented at the 4th International Congress on Personal Construct Psychology, St Catherines, Ontario

De Boeck, P. (1981) 'An Interpretation of Loose Construing in Schizophrenic Thought Disorder' in H. Bonarius, R. Holland and S. Rosenberg (eds.), *Recent Advances in the Theory and Practice of Personal Construct Psychology,* Macmillan, London

De Boeck, P., Van den Bergh, O. and Claeys, W. (1981) 'The Immediacy Hypothesis of Schizophrenia Tested in the Grid Test', *British Journal of Clinical Psychology, 20,* 131-2

Delia, J.G. (1980) 'Some Thoughts Concerning the Study of Interpersonal Relationships and their Development', *The Western Journal of Speech Communication, 44,* 97-103

Delia, J.G. and O'Keefe, B.J. (1976) 'The Interpersonal Constructs of Machiavellians', *British Journal of Social and Clinical Psychology, 15,* 435-6

Dewey, J. (1938) *Experience and Education,* Macmillan, New York

Dingemans, P.M., Space, L.G. and Cromwell, R.L. (1983) 'How General is the Inconsistency in Schizophrenic Behaviour?' in J. Adams-Webber and J. Mancuso (eds.), *Applications of Personal Construct Theory,* Academic Press, Toronto

Dole, V. and Nyswander, M. (1967) 'Heroin Addiction: A Metabolic Disease', *Archives of International Medicine, 120,* 19-24

Duck, S.W. (1973a) *Personal Relationships and Personal Constructs: A Study of Friendship Formation,* Wiley, London

Duck, S.W. (1973b) 'Similarity and Perceived Similarity of Personal Constructs as Influences of Friendship Choice', *British Journal of Social and Clinical Psychology, 12,* 1-6

Duck, S.W. (1977) 'Inquiry, Hypothesis and the Quest for Validation: Personal Construct Systems in the Development of Acquaintance' in S. Duck (ed.), *Theory and Practice in Interpersonal Attraction,* Academic Press, London

Duck, S.W. (1979a) 'The Personal and the Interpersonal in Construct Theory: Social and Individual Aspects of Relationships' in P. Stringer and D. Bannister (eds.), *Constructs of Sociality and Individuality,* Academic Press, London, pp. 279-97

Duck, S.W. (1979b) 'Personal Constructs in the Development and Collapse of Personal Relationships', Paper Presented at the 3rd International Congress on Personal Construct Psychology, Breukelen, Netherlands

Duck, S.W. (1982) 'Two Individuals in Search of Agreement: The Commonality Corollary' in J.C. Mancuso and J.R. Adams-Webber, (eds.), *The Construing Person,* Praeger, New York, pp. 222-34

Duck, S.W. (1983) 'Sociality and Cognition in Personal Construct Theory' in J.

Adams-Webber and J. Mancuso (eds.), *Applications of Personal Construct Theory*, Academic Press, Toronto

Duck, S.W. (1984) 'A Perspective on the Repair of Personal Relationships: Repair of What, When?' in S. Duck (ed.), *Personal Relationship 5: Repairing Personal Relationships*, Academic Press, London

Duck, S.W. and Allison, D. (1978) 'I Liked You But I Can't Live with You: A Study of Lapsed Friendships', *Social Behaviour and Personality, 8,* 43-7

Duck, S.W. and Miell, D. (1984) 'Towards a Comprehension of Friendship Development and Breakdown' in Tajfel, Fraser and Jaspars (eds.), *The Social Dimension: European Perspectives on Social Psychology*, vol. 1, Cambridge University Press, pp. 228-48

Duck, S.W. and Sants, H. (1983) 'On the Origin of the Specious: Are Personal Relationships Really Interpersonal States?' *Journal of Social and Clinical Psychology, 1,* 27-41

Duck, S.W. and Spencer, C. (1972) 'Personal Constructs and Friendship Formation', *Journal of Personality and Social Psychology, 23,* 40-5

Durkheim, E. (1897) *Suicide*, (J.A. Spaulding and G. Simpson, Translators, 1951), The Free Press, Glencoe, Illinois

Eland, F.A., Epting, F.R. and Bonarius, H. (1979) 'Self-Disclosure and the Reptest Interaction Technique (RIT)' in P. Stringer and D. Bannister (eds.), *Constructs of Sociality and Individuality*, Academic Press, London, pp. 177-92

Emmelkamp, P.M.G. and Cohen-Kettenis, P. (1975) 'Relationship of Locus of Control to Phobic Anxiety and Depression', *Psychological Reports, 36,* 390

Epting, F.R. and Amerikaner, M. (1980) 'Optimal Functioning: A Personal Construct Approach' in A.W. Landfield and L.M. Leitner (eds.), *Personal Construct Psychology: Psychotherapy and Personality*, Wiley-Interscience, New York

Epting, F.R. and Neimeyer, G. (1983) *Personal Meanings of Death*, Hemisphere, New York

Erickson, M.H. and Rossi, E.L. (1979) *Hypnotherapy: An Exploratory Casebook*, Irvington, New York

Eysenck, H.J. (1960) *The Structure of Human Personality*, Macmillan, New York

Farrell, P. (1984) 'A Pilot Investigation of Family Hierarchy: Definition and Utility as a Measure of Change', Unpublished Clinical Research Dissertation, Plymouth Polytechnic

Feldman, H.W. (1968) 'Ideological Supports to Becoming a Heroin Addict', *Journal of Health and Social Behaviour, 9,* 131-9

Ferlic, N., Colman, A. and Kennedy, B.J. (1979) 'Group Counselling in Adult Patients with Advanced Cancer', *Cancer, 43,* 760-6

Fielding, J.M. (1975) 'A Technique for Measuring Outcome in Group Psychotherapy', *British Journal of Medical Psychology, 48,* 189-98

Fielding, J.M. (1983) 'Verbal Participation and Group Therapy Outcome', *British Journal of Psychiatry, 142,* 524-8

Fincham, F. (1982) 'Piaget's Theory and the Learning Disabled' in S. and C. Modgil (eds.), *Jean Piaget: Consensus and Controversy*, Holt, Rinehart and Winston, London

Fisch, R., Weakland, J. and Segal, L. (1982) *The Tactics of Change, Doing Therapy Briefly*, Jossey-Bass, San Francisco

Flavell, J.H. and Draguns, J. (1957) 'A Microgenetic Approach to Perception and Thought', *Psychological Bulletin, 54,* 197-217

Foa, U.G. (1961) 'Convergences in the Analysis of the Structure of Interpersonal Behaviour', *Psychological Review, 68*, 341-53

Foulkes, S.H. and Anthony, G.J. (1957) *Group Psychotherapy*, Penguin, Harmondsworth

Fraiberg, S. (1970) 'Intervention in Infancy: A Program for Blind Infants', *Journal of the American Academy of Child Psychiatry, 10*, 381-405

Frank, J.D. (1974) *Persuasion and Healing* (revised edition), Schocken Books, New York

Fransella, F. (1972) *Personal Change and Reconstruction*, Academic Press, London

Fransella, F. (1974) 'Thinking in the Obsessional' in H.R. Beech (ed.), *Obsessional States*, Academic Press, New York

Fransella, F. (1981) 'Nature Babbling to Herself: The Self Characterisation as a Therapeutic Tool' in H. Bonarius, R. Holland and S. Rosenberg (eds.), *Personal Construct Psychology: Recent Advances in Theory and Practice*, Macmillan, London

Fransella, F. (1984) 'Resistance: A Personal Construct Viewpoint', *British Journal of Cognitive Psychotherapy* (in press)

Fransella, F. and Adams, B. (1966) 'An Illustration of the Use of Repertory Grid Technique in the Clinical Setting', *British Journal of Social and Clinical Psychology, 5*, 51-62

Fransella, F. and Bannister, D. (1977) *A Manual for Repertory Grid Technique*, Academic Press, London

Fransella, F. and Button, E.J. (1983) 'The "Construing" of Self and Body Size in Relation to Maintenance of Weight Gain in Anorexia Nervosa' in P.L. Darby, P.E. Garfinkel, D.M. Garner, and D.V. Coscina (eds.), *Anorexia Nervosa: Recent Developments in Research*, Alan Liss Inc., New York

Fransella, F. and Crisp, A.H. (1970) 'Conceptual Organisation and Weight Change', *Psychosomatics and Psychotherapy, 18*, 176-85

Fransella, F. and Crisp, A.H. (1979) 'Comparisons of Weight Concepts in Groups of a) Neurotics, b) Normal and c) Anorexia Females', *British Journal of Psychiatry, 134*, 79-86

Fransella, F. and Joyston-Bechal, M.P. (1971) 'An Investigation of Conceptual Process and Pattern Change in a Psychotherapy Group', *British Journal of Psychiatry, 119*, 199-206

Frazer, H.M. (1980) 'Agoraphobia; Parental Influences and Cognitive Structures', Unpublished PhD Thesis, University of Toronto

Freud, S. (1955) *Mourning and Melancholia*, Standard edn., vol. 18, Hogarth, London

Frith, C.E. and Lillie, F.J. (1972) 'Why Does the Repertory Grid Indicate Thought Disorder?' *British Journal of Social and Clincial Psychology, 11*, 73-8

Gambino, B. and Shaffer, H. (1979) 'The Concept of Paradigm and the Treatment of Addiction', *Professional Psychology, 10*, 207-22

Gartner, A. and Riessman, F. (1977) *Self Help in the Human Services*, Jossey-Bass, San Francisco

Giedt, F.H. (1956) 'Factor Analysis of Roles Patients Take in Therapy Groups', *Journal of Social Psychology, 44*, 165-71

Giorgi, A. (1970) *Psychology as a Human Science: A Phenomenologically Based Approach*, Harper and Row, New York

Girodo, M. (1977) 'Self Talk: Mechanisms in Anxiety and Stress Management' in C.

Spielberger and P. Sarason (eds.), *Stress and Anxiety*, vol. 4, Hemisphere, Washington DC

Glantz, M., Burr, W. and Bosse, R. (1981) 'Constructs Used By Alcoholics, Non Psychotic Out-Patients and Normals', Paper Presented at the 4th International Congress on Personal Construct Psychology, St Catherines, Ontario

Glatt, M.M. (1974) *Drugs, Society and Man: A Guide to Addiction and its Treatment*, Medical and Technical Publishing Company, Lancaster

Glazer, H.I., Clarkin, J.F. and Hunt, J.F. (1981) 'Assessment of Depression' in J.F. Clarkin and H.I. Glazer (eds.), *Depression; Behavioural and Directive Intervention Strategies*, Garland, New York

Gochman, I.R. and Keating, J.P. (1980) 'Misattribution to Crowding: Blaming Crowding for Non-Density-Caused Events', *Journal of Non Verbal Behaviour, 4*, 157-75

Goldstein, A.J. (1982) 'Agoraphobia: Treatment Successes, Treatment Failures and Theoretical Implications' in D.L. Chambless and A.J. Goldstein (eds.), *Agoraphobia: Multiple Perspectives on Theory and Treatment*, Wiley, New York

Gowans, F. and Hulbert, C. (1983) 'Self-Concept Assessment of Mentally Handicapped Adults: A Review', *Mental Handicap, 11*, 121-3

Greaves, G. (1974) 'Toward an Existential Theory of Drug Dependence', *Journal of Nervous and Mental Disease, 150*, 263-73

Green, H. (1964) *I Never Promised You a Rose Garden*, Holt, Rinehart and Winston, New York

Hafner, R.J. (1977a) 'The Husbands of Agoraphobic Women: Assortative Mating or Pathogenic Interaction?' *British Journal of Psychiatry, 130*, 233-9

Hafner, R.J. (1977b) 'The Husbands of Agoraphobic Women and their Influence on Treatment Outcome', *British Journal of Psychiatry, 131*, 289-94

Haley, J. (1959a) 'An Interactional Description of Schizophrenia', *Psychiatry, 22*, 321-32

Haley, J. (1959b) 'The Family of the Schizophrenic: A Model System', *Journal of Nervous and Mental Disease, 129*, 357-74

Haley, J. (1963) *Strategies of Psychotherapy*, Grune and Stratton, New York

Haley, J. (1973) *Uncommon Therapy: The Psychiatric Techniques of Milton H. Erickson*, M.D. Norton, New York

Hamilton, V. (1957) 'Perceptual and Personality Dynamics in Reactions to Ambiguity', *British Journal of Psychology, 48*, 200-15

Hannam, C. (1980) *Parents and Mentally Handicapped Children*, Penguin, Harmondsworth

Harrow, M. and Quinlan, D. (1977) 'Is Disordered Thinking Unique to Schizophrenia?' *Archives of General Psychiatry, 34*, 15-21

Hartman, D. (1969) 'A Study of Drug-taking Adolescents', *The Psychoanalytic Study of the Child, 24*, 385-98

Hayden, B. (1979) 'The Self and Possibilities for Change', *Journal of Personality, 47*, 546-56

Hayden, B., Nasby, W. and Davids, A. (1977) 'Interpersonal Conceptual Structures, Predictive Accuracy and Social Adjustment of Emotionally Disturbed Boys', *Journal of Abnormal Psychology, 86*, 315-20

Haygood, R.C. and Bourne, L.E. (1965) 'Attribute and Rule-Learning Aspects of Conceptual Behaviour', *Psychological Review, 72*, 175-95

Haynes, E.T. and Phillips, J.P.N. (1973) 'Inconsistency, Loose Construing and

Schizophrenic Thought Disorder', *British Journal of Psychiatry, 123*, 209-17

Heather, N. (1976) 'The Specificity of Schizophrenic Thought Disorder: A Replication and Extension of Previous Research Findings', *British Journal of Social and Clinical Psychology, 15,* 131-8

Heather, N., Edwards, S. and Hore, B. (1975) 'Changes in Construing and Outcome of Group Therapy for Alcoholism', *Journal of Studies on Alcohol, 36,* 1238-53

Heber, R. (1959) *Manual on Terminology and Classification in Mental Retardation,* AAMD, Washington DC

Heifetz, L. (1980) 'From Consumer to Middleman: Emerging Roles for Parents in the Network of Services for Retarded Children' in R. Abidin (ed.), *Parent Education and Intervention Handbook,* Thomas, Springfield

Herr, J. and Weakland, J. (1979) *Counselling Elders and their Families,* Springer, New York

Hewstone, M., Hooper, D. and Miller, K. (1981) 'Psychological Change in Neurotic Depression: A Repertory Grid and Personal Construct Theory Approach', *British Journal of Psychiatry, 139,* 47-51

Hill, P., Murray, R. and Thorley, A. (1979) *Essentials of Postgraduate Psychiatry,* Academic Press, London

Hillman, J. (1976) *Suicide and the Soul,* Spring Publication, Zurich

Hinkle, D. (1965) 'The Change of Personal Constructs from the Viewpoint of a Theory of Construct Implications', Unpublished PhD Thesis, Ohio State University

Holland, R. (1977) *Self and Social Context,* St Martins, New York

Hollon, S.D. and Beck, A.T. (1979) 'Cognitive Therapy for Depression' in P.C. Kendall and S.D. Hollon (eds.), *Cognitive-Behavioural Interventions: Theory, Research and Procedures,* Academic Press, New York

Holmes, J. (1982) 'Phobia and Counter-Phobia: Family Aspects of Agoraphobia', *Journal of Family Therapy, 4,* 133-52

Honess, T. (1979) 'Children's Implicit Theories of Their Peers: A Developmental Analysis', *British Journal of Psychology, 70* 417-24

Honess, T. (1982) 'Accounting for Oneself: Meanings of Self-Descriptions and Inconsistencies in Self-Descriptions', *British Journal of Medical Psychology, 55,* 41-52

Honikman, B. (1976) 'Construct Theory as an Approach to Architectural Design', in P. Slater (ed.), *The Measurement of Intrapersonal Space by Grid Technique,* vol. 1 *Explorations of Intrapersonal Space,* Wiley, London

Hoy, R.M. (1973) 'The Meaning of Alcoholism for Alcoholics: A Repertory Grid Study', *British Journal of Social and Clinical Psychology, 12,* 98-9

Jackson, S.R. and Bannister, D. (1984) 'Growing into Self' in D. Bannister (ed.), *Issues and Approaches in Personal Construct Theory,* Academic Press, London

Janis, I.L. and Rodin, J. (1979) 'Attribution Control and Decision Making: Social Psychology and Health' in G.C. Stone, F. Cohen and N.E. Adler (eds.), *Health Psychology: A Handbook,* Jossey Bass, San Francisco

Johnson, J.H. and Sarason, I.G. (1978) 'Life Stress, Depression and Anxiety: Internal-External Control as a Moderator Variable', *Journal of Psychosomatic Research, 22,* 205-8

Jung, C.G. (1959) *Aion: Researches into the Phenomenological Self,* Pantheon Books, Bollingen Foundation Inc., New York

Karst, T.O. (1980) 'The Relationship between Personal Construct Theory and

Psychotherapeutic Techniques' in A.W. Landfield and L.M. Leitner (eds.), *Personal Construct Psychology: Psychotherapy and Personality*, Wiley, New York.

Kelly, G.A. (1955) *The Psychology of Personal Construct*, vols. 1 and 2, Norton, New York

Kelly, G.A. (1961) 'Suicide: The Personal Construct Point of View' in N. Farberow and E. Schneidman (eds.), *The Cry for Help*, McGraw-Hill, New York, pp. 225-80

Kelly, G.A. (1966a) Transcript of a Tape-recorded Conversation with Fay Fransella

Kelly, G.A. (1966b) 'A Brief Introduction to Personal Construct Theory' in D. Bannister and J.M.M. Mair, *The Evaluation of Personal Constructs*, Academic Press, London

Kelly, G.A. (1969a) 'Man's Construction of His Alternativises' in B. Maher (ed.), *Clinical Psychology and Personality: The Selected Papers of George Kelly*, Wiley, New York

Kelly, G.A. (1969b) 'The Autobiography of a Theory' in B. Maher (ed.), *Clinical Psychology and Personality*, Wiley, New York

Kelly, G.A. (1969c) 'Ontological Acceleration' in B. Maher (ed.), *Clinical Psychology and Personality*, Wiley, New York, pp. 7-45

Kelly, G.A. (1969d) 'In Whom Confide: On Whom Depend for What' in B. Maher (ed.), *Clinical Psychology and Personality*, Wiley, New York, pp. 189-206

Kelly, G.A. (1969e) 'Sin and Psychotherapy' in B. Maher (ed.), *Clinical Psychology and Personality* , Wiley, New York, pp. 165-88

Kelly, G.A. (1969f) 'Personal Construct Theory and the Psychotherapeutic Interview' in B. Maher (ed.), *Clinical Psychology and Personality*, Wiley, New York, p. 231

Kelly, G.A. (1969g) 'Psychotherapy and the Nature of Man' in B. Maher (ed.) *Clinical Psychology and Personality,* Wiley, New York, pp. 207-15

Kelly, G.A. (1969h) 'The Psychotherapeutic Relationship' in B. Maher (ed.), *Clinical Psychology and Personality*, Wiley, New York

Kelly, G.A. (1973) 'Fixed Role Therapy' in R.M. Jurjevich (ed.), *Direct Psychotherapy: 28 American Originals*, University of Miami Press, Coral Gables

Kelly, G.A. (1977) 'The Psychology of the Unknown' in D. Bannister (ed), *New Perspectives in Personal Construct Theory*, Academic Press, London

Kelly, G.A. (1980) 'The Psychology of the Optimal Man' in A.W. Landfield and L.M. Leitner (eds.), *Personal Construct Psychology: Psychotherapy and Personality*, Wiley, New York, pp. 18-35

Klein, N. and Safford, P. (1977) 'Application of Piaget's Theory to the Study of Thinking of the Mentally Retarded', *Journal of Special Education, 11*, 201–16

Koch, H.C.H. (1983a) 'Changes in Personal Construing in Three Psychotherapy Groups and a Control Group', *British Journal of Medical Psychology, 56*, 245-54

Koch, H.C.H. (1983b) 'Correlates of Changes in Personal Construing of Members of Two Psychotherapy Groups: Changes in Affective Expression', *British Journal of Medical Psychology, 56*, 323-7

Kornhauser, A.W. (1965) *Mental Health of the Industrial Worker*, Wiley, New York

Koslowsky, M., Kroog, S.H. and LaVoie, L. (1978) 'Perception of the Aetiology of Illness: Causal Attributions in a Heart Patient Population', *Perceptual and Motor Skills, 47*, 475-85

Kremsdorf, R.B. (1985) 'An Extension of Fixed-Role Therapy with a Couple' in F.R. Epting and A.W. Landfield (eds.), *Anticipating Personal Construct Theory*, Nebraska Press, Lincoln, Nebraska

Kuiper, N.A. and Derry, P.A. (1981) 'The Self as a Cognitive Prototype: An Application to Person Perception and Depression' in N. Cantor and J.F. Kihlstrom (eds.), *Personality, Cognition and Social Interaction*, Erlbaum, Hillsdale, New Jersey

Lacey, R. (1984) 'Where Have All the Patients Gone?', *The Guardian*, 4th July, London

Lader, M.H. and Matthews, A.M. (1968) 'A Physiological Model of Phobic Anxiety and Desensitization', *Behaviour Research and Therapy*, 6, 411-21

Laing, R.D. and Esterson, A. (1964) *Sanity, Madness and the Family—Families of Schizophrenics*, Tavistock Publications, London

Landfield, A.W. (1954) 'A Movement Interpretation of Threat', *Journal of Abnormal and Social Psychology*, 49, 529-32

Landfield, A.W. (1955) 'Self Predictive Orientation and the Movement Interpretation of Threat', *Journal of Abnormal and Social Psychology*, 51, 434-8

Landfield, A.W. (1971) *'Personal Construct Systems in Psychotherapy'*, Rand McNally, Chicago

Landfield, A.W. (1976) 'A Personal Construct Approach to Suicidal Behaviour' in P. Slater (ed.), *Explorations of Intrapersonal Space*, Wiley, London, pp. 93-107

Landfield, A.W. (1979) 'Exploring Socialisation through the Interpersonal Transaction Group' in P. Stringer and D. Bannister (eds.), *Constructs of Sociality and Individuality*, Academic Press, London, pp. 133-52

Landfield, A.W. (1980a) 'The Person as Perspectivist, Literalist and Chaotic Fragmentalist' in A.W. Landfield and L.M. Leitner (eds.), *Personal Construct Psychology: Psychotherapy and Personality*, Wiley, New York

Landfield, A.W. (1980b) 'Personal Construct Psychotherapy: A Personal Construction' in A.W. Landfield and L.M. Leitner (eds.), *Personal Construct Psychology: Psychotherapy and Personality*, Wiley, New York

Landfield, A.W. (1982) 'A Construction of Fragmentation and Unity: The Fragmentation Corollary' in J.C. Mancuso and J.R. Adams-Webber, *The Construing Person*, Praeger, New York

Landfield, A.W. and Barr, M.A. (1976) 'Ordination: A New Measure of Concept Organization', Unpublished Manuscript, University of Nebraska-Lincoln, Lincoln, Nebraska

Landfield, A.W. and Leitner, L.M. (1980) *Personal Construct Psychology: Psychotherapy and Personality*, Wiley-Interscience, New York

Landfield, A.W. and Rivers, P.C. (1975) 'An Introduction to Interpersonal Transaction and Rotating Dyads', *Psychotherapy: Theory, Research and Practice*, 12, 366-74

Langer, E.F., Janis, I.L. and Wolfer, J.A. (1975) 'Reduction of Psychological Stress in Surgical Patients', *Journal of Experimental Social Psychology*, 11, 155-65

Lawlor, M. and Cochran, L. (1981), 'Does Invalidation Produce Loose Construing?' *British Journal of Medical Psychology*, 54, 41-50

Lazarus, A. (1976), *Multi-Modal Therapy*, Academic Press, London

Leary, T. (1957) *'Interpersonal Diagnosis of Personality'*, Ronald Press, New York

Leitner, L.M. (1981a) 'Construct Validity of a Repertory Grid Measure of Personality Styles', *Journal of Personality Assessment, 45*, 539-44

Leitner, L.M. (1981b) 'Psychopathology and the Differentiation of Values, Emotions and Behaviours: A Repertory Grid Study', *British Journal of Psychiatry, 138*, 147-53

Leitner, L.M. (1985) 'The Terrors of Cognition: on the Experiential Validity of Personal Construct Theory' in D. Bannister (ed.), *Further Perspectives on Personal Construct Theory*, Academic Press, London

Leitner, L.M. and Klion, R.E. (1984) 'Construct Similarity, Self-Meaningfulness and Interpersonal Attraction', Unpublished Manuscript, Miami University, Oxford, Ohio

Lester, D. (1968) 'Suicide as an Aggressive Act: A Replication with a Control for Neuroticism', *Journal of General Psychology, 79*, 83-6

Lester, D. (1971) 'Cognitive Complexity of the Suicidal Individual', *Psychological Reports, 28*, 158

Levenson, M. and Neuringer, C. (1971) 'Problem-Solving Behaviour in Suicidal Adolescents', *Journal of Consulting and Clinical Psychology, 37*, 433-6

Leventhal, H. (1975) 'The Consequences of Depersonalisation During Illness and Treatment', in J. Howard and A. Strauss (eds.), *Humanizing Health Care*, Wiley, New York

Levine, F.G.M. and Fasnacht, G. (1974) 'Token Rewards May Lead to Token Learning', *American Psychologist, 29*, 816-20

Lewinsohn, P.M. and Libet, J. (1972) 'Pleasant Events, Activity Schedules and Depression', *Journals of Abnormal Psychology, 79*, 291-5

Lewinsohn, P.M., Munoz, R.F., Youngren, M.A. and Zeiss, A.M. (1978) *Control Your Depression*, Prentice-Hall, Englewood Cliffs, New Jersey

Lewis, F.M. and Bloom, J.R. (1978–9) 'Psychosocial Adjustment to Breast Cancer: A Review of Selected Literature', *International Journal of Psychiatry in Medicine, 9*, 1-17

Lidz, T. (1973) *The Origin and Treatment of Schizophrenic Disorders*, Basic Books, New York

Linehan, M. (1981) 'A Social-Behavioural Analysis of Suicide and Parasuicide: Implications for Clinical Assessment and Treatment' in J. Clarkin and H. Glazer (eds.), *Depression: Behavioural and Directive Intervention Strategies*, Garland STPM Press, New York

Lipowski, Z.J. (1970) 'Physical Illness, the Individual and the Coping Process', *Psychiatry in Medicine, 1*, 91-101

Ludwig, A.M. (1969) 'Altered States of Consciousness' in C. Tart (ed.), *Altered States of Consciousness; A Book of Readings*, Wiley, New York

McConachie, H. (1981) 'Evaluation of the Anson House Preschool Project Parent Teaching Course 1979-1981', Unpublished Manuscript

McConachie, H. (1982) 'Fathers of Mentally Handicapped Children', in N. Beail and J. McGuire (eds.), *Fathers: Psychological Perspectives*, Junction, London

McCoy, M. (1977) 'A Reconstruction of Emotion' in D. Bannister (ed.), *New Perspectives in Personal Construct Theory*, Academic Press, London

McCoy, M. (1981) 'Positive and Negative Emotion: A Personal Construct Theory Interpretation' in H. Bonarius, R. Holland and S. Rosenberg (eds.), *Personal Construct Psychology: Recent Advances in Theory and Practice*, Macmillan, London

McGuire, W.J. (1960) 'A Syllogistic Analysis of Cognitive Relationships' in M.J. Rosenberg, C.I. Hovland, W.J. McGuire, R.P. Abelson and J.W. Brehm (eds.), *Attitude Organisation and Change*, Yale University Press, New Haven

McPherson, F.M., Armstrong, J. and Heather, N. (1975) 'Psychological Construing, "Difficulty" and Thought Disorder', *British Journal of Medical Psychology, 48,* 303-15

McPherson, F.M., Blackburn, I.M., Draffan, J.W. and McFayden, M. (1973) 'A Further Study of the Grid Test of Schizophrenic Thought Disorder', *British Journal of Social and Clinical Psychology, 12,* 420-7

McPherson, F.M. and Buckley, F. (1970) 'Thought Process Disorder and Personal Construct Subsystems', *British Journal of Social and Clinical Psychology, 9,* 380-1

McPherson, F.M. and Gray, A. (1976) 'Psychological Construing and Psychological Symptoms', *British Journal of Medical Psychology, 49,* 73-9

McPherson, F.M. and Walton, H.J. (1970) 'The Dimensions of Psychotherapy Group Interaction: An Analysis of Clinicians' Constructs', *British Journal of Medical Psychology, 43,* 280-1

Madden, J.S. (1979 *'A Guide to Alcohol and Drug Dependence'*, John Wright, Bristol

Maddox, G.L., Back, L.K., and Liederman, V. (1968) 'Overweight as Social Deviance and Disability', *Journal of Health and Social Behaviour, 9,* 287-98

Mair, J.M.M. (1970) 'Experimenting with Individuals', *British Journal of Medical Psychology, 43,* 245-56

Mair, J.M.M. (1977a), 'Metaphors for Living', in A.W. Landfield (ed.), *Nebraska Symposium on Motivation 1976,* University of Nebraska Press, Lincoln, Nebraska, pp. 241-90

Mair, J.M.M. (1977b) 'The Community of Self' in D. Bannister (ed.), *New Perspectives in Personal Construct Theory*, Academic Press, London

Mair, J.M.M. (1983) 'The Long Quest to Know', Paper Presented at the 5th International Conference on Personal Construct Psychology, Pine Manor College, Boston, Mass

Makhlouf-Norris, F. and Jones, H.G. (1971) 'Conceptual Distance Indices as Measures of Alienation in Obsessional Neurosis', *Psychological Medicine, 1,* 381-7

Makhlouf-Norris, F., Jones, H.G. and Norris, H. (1970) 'Articulation of the Conceptual Structure in Obsessional Neurosis', *British Journal of Social and Clinical Psychology, 9,* 264-74

Makhlouf-Norris, F. and Norris, H. (1973) 'The Obsessive Compulsive Syndrome as a Neurotic Device for the Reduction of Self-Uncertainty', *British Journal of Psychiatry, 122,* 277-88

Malan, D.H. (1976) *Towards the Validation of Dynamic Psychotherapy*, Plenum Press, New York

Malan, D.H. (1979) *'Individual Psychotherapy and the Science of Psychodynamics'*, Butterworths, London

Mancuso, J.C. (1977) 'Current Motivational Models in the Elaboration of Personal Construct Theory' in A.W. Landfield (ed.), *Nebraska Symposium on Motivation; Personal Construct Psychology*, University of Nebraska Press, Lincoln, Nebraska, pp. 43-97

Mancuso, J.C. and Adams-Webber, J.R. (1982) 'Personal Construct Psychology as Personality Theory: Introduction' in J.C. Mancuso and J.R. Adams-Webber (eds.), *The Construing Person*, Praeger, New York

Mancuso, J. and Handin, K.H. (1980) 'Training Parents to Construe the Child's Construing' in A.W. Landfield and L.M. Leitner (eds.), *Personal Construct Psychology: Psychotherapy and Personality*, Wiley, New York, pp. 271–88

Mann, R.D. (1961) 'Dimensions of Individual Performance in Small Groups Under Task and Social Emotional Conditions', *Journal of Abnormal and Social Psychology, 62*, 682-94

Marcia, J.E. Rubin, B.M. and Efran, J.S. (1969) 'Systematic Desensitisation, Expectancy Change or Counter Conditioning?' *Journal of Abnormal Psychology, 74*, 382-7

Margolius, O. (1980) 'Conflicts in Construing the Self: Differences between Neurotics and Normals', Unpublished MSc Dissertation, N.E. London Polytechnic

Marziali, E.A. Sullivan, J.M. (1980) 'Methodological Issues in the Content Analysis of Brief Psychotherapy', *British Journal of Medical Psychology, 53*, 19-27

Matson, J. and Mulick, J. (1983) *Handbook of Mental Retardation*, Pergamon, New York

Mayer-Gross, W., Slater, E. and Roth, M. (1954) *Clinical Psychiatry*, Cassell and Co. Ltd., London

Mead, G.H. (1934) *Mind, Self and Society*, University of Chicago Press, Chicago

Mechanic, D. (1977) *Medical Psychology*, Free Press, New York

Melzak, R. (1980) 'Psychological Aspects of Pain' in J.J. Bonica (ed.), *Pain*, Raven, New York

Menninger, K. (1938) *Man Against Himself*, Harcourt, Brace and Co., New York

Melzak, R. (1980) 'Psychological Aspects of Pain' in J.J. Bonica (ed.), *Pain*, Raven, New York

Menninger, K. (1938) *Man Against Himself*, Harcourt, Brace and Co., New York

Meyer, V., Levy, R. and Schnurer, A. (1974) 'The Behavioural Treatment of Obsessional States' in H.R. Beech (ed.), *Obsessional States*, Methuen, London

Millar, D.G. (1980) 'A Repertory Grid Study of Obsessionality: Distinctive Cognitive Structure or Distinctive Cognitive Content?', *British Journal of Medical Psychology, 53*, 59-66

Miller, A.D. (1968) 'Psychological Stress as a Determinant of Cognitive Complexity', *Psychological Reports, 23*, 635-9

Miller, G.A. and Chapman, L.J. (1968) 'Response Bias and Schizophrenic Beliefs', *Journal of Abnormal Psychology, 73*, 252-5

Miller, K. and Treacher, A. (1981) 'Delinquency: A Personal Construct Theory Approach' in H. Bonarius, R. Holland and S. Rosenberg (eds.), *Personal Construct Psychology: Recent Advances in Theory and Practice*, Macmillan, London, pp. 241-50

Milner, A.D., Beech, H.R. and Walker, V. (1971) 'Decision Processes and Obsessional Behaviour', *British Journal of Social and Clinical Psychology, 10*, 88-9

Mintz, R. (1968) 'The Psychotherapy of the Suicidal Patient' in H.L.P. Resnick (ed.), *Suicidal Behaviours*, Little and Brown, Boston, pp. 271-96

Motti, F., Cichetti, D. and Sroufe, L. (1983) 'From Infant Affect Expression to Symbolic Play: The Coherence of Development in Down's Syndrome Children', *Child Development 54*, 1168-75

Mowrer, O.H. (1950) *Learning Theory and Personality Dynamics,* Ronald Press, New York

Munden, A. (1982) 'Eating Problems Amongst Women in a University Population', Unpublished Dissertation, Faculty of Medicine, University of Southampton

Myatt, R. (1983) 'Evaluating Parental Intervention Projects', Paper Presented at the London Conference of the British Psychological Society

Nathan, P.E. and Lansky, D. (1978) 'Common Methodological Problems in Research on the Addictions', *Journal of Consulting and Clinical Psychology, 46,* 712-26

Neimeyer, G.J. (1984) Personal Communication

Neimeyer, G.J. (1985a) 'Cognitive Complexity and Marital Satisfaction', *Journal of Social and Clinical Psychology*

Neimeyer, G.J. (1985b) 'Personal Constructs in Couples' Counselling' in F.R. Epting and A.W. Landfield (eds.), *Anticipating Personal Construct Theory,* Nebraska Press, Lincoln, Nebraska

Neimeyer, G.J. and Banikiotes, P.G. (1980) 'Flexibility of Disclosure and Measures of Cognitive Integration and Differentiation', *Perceptual and Motor Skills, 50,* 907-10

Neimeyer, G.J. and Banikiotes, P.G. (1981) 'Self-Disclosure, Flexibility, Empathy and Perceptions of Adjustment and Attraction', *Journal of Counselling Psychology, 28,* 272-5

Neimeyer, G.J., Banikiotes, P.G. and Ianni, L.E. (1979) 'Self-Disclosure and Psychological Construing: A Personal Construct Approach to Interpersonal Perceptions', *Social Behaviour and Personality, 7,* 161-5

Neimeyer, G.J. and Hudson, J.E. (1985) 'Couples' Constructs: Personal Systems in Marital Satisfaction' in D. Bannister (ed.), *Issues and Approaches in Personal Construct Theory,* Wiley, London

Neimeyer, G.J. and Neimeyer, R.A. (1981a) 'Functional Similarity and Interpersonal Attraction', *Journal of Research in Personality, 15,* 427–35

Neimeyer, G.J. and Neimeyer, R.A. (1981b) 'Personal Construct Perspectives on Cognitive Assessment' in T. Merluzzi, C. Glass and M. Gesest (eds.), *Cognitive Assessment,* Guildford, New York, pp. 188-232

Neimeyer, R.A. (1980) 'George Kelly as Therapist: A Review of his Tapes' in A.W. Landfield and L.M. Leitner (eds.),*Personal Construct Psychology: Psychotherapy and Personality,* Wiley, New York

Neimeyer, R.A. (1984), 'Toward a Personal Construct Conceptualization of Depression and Suicide' in F.R. Epting and R.A. Neimeyer (eds.), *Personal Meanings of Death: Applications of Personal Construct Theory to Clinical Practice.* Hemisphere/McGraw-Hill, New York, pp. 127-73

Neimeyer, R.A. (1985a) 'Personal Constructs in Clinical Practice', in P. Kendall (ed.), *Advances in Cognitive-Behavioural Research and Therapy,* vol. 4, Academic Press, New York

Neimeyer, R.A. (1985b) International Journal of Mental Health: *Special Issue on Group Therapies for Depression*

Neimeyer, R.A. (1985c) *The Development of Personal Construct Psychology,* Nebraska Press, Lincoln, Nebraska

Neimeyer, R.A., Heath, A.E. and Strauss, J. (1985) 'Personal Reconstruction During Cognitive Therapy for Depression' in F.R. Epting and A.W. Landfield (eds.), *Anticipating Personal Construct Theory,* Nebraska Press, Lincoln,

Nebraska

Neimeyer, R.A., Klein, M.H., Gurman, A.S. and Griest, J.H. (1983) 'Cognitive Structure and Depressive Symptomatology', *British Journal of Cognitive Psychotherapy, 1,* 65-73

Neimeyer, R.A. and Neimeyer, G.J. (1982) 'Interpersonal Relationships and Personal Elaboration; a Personal Construct Theory Model', Paper Presented at the International Conference on Personal Relationships, Madison, Wisconsin

Neimeyer, R.A. and Neimeyer, G.J. (1983) 'Structural Similarity in the Acquaintance Process', *Journal of Social and Clinical Psychology, 1,* 146-54

Neimeyer, R.A., Neimeyer, G.J. and Landfield, A.W. (1983) 'Conceptual Differentiation, Integration and Empathic Prediction', *Journal of Personality, 51,* 185-91

Neuringer, C. (1961) 'Dichotomous Evaluation in Suicidal Individuals', *Journal of Consulting Psychology, 25,* 445-9

Neuringer, C. (1964) 'Rigid Thinking in Suicidal Individuals', *Journal of Consulting Psychology, 28,* 54-8

Neuringer, C. (1974) 'Attitude Towards Self in Suicidal Individuals', *Suicide and Life-Threatening Behaviour, 4,* 96-196

Neuringer, C. and Lettieri, D. (1971) 'Cognition, Attitude and Affect in Suicidal Individuals', *Suicide and Life-Threatening Behaviour, 1,* 106-24

Nooe, R. (1977) 'Measuring Self-Concepts of Mentally Retarded Adults', *Social Work, 22,* 320-2

Norris, H. and Makhlouf-Norris, F. (1976) 'The Measurement of Self-Identity' in P. Slater (ed.), *The Measurement of Intrapersonal Space by Grid Technique,* vol. 1, Wiley, London

Nylander, I. (1971) 'The Feeling of Being Fat and Dieting in a School Population', *Acta Sociomedica Scandinavica, 3,* 17-26

Oliver, C. (1980) 'Repertory Grid Technique and Mentally Handicapped Children: An Exploratory Study', Unpublished BSc Dissertation, Loughborough University of Technology

Olsen, J.M. and Partington, J.T. (1977) 'An Integrative Analysis of Two Cognitive Models of Interpersonal Effectiveness', *British Journal of Social and Clinical Psychology, 16,* 13-14

O'Reilley, J. (1977) 'The Interplay Between Mothers and their Children: A Construct Theory Viewpoint' in D. Bannister (ed.), *New Perspectives in Personal Construct Theory,* Academic Press, London, pp. 195-219

Ornstein, R.E. (1972) *The Psychology of Consciousness,* W.H. Freeman, Chicago

Palazzoli, M.S., Boscolo, L., Cecchin, G. and Prata, G. (1978) *Paradox and Counter Paradox: A New Model of the Therapy of the Family in Schizophrenic Transaction,* Jason Aranson, New York

Palazzoli, M.S., Boscolo, L., Cecchin, G. and Prata, G. (1980) Hypothesising, Circularity and Neutrality — Three Guidelines for the Conductor of the Session', *Family Process, 19,* 2-12

Palmer, R.L. (1979) 'Dietary Chaos Syndrome: A Useful New Term?', *British Journal of Medical Psychology, 52,* 187-90

Parker, A. (1981) 'The Meaning of Attempted Suicide to Young Parasuicides: A Repertory Grid Study', *British Journal of Psychiatry, 139,* 306-12

Partington, J. (1970) 'Dr Jeckyll and Mr High: Multidimensional Scaling of Alcholics' Self-Evaluation', *Journal of Abnormal Psychology, 75,* 131-8

Paykel, E.S., Myers, J.K., Dienelt, M.N., Klerman, G.L., Lindenthal, J.J. and Pepper, M.P. (1969) 'Life Events and Depression: A Controlled Study', *Archives of General Psychiatry, 21,* 753-60

Paykel, E.S., Prusoff, B.A. and Uhlenhuth, E.H. (1971) 'Scaling of Life Events', *Archives of General Psychiatry, 25,* 340-7

Payne, R.W. (1961) 'Cognitive Abnormalities' in H.J. Eysenck (ed.), *Handbook of Abnormal Psychology,* Basic Books, New York, pp. 193-261

Penrod, J.H. and Epting, R.F. (1981) 'Interpersonal Cognitive Differentiation and Drug of Choice', *Psychological Reports, 49,* 752-6

Peres, R. (1947) *Trends in Psychotherapy,* Columbia University Press, Columbia

Perry, W.R. (1978) 'Construing Interpersonal Construction Systems: Conjectures of Sociality' in F. Fransella (ed.), *Personal Construct Psychology 1977,* Academic Press, London, pp. 181-91

Plant, R.D. (1984) 'Belief and Illness: A Study of Patients with Rheumatoid Arthritis', Unpublished MSc Dissertation, Faculty of Medicine, University of Southampton

Plutchik, R., Jerrett, I., Karasu, T.B. and Skodol A. (1979) 'Appearance of New Symptoms in Hospitalised Patients: An Instance of Institutional Iatrogenesis?' *Journal of Clinical Psychiatry, 40,* 276-9

Poole, A. (1976) 'A Further Attempt to Cross-Validate the Grid Test of Schizophrenic Thought Disorder', *British Journal of Social and Clinical Psychology, 15,* 179-88

Pope, M. and Keen, T. (1981) *Personal Construct Psychology and Education,* Academic Press, London

Procter, H.G. (1978) 'Personal Construct Theory and the Family: A Theoretical and Methodological Study'. Unpublished PhD Thesis, University of Bristol

Procter, H.G. (1981) 'Family Construct Psychology: An Approach to Understanding and Treating Families' in S. Walrond-Skinner (ed.), *Developments in Family Therapy,* Routledge and Kegan Paul, London

Procter, H.G. and Dallos, R. (in press) *Family Processes: The Interactional View,* D307 Social Psychology Course, Unit 2, Open University Press, Milton Keynes

Procter, H.G. and Stephens, T. (1984) 'Developing Family Therapy in the Day Hospital' in A. Treacher and J. Carpenter, *Using Family Therapy,* Blackwell, Oxford

Rachman, S. (1983) 'The Modification of Agoraphobic Avoidance Behaviour: Some Fresh Possibilities', *Behaviour Research and Therapy, 21,* 567-74

Radley, A.R. (1974) 'Schizophrenic Thought Disorder and the Nature of Personal Constructs', *British Journal of Social and Clinical Psychology, 13,* 315-28

Raps, C.S., Peterson, C., Jonas, M. and Seligman, M.E.P. (1982) 'Patient Behaviour in Hospitals: Helplessness, Reactance or Both?' *Journal of Personality and Social Psychology, 42,* 1036-41

Rathod, P. (1981) 'Methods for the Analysis of Repgrid Data', in H. Bonarius, R. Holland, and S. Rosenberg (eds.), *Personal Construct Psychology: Recent Advances in Theory and Practice,* Macmillan, London, pp. 117-46

Ravenette, A.T. (1977) 'Personal Construct Theory; an Approach to the Psychological Investigation of Children and Young People' in D. Bannister (ed.), *New Perspectives in Personal Construct Theory,* Academic Press, London, pp. 251-80

Ravenette, A.T. (1980) 'The Exploration of Consciousness: Personal Construct Intervention with Children' in A.W. Landfield and L.M. Leitner (eds.), *Personal*

Construct Psychology: Psychotherapy and Personality, Wiley, New York, pp. 36-51

Reed, G.F. (1969a) 'Under-Inclusion: A Characteristic of Obsessional Personality Disorder: 1', *British Journal of Psychiatry, 115*, 781-5

Reed, G.F. (1969b) 'Under-Inclusion: A Characteristic of Obsessional Personality Disorder: 2', *British Journal of Psychiatry, 115*, 787-90

Reid, F. (1979) 'Personal Constructs and Social Competence' in P. Stringer and D. Bannister (eds.), *Constructs of Sociality and Individuality,* Academic Press, London, pp. 233-54

Rigdon, M.A. and Epting, F.R. (1983) 'A Personal Construct Perspective on the Obsessional Client' in J.R. Adams-Webber and J.C. Mancuso (eds.), *Applications of Personal Construct Theory,* Academic Press, Toronto

Roberts, J.M. (1980) *History of the World,* Penguin

Robertson, I.T. and Molloy, K.J. (1982) 'Cognitive Complexity, Neuroticism and Research Ability', *British Journal of Educational Psychology, 52*, 113-18

Rodda, B.E., Miller, M.C. and Bruhn, J.G. (1971) 'Prediction of Anxiety and Depression Patterns Among Coronary Patients Using a Markov Process Analysis', *Behavioural Science, 16*, 482-9

Rogers, C.R. (1956) 'Intellectualized Psychotherapy', *Contemporary Psychology, 1*, 335-8

Rollnick, S. and Heather, N. (1980) 'Psychological Change Among Alcoholics During Treatment', *British Journal of Alcohol and Alcoholism, 15*, 118-23

Rosch, E.H. (1973) 'Natural Categories', *Cognitive Psychology, 4*, 328-50

Rosen, N.A. and Wyer, R.S. (1972) 'Some Further Evidence for the "Socratic Effect" Using a Probability Model of Cognitive Organisation', *Journal of Personality and Social Psychology, 24*, 420-4

Ross, M.V. (1985) 'Depression, Self Concept and Personal Constructs' in F.R. Epting and A.W. Landfield (eds.), *Anticipating Personal Construct Theory,* Nebraska Press, Lincoln, Nebraska

Rounsaville, B.J., Weissman, M.M., Wilber, C.H. and Kleber, H.D. (1982) 'Pathways to Opiate Addiction: An Evaluation of Differing Antecedents', *British Journal of Psychiatry, 141*, 437-46

Rowe, D. (1971) 'Poor Prognosis in a Case of Depression as Predicted by the Repertory Grid', *British Journal of Psychiatry, 118*, 297-300

Rowe, D. (1978) *The Experience of Depression,* Wiley, London

Rowe, D. (1982) *The Construction of Life and Death,* Wiley, New York

Rowe, D. (1983) *Depression: The Way Out of Your Prison,* Routledge and Kegan Paul, London

Rowe, D. (1984) 'Constructing Life and Death' in F.R. Epting and R.A. Neimeyer (eds.), *Presonal Meanings of Death,* Hemisphere, New York

Rudestam, K.E. (1980) *Methods of Self Change,* Brooks/Cole, Belmont, California

Rush, A.J. (1982) 'Diagnosing Depressions', in A.J. Rush (ed.), *Short-Term Psychotherapies for Depression,* Guildford, New York

Ryle, A. (1967) 'A Repertory Grid Study of the Meaning and Consequences of a Suicidal Act', *British Journal of Psychiatry, 113*, 1393-403

Ryle, A. (1975) *Frames and Cages: The Repertory Grid Approach to Human Understanding,* Sussex University Press, London. Also International Universities Press, New York

Ryle, A. (1978) 'A Common Language for the Psychotherapies?' *British Journal of*

Psychiatry, 132, 585-94

Ryle, A. (1979a) 'The Focus in Brief Interpretive Psychotherapy: Dilemmas, Traps and Snags as Target Problems', *British Journal of Psychiatry, 134,* 46-54

Ryle, A. (1979b) 'Defining Goals and Assessing Change in Brief Psychotherapy: A Pilot Study Using Target Ratings and the Dyad Grid', *British Journal of Medical Psychology, 52,* 223-33

Ryle, A. (1980) 'Some Measures of Goal Attainment in Focussed Integrated Active Psychotherapy: A Study of 15 Cases', *British Journal of Psychiatry, 137,* 475-86

Ryle, A. (1981) 'Dyad Grid Dilemmas in Patients and Control Subjects,' *British Journal of Medical Psychology, 54,* 353-8

Ryle, A. and Breen, D. (1971) 'The Recognition of Psychopathology on the Repertory Grid', *British Journal of Psychiatry, 119,* 319-22

Ryle, A. and Breen, D. (1972a) 'A Comparison of Adjusted and Maladjusted Couples Using the Double Dyad Grid', *British Journal of Medical Psychology, 45,* 375-82

Ryle, A. and Breen, D. (1972b) 'The Use of the Double Dyad Grid in the Clinical Setting', *British Journal of Medical Psychology, 45,* 383-9

Ryle, A. and Breen, D. (1972c) 'Some Differences in the Personal Constructs of Neurotic and Normal Subjects', *British Journal of Psychiatry, 120,* 483-9

Ryle, A. and Lipshitz, S. (1975) 'Recording Change in Marital Therapy with the Reconstruction Grid', *British Journal of Medical Psychology, 48,* 39-48

Ryle, A. and Lipshitz, S. (1976a) 'Repertory Grid Elucidation of a Difficult Conjoint Therapy', *British Journal of Medical Psychology, 49,* 281-5

Ryle, A. and Lipshitz, S. (1976b) 'An Intensive Case Study of a Therapeutic Group', *British Journal of Psychiatry, 128,* 581-7

Ryle, A. and Lipshitz, S. (1981) 'Recording Change in Marital Therapy with the Reconstruction Grid' in S. Walrond Skinner (ed.), *Developments in Family Therapy,* Routledge and Kegan Paul, London, pp.246-57

Ryle, A. and Lunghi, M.W. (1969) 'The Measurement of Relevant Change After Psychotherapy: Use of Repertory Grid Testing', *British Journal of Psychiatry, 115,* 1297-304

Ryle, A. and Lunghi, M.W. (1970) 'The Dyad Grid: A Modification of Repertory Grid Technique', *British Journal of Psychiatry, 117,* 323-7

Salmon, P. (1970) 'A Psychology of Personal Growth' in D. Bannister (ed.), *Perspectives in Personal Construct Theory,* Academic Press, London, pp. 197-221

Salmon, P. (1976) 'Grid Measures with Child Subjects', in P. Slater (ed.), *The Measurement of Intrapersonal Space by Grid Technique, vol. 1: Explorations of Intrapersonal Space,* Wiley, London, pp. 15-46

Salmon, P. (1979) 'Children as Social Beings' in P. Stringer and D. Bannister (eds.), *Constructs of Sociality and Individuality,* Academic Press, London, pp. 221-32

Salzinger, K. (1971) 'The Immediacy Hypothesis and Schizophrenia' in H.M. Yaker, H. Osmond and F. Cheek (eds.), *The Future of Time,* Doubleday Doran, New York

Sarason, I.G. (1979) 'Three Lacunae of Cognitive Therapy and Research', *3, 223-35*

Schachter, S. and Singer, J.C. (1962) 'Cognitive, Social and Physiological Determinants of Emotional State', *Psychological Review, 69,* 379-99

Schilder, P. (1951) 'On The Development of Thoughts' in D. Rapaport (ed.), *Organization and Pathology of Thought,* Columbia University Press, New York

Schmitt, F.E. and Wooldridge, P.J. (1973) 'Psychological Preparation of Surgical

Patients', *Nursing Research, 22,* 108-116

Schneidman, E.S. (1968) 'Orientation Toward Death' in H.L. Resnick (ed.), *Suicidal Behaviour,* Little and Brown, Boston

Schoolar, J.C., White, E.H. and Cohen, C.P. (1972) 'Drug Abusers and Their Clinical Counterparts: A Comparison of Personality Dimensions', *Journal of Consulting and Clinical Psychology, 29,* 9-14

Schurr, K., Joiner, L. and Towne, R. (1970) 'Self-Concept Research on the Mentally Retarded', *Mental Retardation, 8,* 39-43

Schutz, W.C. (1958) *'F.I.R.O: A Three-Dimensional Theory of Interpersonal Behaviour',* Holt, Rinehart and Winston, New York

Scott, R.D. and Ashworth, P.L. (1969) 'The Shadow of the Ancestor: a Historical Factor in the Transmission of Schizophrenia', *British Journal of Medical Psychology, 42,* 13-32

Sechehaye, M.A. (1950) *Journal d'un Schizophrene,* Presse Universitaire de France, Paris

Secunda, S.K., Katz, M.N., Friedman, R.J. and Schuyler, D. (1973) *Special Report: 1973 The Depressive Disorders',* US Government Printing Office, Washington DC

Seligman, M. (1979) *Strategies for Helping Parents of Exceptional Children,* Free Press, New York

Seligman, M.E.P., and Johnston, J. (1973) 'A Cognitive Theory of Avoidance Learning' in F.S. McGuigan and D. Lumsden (eds.), *Contemporary Approaches to Conditioning and Learning,* Winston, Washington

Sells, S.B. and Simpson, D.D. (1976) *The Effectiveness of Drug Abuse Treatment: Evaluation of Treatment Outcomes for 1971-1972. DRAP Admission Cohort,* Ballinger Publishing Co., Cambridge, Massachusetts

Seltzer, G. (1983) 'Systems of Classification' in J. Matson and J. Mulick (eds.), *Handbook of Mental Retardation,* Pergamon, New York

Shakow, D. (1963) 'Psychological Deficit in Schizophrenia', *Behavioural Science, 8,* 275-305

Shean, G. (1978) *Schizophrenia: An Introduction to Research and Theory,* Winthrop Publishers, Cambridge, Massachusetts

Sheehan, M.J. (1981) 'Constructs and "Conflict" in Depression', *British Journal of Psychology, 72,* 197-209

Sheehan, M.J. (1984) 'Personal Constructs and Depression: A Process Study', Unpublished PhD Thesis, University of London

Shibutani, T. (1955) 'Reference Groups as Perspectives,' *American Journal of Sociology, 60,* 562-9

Silverman, G. (1977) 'Aspects of Intensity of Affective Constructs in Depressed Patients', *British Journal of Psychiatry, 130,* 174-76

Simonton, O.C., Matthews-Simonton, S. and Creighton, J. (1978) *Getting Well Again,* Torcher, Los Angeles

Slade, P.D. and sheehan, M.J. (1981) 'Modified Conflict Grid Programme', Royal Free Hospital,London

Slater, P. (1964) *The Principal Components of a Repertory Grid,* Vincent Andrews, London

Slater, P. (1972) *Notes on INGRID 72,* St Georges Hospital, London

Slater, P. (1976) *The Measurement of Intrapersonal Space by Grid Technique, vol. 1: Explorations of Intrapersonal Space,* Wiley, London

Slater, P. (1977) *The Measurement of Intrapersonal Space by Grid Technique, vol. 2: Dimensions of Intrapersonal Space,* Wiley, London

Slater, P. (1983) 'An Interviewing Procedure for Analysing Disagreements', Paper Presented at the 5th International Congress on Personal Construct Psychology, Boston, Massachusetts

Sluzki, C.E. and Ransom, D.C. (eds.), (1976) *Double Bind: The Foundations of the Communicational Approach to the Family,* Grune and Stratton, New York and London

Smail, D.J. (1970) 'Neurotic Symptoms, Personality and Personal Constructs', *British Journal of Psychiatry, 117,* 645-8

Smail, D.J. (1984) *Illusion and Reality: The Meaning of Anxiety,* Dent, London

Smedlund, J. (1977) 'Piaget's Psychology in Practice', *British Journal of Educational Psychology, 47,* 1-6

Smith, A. and Evans, D. (1980) 'Construct Structure Associated with Alcohol Dependent Behaviour in Males', *Psychological Reports, 47,* 87-99

Snow, C. (1972) 'Mothers' Speech to Children Learning Language', *Child Development, 43,* 549-55

Solnit, A. and Stark, M. (1961) 'Mourning and the Birth of a Defective Child', Psychoanalytic Study of the Child, *16,* 513-37

Sontag, S. (1977) *Illness as Metaphor,* Allen Lane, London

Space, L.G. (1976) 'Cognitive Structure Comparison of Depressives, Neurotics and Normals', Unpublished PhD Thesis, Wayne State University

Space, L.G. and Cromwell, R.L. (1977) 'Personal Constructs Among Schizophrenic Patients' in S. Schwartz (ed.), *Language and Cognition in Schizophrenia,* Lawrence Erlbaum, Hillsdale, New Jersey

Space, L.G. and Cromwell, R.L. (1980) 'Personal Constructs Among Depressed Patients', *Journal of Nervous and Mental Disease, 168,* 150-8

Space, L.G. Dingemans, P. and Cromwell, R.L. (1983) 'Self-Construing and Alienation in Depressives, Schizophrenics and Normals' in J. Adams-Webber and J. Mancuso (eds.), *Applications of Personal Construct Theory,* Wiley, Toronto

Spence, S. and Shephard, G. (1983) *Developments in Social Skills Training,* Academic Press, London

Spencer, J.A. and Fremouw, W.J. (1979) 'Binge-Eating as a Function of Restraint and Weight Classification', *Journal of Abnormal Psychology, 8,* 262-7

Sperlinger, D.J. (1976) 'Aspects of Stability in the Repertory Grid', *British Journal of Medical Psychology, 49,* 341-7

Staffieri, J.R. (1967), 'A Study of Social Stereotypes of Body Image in Children', *Journal of Personality and Social Psychology, 7,* 101-4

Stefan, C. and Linder, H. (in press) 'Suicide. An Experience of Chaos or Fatalism: Perspectives from Personal Construct Theory' in D. Bannister (ed.), *Further Perspectives in Personal Construct Theory,* Academic Press, London

Stewart, V. and Stewart, A. (1981) *Business Applications of Repertory Grid Technique,* McGraw-Hill, New York

Straus, A.L. (1975) *Chronic Illness and the Quality of Life,* Mosby, St Louis

Stringer, P. (1979) 'Individuals, Roles and Persons', in P. Stringer and D. Bannister (eds.), *Constructs of Sociality and Individuality,* Academic Press, London, pp. 91-112

Stringer, P. and Bannister, D. (1979a) *Constructs of Sociality and Individuality,*

Academic Press, London

Stringer, P. and Bannister, D. (1979b) 'Introduction' in P. Stringer and D. Bannister (eds.), *Constructs of Sociality and Individuality,* Academic Press, London

Stuart, R. (1980) *Helping Couples Change,* Guildford, New York

Sugarman, B. (1974) *Daytop Village: A Therapeutic Community,* Holt, Rinehart and Winston, New York

Sypher, H.E., Nightingale, J.P., Vielhaber, M.E. and Sypher, B.D. (1981) 'The Interpersonal Constructs of Machiavellians: A Reconsideration', *British Journal of Social Psychology, 20,* 219-20

Tart, C.T. (1971) *On Being Stoned: A Psychological Study of Marijuana Intoxication,* Science of Behaviour Books, Palo Alto

Taylor, S.E. (1979) 'Hospital Patient Behaviour: Reactance, Helplessness or Control', *Journal of Social Issues, 35,* 156-84

Thomas, L.F. (1979) 'Construct, Reflect and Converse: The Conversational Reconstruction of Social Realities' in P. Stringer and D. Bannister (eds.), *Constructs of Sociality and Individuality,* Academic Press, London, pp. 49-72

Thomas, L.F. and Shaw, M.L.G. (1976) '*FOCUS*', Centre for the Study of Human Learning, Brunel University, Uxbridge, Middlesex

Thomas, L.F. and Shaw, M.L.G. (1977) '*PEGASUS*', Centre for the Study of Human Learning, Brunel University, Uxbridge, Middlesex

Tripodi, T. and Bieri, J. (1964) 'Information Transmission in Clinical Judgement as a Function of Stimulus Dimensionality and Cognitive Complexity, *Journal of Personality, 32,* 119-37

Trower, P., Bryant, B. and Argyle, M. (1978) *Social Skills and Mental Health,* Methuen, London

Tschudi, F. (1977) 'Loaded and Honest Questions: A Construct Theory View of Symptoms and Therapy' in D. Bannister (ed.), *New Perspectives in Personal Construct Theory,* Academic Press, London

Tschudi, F. (1983) 'Constructs are Hypotheses' in J. Adams-Webber and J. Mancuso (eds.), *Applications of Personal Construct Theory,* Academic Press, Toronto, pp. 115-25

Tuckman, B. (1965) 'Developmental Sequence in Small Groups', *Psychological Bulletin, 63,* 384-99

Van Den Bergh, J.H. (1980) *The Psychology of the Sick Bed,* Humanities Press, New York

Van den Bergh, O., De Boeck, P. and Claeyes, W. (1981) 'Research Findings on the Nature of Constructs in Schizophrenics', *British Journal of Clinical Psychology, 20,* 123-30

van der Kloot, W.A. (1981) 'Multidimensional Scaling of Repertory Grid Responses: Two Applications of HOMALS' in H. Bonarius, R. Holland, and S. Rosenberg (eds.), *Personal Construct Psychology: Recent Advances in Theory and Practice,* Macmillan Press, London, pp. 177-86

Vernon, D.T.A. and Bigelow, D.A. (1974) 'Effect of Information About a Potentially Stressful Situation on Response to Stress Impact' *Journal of Personality and Social Psychology, 29,* 50-9

Viney, L.L. (1983a) 'Experiencing Chronic Illness: A Personal Construct Commentary' in J. Adams-Webber, and J. Mancuso (eds.), *Applications of Personal Construct Theory,* Academic Press, London

Viney, L.L. (1983b) *Images of Illness,* Krieger, Malabar

Viney, L.L. (in press, a) 'Concerns About Death Among Severely Ill People', *Death Education*

Viney, L.L. (in press, b) 'Loss of Life and Loss of Bodily Integrity: Two Different Sources of Threat for People Who are Ill', *Omega*

Viney, L.L. and Benjamim, Y. (in press) 'A Hospital-Based Counselling Service for Medical and Surgical Patients', *Journal of Applied Rehabilitation Counselling*

Viney, L.L., Clarke, A.M., Bunn, T.A. and Tech, H.Y. (1983) *Crisis Counselling for Ill or Injured Patients Who are Hospitalised: Report to the Commonwealth Department of Health*, University of Wollongong, Wollongong, Australia

Viney, L.L. and Westbrook, M.T. (1981) 'Psychological Reactions to Chronic Illness-Related Disability as a Function of its Severity and Type, *Journal of Psychosomatic Medicine*, 35, 513-23

Viney, L.L. and Westbrook, M.T. (1982a) 'Patterns of Anxiety in the Chronically Ill', *British Journal of Medical Psychology*, 55, 87-95

Viney, L.L. and Westbrook, M.T. (1982b) 'Psychological Reactions to Chronic Illness: Do They Predict Rehabilitation?', *Journal of Applied Rehabilitation Counselling*, 13, 38-44

Viney, L.L. and Westbrook, M.T. (1983) 'Psychological Reactions to Chronic Illness: Do They Predict Death?' Unpublished Paper, University of Wollongong, Wollongong, Australia

Viney, L.L., Westbrook, M.T. and Preston, C. (1984) 'The Addiction Experience as a Function of the Addict's History', *British Journal of Clinical Psychology*, in press

Von Domarus, E. (1964) 'The Specific Laws of Logic in Schizophrenia' in J.S. Kasanin (ed.), *Language and Thought in Schizophrenia*, Norton, New York, pp. 104-14

Waisbren, S. (1980) 'Parents' Reactions After the Birth of a Developmentally Disabled Child', *American Journal of Mental Deficiency*, 84, 345-51

Warner, R. (1976-7) 'The Relationship Between Language and Disease concepts', *International Journal of Psychiatry in Medicine*, 7, 57-68

Watson, J.P. (1970a) 'The Relationship Between a Self-Mutilating Patient and Her Doctor,' *Psychotherapy and Psychosomatics*, 18, 67-73

Watson, J.P. (1970b) 'A Repertory Grid Method of Studying Groups', *British Journal of Psychiatry*, 117, 309-18

Watson, J.P. (1972) 'Possible Measures of Change During Group Psychotherapy', *British Journal of Medical Psychology*, 45, 71-7

Watson, J.P. (1984), Personal Communication

Watzlawick, P., Beavin, J. and Jackson, D.D. (1967) *Pragmatics of Human Communication*, Norton, New York

Watzlawick, P., Weakland, J. and Fisch, R. (1974) *Change: Principles of Problem Formation and Problem Solving*, Norton, New York

Weil, A. (1975) *The Natural Mind*, Penguin, Harmondsworth

Weiss, R.S. (1975) *Marital Separation*, Basic Books, New York

Weissman, M.M. (1984) 'The Psychological Treatment of Depression; an Update of Clinical Trials' in J. Williams and R.L. Spitzer (eds.), *Psychotherapy Research: Where are We and Where Should We Go?*, Guildford, New York

Wellisch, D.K. (1981) 'Intervention with the Cancer Patient' in C.K. Prokop and L.A. Bradley (eds.), *Medical Psychology*, Academic Press, New York

Westbrook, M.T. and Viney, L.L. (1982) 'Psychological Reaction to the Onset of

Chronic Illness', *Social Science and Medicine, 16*, 220-30

Whitaker, D.S. and Lieberman, M.A. (1965) *Psychotherapy Through the Group Process*, Allerton Press, New York

Widom, C.S. (1976) 'Interpersonal and Personal Construct Systems in Psychopaths', *Journal of Consulting and Clinical Psychology, 44*, 614-23

Wieder, H. and Kaplan, E.H. (1969) 'Drug Use in Adolescents: Psychodynamic Meaning and Pharmacogenic Effect', *The Psychoanalytic Study of the Child, 24*, 399-431

Wikler, A. (1965) 'Conditioning Factors in Opiate Addiction' in D. Wilner and G. Kanenbaum (eds.), *Narcotics*, McGraw-Hill, New York

Williams, S.H. and Neimeyer, G.J. (1984) 'Personal Identities and Personal Constructs', Unpublished Manuscript, University of Florida, Gainesville, Florida

Wink, C. (1963) 'Mental Retardation and Leaning Under Symbolic Reinforcement in View of Self-Acceptance', *Dissertation Abstracts, 23*, 2430-1

Winokur, G. (1981) *Depression: the Facts*, Oxford University Press, Oxford

Winter, D.A. (1979) 'Repertory Grid Technique in Research in the Psychological Therapies', Unpublished PhD Thesis, University of Durham

Winter, D.A. (1981) 'Dilemmas and Their Resolution During Therapy: Problems of Repertory Grid Assessment', Paper Presented at the 4th International Congress on Personal Construct Psychology, Brock University of Ontario

Winter, D.A. (1982) 'Construct Relationships, Psychological Disorder and Therapeutic Change', *British Journal of Medical Psychology, 55*, 257-69

Winter, D.A. (1983a) 'Logical Inconsistency in Construct Relationships: Conflict or Complexity?' *British Journal of Medical Psychology, 56*, 79-87

Winter, D.A. (1983b) 'Constriction and Construction in Agoraphobia', Paper Presented at the 5th International Congress on Personal Construct Psychology, Pine Manor College, Boston, Massachussetts

Winter, D.A. and Trippett, C.J. (1977) 'Serial Change in Group Psychotherapy', *British Journal of Medical Psychology, 50*, 341-8

Woodfield, R. and Viney, L.L. (in press) 'A Personal Construct Approach to Bereavement', *Omega*

Wooster, D. (1970) 'Formation of Stable and Discrete Concepts of Personality by Normal and Mentally Retarded Boys', *Journal of Mental Subnormality, 16*, 24-8

Worchel, T. and Worchel, P. (1961) 'The Parental Concept of the Mentally Retarded Child', *American Journal of Mental Deficiency, 65*, 782-8

Worden, V.W. and Sobel, H.J. (1978) 'Ego Strength and Psychosocial Adaptation to Cancer,' *Psychosomatic Medicine, 40*, 585-91

Wortman, C.B. and Dunkel-Schetter, C. (1979) 'Interpersonal Relationships and Cancer: A Theoretical Analysis', *Journal of Social Issues, 35*, 120-55

Wright, K.J.T. (1970) 'Exploring the Uniqueness of Common Complaints', *British Journal of Medical Psychology, 43*, 221-32

Wurmser, L. (1972) 'Drug Abuse: Nemesis of Psychiatry', *International Journal of Psychiatry, 10*, 94-107

Wylie, R. (1961) *The Self Concept*, University of Nebraska Press, Lincoln, Nebraska

Yalom, I.D. (1970) *The Theory and Practice of Group Psychotherapy*, Basic Books, New York

Yorke, M. (1983) 'Straight or Bent? An Inquiry Into Rating Scales in Repertory Grids', *British Educational Research Journal, 9*, 141-51

Yule, W. and Carr, J. (1980) *Behavioural Modification for the Mentally Handi-*

capped, Croom Helm, Beckenham
Zigler, R. (1966) 'Research on Personality Structure in the Retardate' in N. Ellis, (ed.), *International Review of Research in Mental Retardation*, vol. 1, Academic Press, New York
Zukav, G. (1980) *The Dancing Wu Li Masters: An Overview of the New Physics*, Fontana, London

INDEX